IMMUNOLOGY
FOR MEDICAL STUDENTS

IMMUNOLOGY
FOR MEDICAL STUDENTS

RODERICK NAIRN, PhD
Executive Vice President for Academic Affairs,
Dean, Graduate School of Biomedical Sciences,
Professor, Microbiology & Immunology,
Texas Tech University Health Sciences Center
Lubbock, Texas, USA

MATTHEW HELBERT, MBChB FRCP FRCPath PhD
Consultant Immunologist,
Manchester Royal Infirmary
Manchester, UK

Illustrations by Ethan Danielson

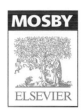

MOSBY

ELSEVIER

1600 John F. Kennedy Blvd.
Ste 1800
Philadelphia, PA 19103-2899

IMMUNOLOGY FOR MEDICAL STUDENTS   ISBN-13: 978-0-323-04331-1

Notice

Knowledge and best practice in this field are constantly changing. As new research and experience broaden our knowledge, changes in practice, treatment and drug therapy may become necessary or appropriate. Readers are advised to check the most current information provided (i) on procedures featured or (ii) by the manufacturer of each product to be administered, to verify the recommended dose or formula, the method and duration of administration, and contraindications. It is the responsibility of the practitioner, relying on their own experience and knowledge of the patient, to make diagnoses, to determine dosages and the best treatment for each individual patient, and to take all appropriate safety precautions. To the fullest extent of the law, neither the Publisher nor the [Editors/Authors] [delete as appropriate] assumes any liability for any injury and/or damage to persons or property arising out or related to any use of the material contained in this book.

The Publisher

First edition 2002
Second edition 2007
 Reprinted 2007, 2008, 2009, 2011, 2012

Previous editions copyrighted 2002
Library of Congress Cataloging-in-Publication Data
Nairn, Roderick.
   Immunology for medical students/Roderick Nairn, Matthew Helbert. —2nd ed.
      p. cm.
   Include index.
   ISBN 0-323-04331-3
   1. Immunology. I. Helbert, Matthew. II. Title.

QR181.N357 2007
616.07'9—dc22

                                              2006044964

Acquisitions Editor: Inta Ozols
Developmental Editor: Katie DeFrancesco
Publishing Services Manager: Linda Van Pelt
Project Manager: Francisco Morales
Design Direction: Louis Forgione

Working together to grow
libraries in developing countries

www.elsevier.com | www.bookaid.org | www.sabre.org

ELSEVIER   BOOK AID International   Sabre Foundation

Printed in China

Last digit is the print number: 9 8 7 6

■ PREFACE TO THE SECOND EDITION

In preparing this edition, we have made improvements throughout to improve the clarity and accessibility of the material. We have updated all the sections, particularly the material dealing with Toll-like receptors, dendritic cells, regulatory T cells, and HIV. We have also introduced a final chapter on therapeutic immunomodulation, which is being increasingly utilized in clinical practice. This chapter also aims to review what readers will have learned about the immunopathogenesis of several diseases covered in earlier chapters. In response to user feedback, we have also enhanced the clinical vignettes, which form the final pages of most chapters. Although some of these vignettes describe rare diseases, we hope that this helps readers link their studies of immunology with real clinical experience.

■ PREFACE TO THE FIRST EDITION

We have recognized the need for an immunology book that is primarily focused on the needs of medical students for as long as we have been teachers of immunology. This book has been written to fill this need. Immunology can fall into different medical school courses or modules. Often, the immunology is taught in the Host Defense course, which integrates basic and clinical immunology (including allergy, immunopathology, etc.). Some medical schools, however, teach basic immunology and clinical immunology in two separate courses. This book should be useful for either curriculum organization.

We have concentrated on a simple, straightforward treatment of the subject. The book is relatively short and contains the topics we considered important to understand the human immune system and its role in protecting us from disease. This reflects our acknowledgment of the time constraints on today's medical student. With new topics and a growing amount of information considered to be essential, there are increasing demands on students. It is therefore important to have a concise, readable textbook, and that has been our primary aim. Most chapters contain the information needed for a typical 50-minute large class or small-group teaching/learning session. This, of course, means that details dear to the hearts of some immunologists are not covered!!

We are aware of two specific problems that medical students have with immunology. First, the immune system is complex, because it has evolved to respond to the wide range of pathogens. Many students find themselves bogged down in the complexities of the molecules and cells of the immune system, without having an understanding of how these components work together to fight infection. We begin our book with two overview chapters that explain what the immune system does and then how the components fit together. We recommend that students begin by reading these chapters. Further on in the text, there are more short, integrating overview chapters. These are not just for revision, but are there to make sure that the student understands how the material that they have read fits into the overall system. The second problem is that medical students do not always immediately see the relevance of immunology to day-to-day clinical practice. We have included clinical correlations throughout the text, which explain how understanding the science of immunology can translate into understanding real clinical problems.

The book is a concise description of the science of immunology, a topic that defies a final complete description, because there is much still to be learned. Hopefully, we will have succeeded in inducing an interest and appreciation of the relevance of immunology to medical students, to form the basis for a lifetime of learning about the immune system and its potential for use in improving the human condition. Most medical students today could still be practicing medicine in 40 to 50 years. Approximately 50 years ago, immunology was still in its infancy. For example, we did not know the chemical structure of antibody molecules in any detail, and treatments such as organ transplantation had not been carried out. The next 50 years will likely bring equally important advances in the field. History suggests that we would be foolish to try to predict what they will be. We hope that you enjoy participating in these advances in immunology and their application to human disease as much as we have in those that we have been privileged to observe in our careers.

2002   R.N. & M.H.

ACKNOWLEDGMENTS

Once again I am indebted to my wife, Morag, for her help in preparing my chapters for this book. This edition is dedicated to my family and to all the medical students I have had the opportunity to teach and learn from.

R.N.

My colleagues' generosity has kept me abreast of a rapidly changing subject and provided me with invaluable material for publication. I would not have been able to write this book without the support and patience of my family, to whom I am indebted.

M.H.

Immunology for Medical Students is organized to be read comprehensively. The flow of the book is from genes and molecules to cells and organs, and finally to the immune system as an integrated system protecting the body from infection and helping to maintain the health of the body.

Section 1 introduces the basic concepts and is essential for an understanding of the language of immunology.

Section 2 continues with a discussion of the antigen-recognition molecules, that is, antibodies, T-cell receptors, and the molecules encoded by the major histocompatibility complex.

Section 3 deals with immune physiology, the role of the cells and organs of the immune system in the response to a pathogen.

Section 4 discusses the innate immune system and its connections to the adaptive immune system.

Section 5 considers hypersensitivity, allergy/asthma, autoimmunity, immunodeficiency, transplantation, among others, and includes a new chapter on therapeutic immunomodulation.

Throughout the book, the core knowledge objectives are listed as Learning Points at the ends of chapters to aid in review. There are also several integrating overview chapters (e.g., Review of antigen recognition, Review of immune physiology), and these focus the student on the major points. Each section is relatively freestanding. For example, Section 5, Immune System in Health and Disease, could be used in a clinical correlations course, independent of the remainder of the book. *Immunology for Medical Students* will be most useful in the comprehensive Host Defense-type courses that are growing in popularity in medical schools.

The icons used throughout are illustrated overleaf. You should become familiar with them immediately to follow the illustrations. We have selected several pathogens (listed in the figure overleaf) to use throughout the book as examples. As a reminder, some basic aspects of the structure and mechanism of action of these organisms are described. You should re-acquaint yourself with these organisms, undoubtedly encountered in microbiology or infectious disease courses, and use the figure as a convenient reference as you encounter these pathogens in the examples in this book.

In general, boxes have been clustered at the end of chapters in the second edition to aid in the flow of the text and in understanding of the material.

CLINICAL BOX

Clinical boxes, throughout the text, put immunology into a clinical context. The clinical material selected is current and relevant.

TECHNICAL BOX

Technical boxes show how advances in the field have expanded our knowledge of how the immune system works, and provided new means of preventing disease.

Icons in Immunology

Key molecules

   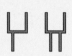

| DNA | Signaling molecule | Cytokine, Chemokine, etc. | Receptor, Surface molecule, Ligand | MHC I | MHC II | Antigen | T cell receptor (TCR) | Immunoglobulin (Ig) | Complement (C′) |

Key cells

  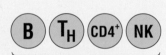

| Professional antigen-presenting cell (APC) | Neutrophil, Eosinophil, Mast cell | Lymphocytes |

Key colours

| Adaptive immune response | Innate immune response | Antigen, micro-organism, tumor, etc. |

Key tissues

| Bone marrow | Thymus | Lymph node | Other (peripheral) tissue | In vitro | Medical intervention |

This figure shows some of the different types of infection the immune system has to cope with. The mechanisms used by the immune system in response to each of these infections is described in detail in different chapters of this book.

Pathogen	Type of Organism	
Human immunodeficiency virus (HIV)	RNA virus	HIV infection requires intimate sexual contact or exposure to blood. HIV has a small genome that frequently mutates, allowing escape from the immune response. Most infected individuals do not develop adequate immunity to clear the virus. Infection frequently results in AIDS. No vaccine exists.
Influenza virus	RNA virus	Influenza causes global epidemics. Casual contact can result in infection of the respiratory tract, causing influenza. Influenza is also a small virus, and annual epidemics reflect the emergence of mutant strains that are not recognized by the populations' immune system. Vaccines exist, but have to be changed every year to overcome mutations. A new avian influenza virus has recently emerged, which would cause a large-scale epidemic if it exchanged genes with the human virus and acquired the ability to easily infect humans.
Epstein-Barr virus (EBV)	DNA virus	EBV infects the pharynx causing glandular fever or "infectious mononucleosis." B lymphocytes of the immune system are also infected, and their uncontrolled growth can sometimes lead to lymphoma (a type of malignancy). EBV has a large genome that does not mutate frequently. The genome encodes proteins that help EBV evade the immune system.
Hepatitis B virus (HBV)	DNA virus	HBV infects liver cells. In many individuals, there is only transient liver damage. In others, there is chronic, severe liver damage, possibly as a result of the immune response to HBV.
Bordetella pertussis	Bacterium	B. pertussis infects the airways and causes whooping cough, which can be life-threatening. A very effective vaccine exists, and whooping cough has become rare in the developed world.
Escherichia coli	Bacterium	E. coli is a normally harmless bacterium living in the colon. If it enters the bloodstream in small numbers, phagocytes usually destroy such bacteria. When E. coli survives in the bloodstream, septic shock may occur.
Mycobacterium tuberculosis	Bacterium	M. tuberculosis also infects the airways. It is able to survive inside phagocytes. Because of this intracellular site, it is difficult for the immune system to clear infection, and tuberculosis may result. Tuberculosis is a major threat to global health, in part because patients with AIDS are particularly unable to clear mycobacterial infection.
Schistosoma	Helminth	This worm invades the gut and urinary tract. A special part of the immune system, involving mast cells, has a role in eradicating such infections.

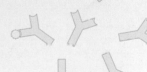

CONTENTS

CONTENTS

CONTENTS

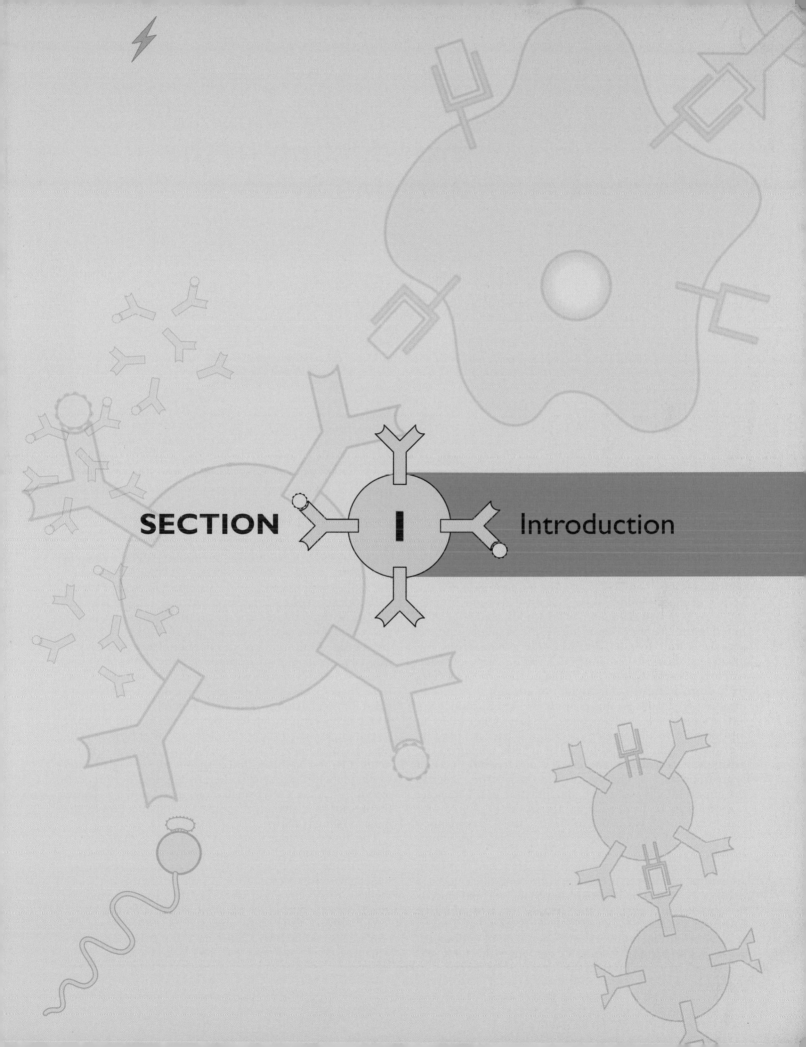

SECTION I Introduction

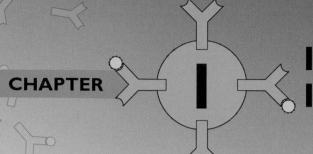

CHAPTER 1

Introduction to the Immune System

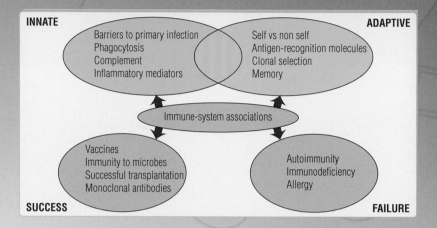

In this chapter, we briefly introduce the major components of the human immune system, what they do, and how they accomplish their host defense role.

We inhabit a world dominated by microbes, many of which can cause harm (Box 1.1). The immune system is the body's primary defense system against invasion by microbes. As you will read later in this book, and as is illustrated in the overview figure above, the immune system is organized into **innate** and **adaptive** components. The innate system is the first line of defense for the body, and it employs nonspecific cells (e.g., **phagocytes**) and molecules (e.g., **complement** components) to attempt to eliminate invading organisms. In this chapter, we first introduce the innate system and its characteristics. This is followed by an introduction to the antigen-specific mechanisms used by the adaptive immune system, which include, among others, **antigen recognition molecules** and specific sets of **lymphocytes**. This chapter also introduces the reader to the important ways in which manipulation of the immune response can aid us in ensuring the health of people—for example, through **vaccination**—and to the diseases caused by "failure" of the immune system—for example, **autoimmunity**.

The human body has evolved in such a way that there are natural barriers to prevent entry by microbes (see also Chapter 2 and Section IV). For example, the skin and mucous membranes are part of the **innate** or **nonadaptive immune system**. However, if these barriers are broken (e.g., after cutting a finger), microbes, including potential **pathogens** (harmful microbes), can enter the body and

begin to multiply rapidly in the warm, nutrient-rich systems, tissues, and organs.

One of the first features of the immune defense system that a foreign organism encounters after being introduced through a cut in the skin is the **phagocytic white blood cells** (leukocytes, e.g., macrophages, Fig. 1.2), which congregate within minutes, and begin to attack the invading, foreign, microbes (see Chapters 2 and 20). Later, neutrophils are recruited into the area of infection. These phagocytic cells bear molecules (pattern-recognition molecules) that detect structures commonly found on the surface of bacteria. Phagocytosis, the ingestion of particulate matter into cells for degradation, is a fundamental mechanism by which many creatures defend themselves against invading foreign organisms (Chapter 20). Various other protein components of serum, including the **complement** components (Chapter 19), may bind to the invader organisms and facilitate their phagocytosis, thereby limiting the source of infection/disease. Other small molecules, known as **interferons**, mediate an early response to viral infection by the innate system (Chapter 19).

The innate immune system is often sufficient to destroy invading microbes. If it fails to clear infection rapidly, it activates the **adaptive** or **acquired immune response**, which takes over. Messenger molecules known as cytokines mediate the connection between the two systems. The interferons are part of the cytokine family (Chapter 23).

The effector cells of the adaptive immune defense system are also white blood cells: the **T** and **B lymphocytes** (Chapters 2, 12, 14, and 15). The B and T cells of the

BOX 1.1 A Young Baby with Her Mother in India

This baby was born a few weeks ago. Her mother is able to provide her with food, warmth, and shelter. However, she has left the safe environment of the uterus and is now exposed to a wide range of harmful bacteria, viruses, fungi, and worms. Her mother is barely able to protect her from these pathogens, particularly in the environment of the developing world where drinking water is often contaminated with human feces. Over the next 5 years, she has a 1 in 8 chance of dying from infections. The largest threat is from water-borne infections causing severe diarrhea. Measles virus infects through the respiratory tract and kills up to 1 in 20 children in the developing world. In addition, this child will encounter parasites that are transmitted through insect bites and worms that can burrow through the skin.

What is remarkable is that seven out of eight children born in this hostile environment survive. What is the nature of the systems that protect children from such a wide range of infections?

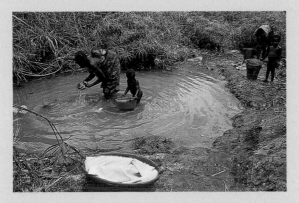

Figure 1.1 A young baby. (With permission from Andy Crump, TDR, WHO, and the Science Photo Library.)

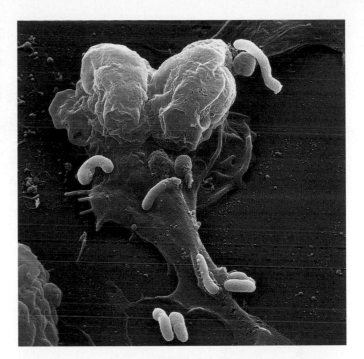

Figure 1.2 Scanning electron micrograph of a macrophage *(red)* engulfing bacteria *(yellow)*. (With permission from Juergen Berger, Max-Planck Institute, and the Science Photo Library.)

adaptive immune system are normally at rest, but they become activated (see Chapters 2 and 11) on encountering a foreign (nonself) entity referred to as an **antigen**. Adaptive immune responses are highly effective, but they can take 7 to 10 days to mobilize completely. A very important aspect of the adaptive immune response is the molecular mechanism used to generate specificity in the response. The immune system as a whole distinguishes *self* from *nonself*. It is able to cope with the great diversity in nonself structures by anticipating these different structures (foreign antigens) and creating a diverse repertoire of antigen receptors or **antigen-recognition molecules**. These receptors bind to small areas of the molecular structures of the nonself entities (e.g., foreign pathogens) called **epitopes**. The genetic mechanisms used for generation of this diverse range of antigen-recognition molecules are described in Chapters 6, 7, 8, 14, and 15. Several versions of these antigen receptors are used by the immune system; these are **antibodies** (B-cell antigen receptors), **T-cell antigen receptors**, and the protein products of a genetic region referred to as the **major histocompatibilty complex (MHC)**. All vertebrates appear to possess an MHC. The MHC genes of humans are referred to as human

leukocyte antigen (HLA) genes and their products as HLA molecules (Chapter 8).

Antibodies, in addition to being antigen receptors on B cells, are also found as soluble antigen-recognizing molecules in the blood (**immunoglobulin or antibody**). Both the B-cell and T-cell antigen receptors are **clonally distributed** (see Fig. 1.3 for B cells and antibodies), which means that a unique antigen receptor is found on each lymphocyte. When a foreign antigen enters the body, it eventually encounters a lymphocyte with a matching receptor. This lymphocyte divides and, in the case of B cells, the daughter clones produce large amounts of soluble receptor. In the case of T cells, large numbers of specific effector cells bearing the appropriate receptor on their cell surface are generated. B-cell and T-cell antigen receptors differ in one very important way: B-cell antigen receptors can interact directly with antigen, whereas T-cell antigen receptors only recognize antigen when it is presented to them on the surface of another cell by MHC molecules (Chapters 2, 7, and 8).

In addition to recognizing nonself antigens, the cells of the immune system also recognize alterations of self that result from certain disease processes—for example, modified self antigens found on tumor cells—and may eliminate the tumor cell once it is recognized (Fig. 1.4 and Chapter 34). The ability to recognize self antigen can, if unregulated, lead to disease—for example, some forms of diabetes mellitus.

A critically important feature of the adaptive immune response is that it displays memory of a previous encounter with a microbe (or antigen). This is the basis of protection from disease by vaccination with an attenuated form

 MHC II   Cytokine, Chemokine, etc.   Complement (C′)   Signaling molecule

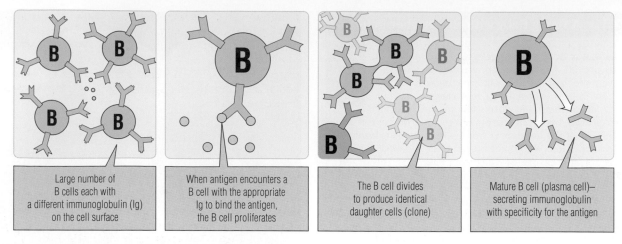

| Large number of B cells each with a different immunoglobulin (Ig) on the cell surface | When antigen encounters a B cell with the appropriate Ig to bind the antigen, the B cell proliferates | The B cell divides to produce identical daughter cells (clone) | Mature B cell (plasma cell)— secreting immunoglobulin with specificity for the antigen |

Figure 1.3 Clonal selection with B cells.

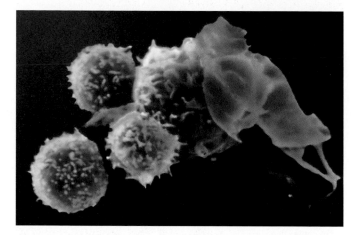

Figure 1.4 Scanning electron micrograph of T cells *(blue)* and a tumor cell *(red)*. (With permission from BSIP Lecaque and the Science Photo Library.)

of the pathogen (see Box 1.2 and Box 2.1), but it is also the way in which the body is protected from re-infection. For example, we are regularly exposed to influenza viruses (Box 1.3). If we re-encounter the same antigenic form of influenza virus, or even an antigenically similar (i.e., cross-reactive) form, the response is faster and greater in magnitude, and infection is limited or prevented. Unfortunately, because influenza virus is one of a class of organisms capable of radically changing its genetic structure (and antigenic makeup), there are always *new* viruses around to cause new infections.

Several overall characteristics of the innate and adaptive immune systems are summarized in Figure 1.7.

The medical successes associated with advances in knowledge about the host defense system include improvements in public health arising from vaccination against communicable diseases (see Box 1.2 and Chapters 4 and 24); success with organ transplantation such as with kidneys and hearts (see Box 1.4 and Chapters 8 and 33); treatments to alleviate hereditary defects in the immune system (Chapter 31); drugs to control the symptoms of allergy

BOX 1.2 Young Person with Jaundice

This medical student has been infected with hepatitis B virus, following a needlestick injury from an infected patient. Hepatitis B is also spread sexually, and in the developing world it is a leading cause of death in adults. Hepatitis B virus multiplies in the liver. The immune response to hepatitis B virus causes inflammation (hepatitis), and in most patients this process can eliminate the virus. If the virus persists, however, cirrhosis or even cancer (hepatoma) can develop.

However, hepatitis B infection is preventable. In recent years, hepatoma is no longer the problem it was in some parts of the world. This has been achieved through vaccines preventing transmission of hepatitis B. This book will help you to answer the question: How can such a safe, simple intervention have such a major impact on health?

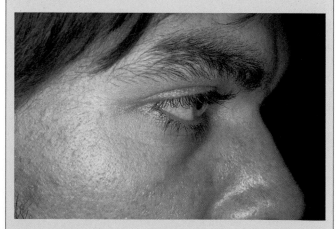

Figure 1.5 Jaundice. (Reproduced with permission from Savin JA, Hunter JAA, Hepburn NC: Skin signs in clinical diagnosis. Diagnosis in color. Mosby-Wolfe; London; 1997.)

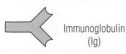 T cell receptor (TCR)   Immunoglobulin (Ig)   Antigen   MHC I

(Chapter 26) or hypersensitivity (Chapters 25, 28–30); and a variety of technologic developments coupled with the ability to manufacture antibodies with precise specificities (**monoclonal antibodies**)—these are used for everything from pregnancy tests to diagnosing cancer (Chapters 4 and 5).

Information obtained about the immune system has had an important role in our understanding and treatment of communicable diseases. Therefore, this is a subject deserving of study in medical school. Moreover, the potential for studies of the immune system to result in therapies for diseases such as cancer, or diseases with an autoimmune component, such as diabetes mellitus, rheumatoid arthritis, and multiple sclerosis, strongly requires the attention of future physicians.

BOX 1.3 A Man Sneezing

Everyone knows what it is like to have influenza. Most people have attacks every few years or so. In the 1990s, influenza killed approximately 1 out of 200 people that it infected. In 1918, there was an influenza epidemic that killed more than 40 million people around the world. When you have finished this book, you should be able to answer questions such as: How is it that we fail to build up life-long immunity to influenza, and why are some outbreaks of infectious agents such as influenza virus so lethal? What can be done to protect people against influenza? Given concerns about a possible avian flu pandemic, it is important that you can answer questions such as: Why does the current flu vaccine not protect people from viruses such as avian flu?

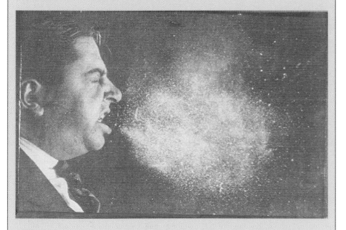

Figure 1.6 Sneezing spreads influenza virus. (With permission of the American Association for the Advancement of Science.)

BOX 1.4 Man with Kidney Failure

This man has irreversible kidney failure. Three times a week, he must undergo dialysis. As a consequence, he is unable to work. His relationship has broken up as a result of his constant ill health. He recently read that his treatment costs more than $40,000 (£20,000) per year. Every year, several thousand people die in car accidents. Many of these people have perfectly healthy kidneys that could be transplanted into our patient. He wants to know why he is waiting so long for a transplant. He is worried about the medication that he will need to take after the transplant. He has heard that these drugs will suppress his immune system and that they will predispose him to certain infections. Would you be able to answer his questions about his treatment? This book will help you to respond to such questions from your patients.

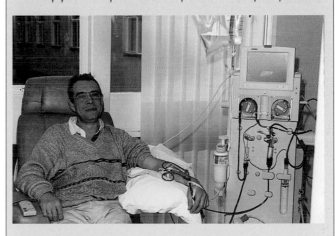

Figure 1.8 Kidney failure. (Courtesy of Dr. H.R. Dalton, Royal Cornwall Hospital, UK.)

 MHC II

 Cytokine, Chemokine, etc.

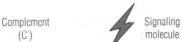 Complement (C')   Signaling molecule

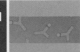

FIG. 1.7 Comparison of Some Overall Features of the Innate and Adaptive Immune Systems*

	Innate	Adaptive
Characteristics	Non-specific response	Very specific
	Fast response (minutes)	Slow response (days)
	No memory	Memory
Components	Natural barriers, phagocytes and secreted molecules	Lymphocytes and secreted molecules
	Few Pattern recognition molecules	Many Antigen-recognition molecules

*See also Fig 19.1

LEARNING POINTS Can You Now ...

1. List the main characteristics of the innate and adaptive immune systems?
2. List at least three examples of antigen-recognition molecules?
3. Define clonal distribution with respect to antigen receptors on B and T cells?
4. Compare antigen recognition by T and B cells?
5. Compare the primary and the secondary immune response to an antigen?
6. List at least three reasons why the study of the immune system is important to you as a physician in training?

 T cell receptor (TCR)   Immunoglobulin (Ig)   Antigen   MHC I

2

Basic Concepts and Components of the Immune System

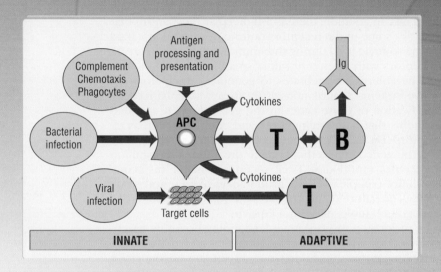

The essential features of the host defense system comprise an innate component that functions as a first line of defense and an adaptive component that takes longer to mobilize, but confers specificity and exhibits memory. As shown in the overview figure above, the two components are not independent but are functionally interrelated in various critical ways, for example through the actions of soluble effector molecules called **cytokines**.

■ INNATE IMMUNITY

An innate immune system exists in some form in most organisms. There are several important principles about the operation of the innate system. First, it is fast! Unlike the adaptive system, which may take days to mobilize, aspects of the innate system are extremely quickly mobilized. For example, phagocytic cells, particularly macrophages resident in tissues, will recognize infection via pattern-recognition molecules that detect structural motifs on invading bacteria. Another pattern-recognition molecule is the mannan-binding lectin (MBL) of the complement system, which recognizes molecules containing mannose on the surface of bacteria and helps to activate the complement cascade (Chapter 19). This use of non-pathogen-

specific recognition molecules is another feature of the innate system.

The innate system uses phagocytic cells, chiefly neutrophils and macrophages, and molecules such as the serum proteins of the complement system, which can interact directly with certain microbes to protect the host. Other cells important in the innate response are the **natural killer** (NK) cells (Chapter 21), which can detect certain virally infected cells and lyse them. Another group of important soluble molecules that is part of the innate defense system is the interferons (Chapter 19). Viral infection triggers interferon production by the infected cell. Interferon will inhibit the replication of many viruses and is not pathogen-specific.

Many innate system components, for example complement, interferon, and other mediator molecules or cells (such as macrophages), can affect cells of the specific adaptive system. This is another important observation. The innate and adaptive systems are interconnected and overlapping. The adaptive system is usually triggered by the innate system, and it only comes into play if the innate system fails to overwhelm the invading microbes, or if the invading microbe has found a way to avoid interaction with the innate system. The innate and adaptive systems are compared throughout this book, and the mechanisms that pathogens use to avoid detection by the immune system are also the subject of a later discussion.

■ ADAPTIVE IMMUNITY

An adaptive immune system is first observed in the evolutionary tree at the level of vertebrates. The adaptive immune system is capable of specifically distinguishing self from non self. This is accomplished by creating an anticipatory defense system of recognition molecules that interact with foreign, nonself antigen. Vertebrate genomes contain several genes encoding many antigen-recognition molecules. These gene families include antigen receptors that are capable of recognizing any given antigen (Fig. 2.1), including self-antigens. In addition, there is a molecular mechanism that enables some of the receptors (antibodies) to be modified at the somatic level during the immune response to create receptors with a better fit (more specific binding).

The ability of vertebrates to generate anticipatory defense systems against nonself entities was enhanced by duplication of those genes in the germline that encoded proteins that had binding **sites** and could function as receptors (Fig. 2.2). The products of these gene duplications are the gene families that encode the antigen-recognition molecules (antibodies, T-cell receptors, major histocompatibility complex [MHC] proteins) we know and study today. The nature of the original function of the primordial recognition molecules is not known.

A major step forward in understanding how this system works came with the idea that each lymphocyte expresses a unique antigen receptor. Once an antigen encounters a lymphocyte bearing the receptor that best fits the antigen, this pre-existing cell divides and gives rise to many daughter cells (clones). Thus, the lymphocyte is clonally expanded,

making available more of the receptor specific for the antigen encountered (Fig. 2.1). In other words, the repertoire of receptors is expressed clonally on lymphocytes, and "on binding antigen" a pre-existing clone is selectively

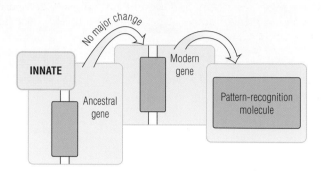

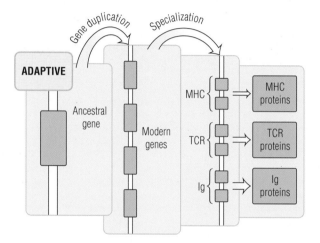

Figure 2.2 Evolution of antigen-recognition molecules and pattern-recognition molecules. Ig, immunoglobulin; MHC, major histocompatibility complex; TCR, T-cell receptor.

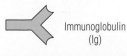

Figure 2.1 Lymphocytes with specific antigen receptors exist before an encounter with antigen.

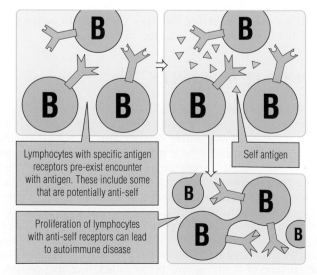

Figure 2.3 Proliferation of anti-self response.

 T cell receptor (TCR)   Immunoglobulin (Ig)   Antigen   MHC I

to generate more of the precise receptor required to interact with the antigen encountered (Fig. 2.1).

One complication of an anticipatory system with pre-existing receptors is, however, that anti-self receptors can be generated (Fig. 2.3), and the cells carrying these potentially damaging receptors must be deleted or inactivated. When mistakes occur and potentially anti-self cells are allowed to remain active, autoimmune (anti-self) disease can occur (Chapter 27).

This model for understanding the development of the capacity to recognize and respond specifically to non self is known as the **clonal selection theory** (Fig. 1.3). Aspects of the theory are developed further in Chapters 6, 7, 14, and 15.

■ COMPONENTS OF THE IMMUNE SYSTEM

The major features of an adaptive immune response are specificity, diversity, and memory. The response is specific in that it discriminates among various molecular entities; it is diverse in that it has the capacity to respond to almost any antigen that may be encountered, and it has memory in that it can recall previous contact with antigen and show a stronger response the second time. The last feature is the basis of vaccination, illustrated in Box 2.1.

The immune system uses cells (Fig. 2.5) and soluble molecules as effectors to protect the host. There are a number of different cell types, all leukocytes, which have

---

BOX 2.1 Vaccination with Hepatitis B

Hepatitis B viral (HBV) infection can cause short-term illness, typically jaundice, or chronic illness, such as cirrhosis, liver cancer, or death. In the United States, approximately 1.25 million people are infected with chronic hepatitis B every year, and approximately 5000 people die from it. Also in the United States, hepatitis B is spread through contact with the bodily fluids of an infected person. A vaccine is available. The vaccine is a recombinant protein (hepatitis B surface antigen: HBsAg) expressed from a plasmid in yeast cells.

The typical vaccination schedule is three intramuscular injections. The second dose is given 1 to 2 months after the first dose, and the third dose is given 4 to 6 months after the first dose. There is an alternative two-dose schedule for adolescents that appears to be just as effective. To assess protection, blood samples are taken after vaccination to ensure that sufficient antibody to HBsAg is present in the vaccine recipient's blood. A level of 10 milli-international units per milliliter (10 mIU/mL) of antibody to HBsAg is thought to be necessary for protection. Figure 2.4 shows a graph of conversion to protected status after the three-dose schedule. If an individual does not have ≥10 mIU/mL of antibody to HBsAg then the vaccine schedule is repeated.

Figure 2.4 also illustrates the difference in antibody response between a primary and a secondary (or subsequent) exposure to antigen. The initial, primary response is relatively slow and low-level. On subsequent immunization, the response is faster and of greater magnitude.

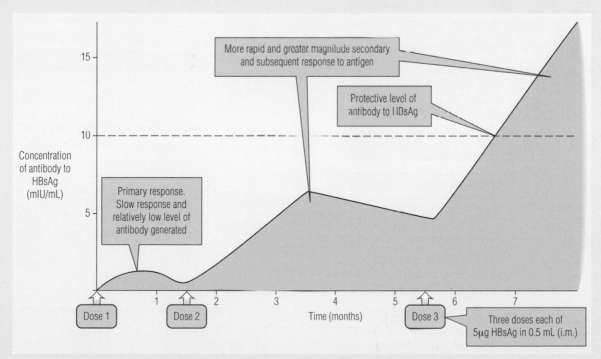

Figure 2.4 Vaccination with hepatitis B surface antigen (HBsAg). i.m., intramuscularly.

 MHC II   Cytokine, Chemokine, etc.   Complement (C')   Signaling molecule

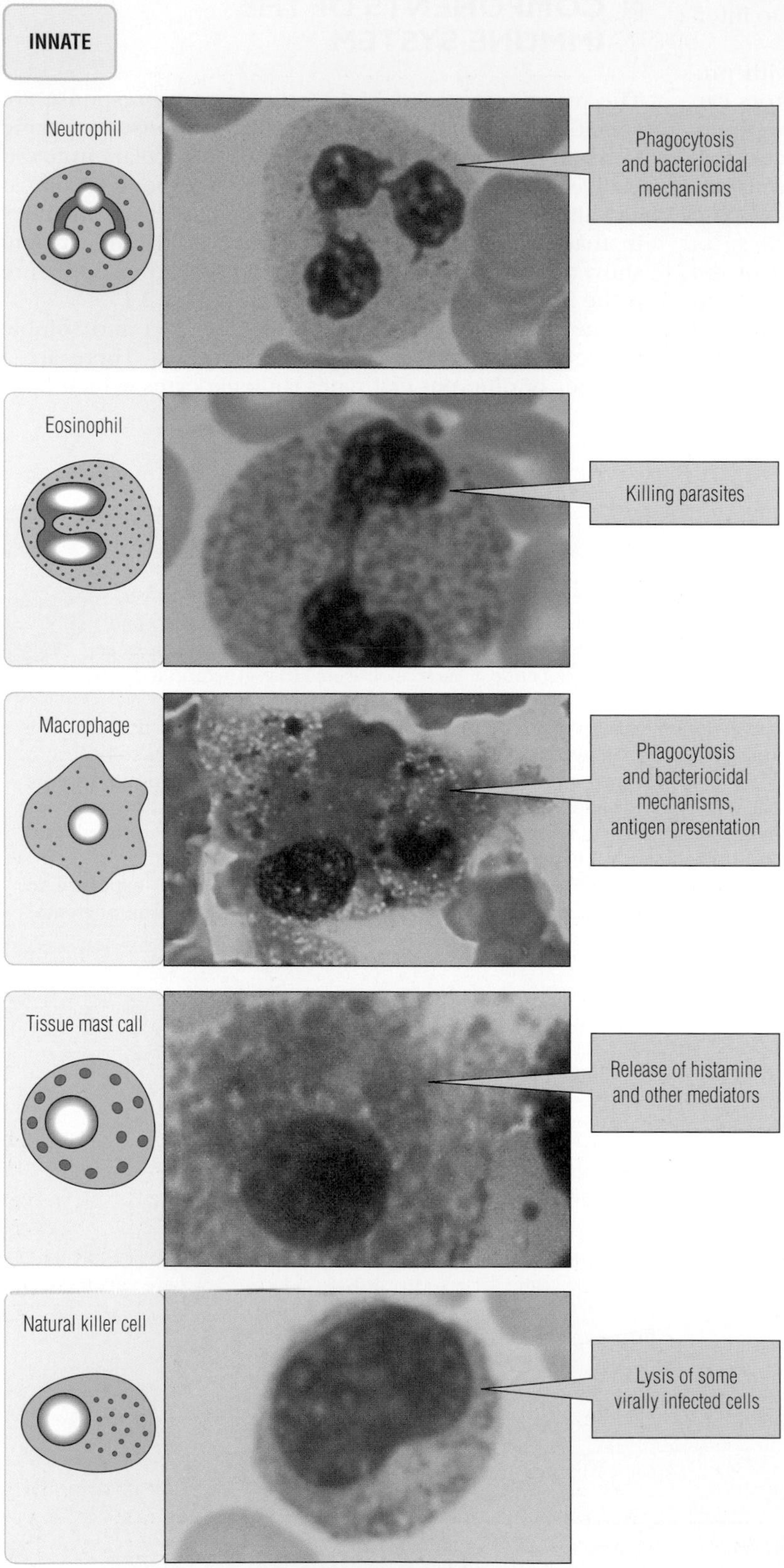

INNATE

Neutrophil

Phagocytosis and bacteriocidal mechanisms

Eosinophil

Killing parasites

Macrophage

Phagocytosis and bacteriocidal mechanisms, antigen presentation

Tissue mast call

Release of histamine and other mediators

Natural killer cell

Lysis of some virally infected cells

Figure 2.5 Major cells of the immune system.

 T cell receptor (TCR)

 Immunoglobulin (Ig)

 Antigen

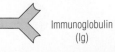 MHC I

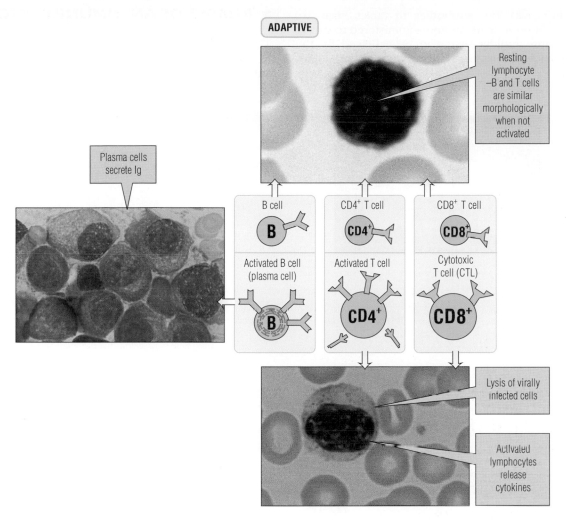

ADAPTIVE

Resting lymphocyte —B and T cells are similar morphologically when not activated

Plasma cells secrete Ig

B cell

Activated B cell (plasma cell)

CD4$^+$ T cell

Activated T cell

CD8$^+$ T cell

Cytotoxic T cell (CTL)

Lysis of virally infected cells

Activated lymphocytes release cytokines

Figure 2.5b (cont'd)

specialized to have different functions. For example, phagocytic cells such as neutrophils and macrophages are used nonspecifically to destroy invading microbes. Mature cells can occur in blood or in tissues—for example, lymphocytes in blood and dendritic cells in tissue. Lymphocytes (B and T cells) provide *specific* immunity. The products of B cells, antibodies, are soluble molecules, sometimes referred to as the humoral immune system. Extracellular pathogens are eliminated chiefly by antibodies, whereas intracellular pathogens require T cells (and macrophages) for elimination. The function of T cells is sometimes referred to as **cell-mediated immunity** in contrast to **humoral** or antibody-mediated immunity. Antigen presenting cells (APCs), such as dendritic cells in the skin and macrophages (Fig. 2.6), are critical in initiating the activation of B and T cells.

Antigen processing and presentation is presented in Chapter 10. Briefly, APCs, such as macrophages, take up antigens and subject them to proteolytic degradation in various compartments of the cell. These events are called

antigen processing, and they are required because, although B-cell antigen receptors bind directly to antigen, T-cell receptors for antigen only recognize *processed* antigen that is displayed on APCs. The peptide antigens are displayed in the peptide-binding groove of MHC molecules (Chapter 8).

Some organisms try to evade the immune system, but the immune system has developed methods of fighting back (Box 2.2).

■ ACTIVE AND PASSIVE IMMUNITY

Two further divisions of immunity exist. **Active immunity** is where the individual plays a direct role in responding to the antigen—for example, after an encounter with a virus (see Box 4.1). This is in contrast to **passive immunity**, wherein immunity is transferred from one individual to another by transferring immune cells or serum from an immunized individual to an unimmunized individual—for example, when anti-rabies antibody is provided after a dog

 MHC II

 Cytokine, Chemokine, etc.

 Complement (C')

 Signaling molecule

bite (see Box 4.2). The antibodies to rabies virus are developed in other individuals and administered to confer protection more rapidly than can be achieved by the injured individuals making the necessary antibodies themselves.

■ PHASES OF AN IMMUNE RESPONSE

There are several steps or phases in an active immune response (Fig. 2.7). First is the **cognitive phase**, when antigen is recognized. Antigen encounters a cell bearing a

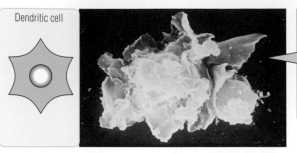

Dendritic cell

Scanning electron micrograph of a dendritic cell as found in lymphoid tissues and in skin. Critical in uptake and presentation of antigen to T cells

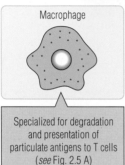

Macrophage

Specialized for degradation and presentation of particulate antigens to T cells (*see* Fig. 2.5 A)

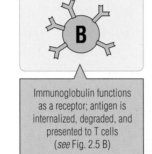

B cell

Immunoglobulin functions as a receptor; antigen is internalized, degraded, and presented to T cells (*see* Fig. 2.5 B)

Figure 2.6 Antigen-presenting cells. Scanning electron micrograph of dendritic cell provided by Dr. Stella Knight, London, UK.

BOX 2.2 Dealing with Sneaky Pathogens

There are many ways in which organisms evolve to evade the immune system and equally numerous ways in which the immune system has developed to fight back. The innate immune system includes two populations of cells, which combat special types of evasion mechanisms.

Parasitic worms have adapted to live inside the host at mucosal surfaces, notably the gut. These surfaces are out of reach of many immune system mechanisms, and the large, multicellular worms are difficult to attack. Mast cells and eosinophils are innate immune system cells that reside or are recruited to mucosal surfaces and can recognize worms. In doing so, they stimulate secretion of mucus and smooth muscle contraction In the affected organ. The worm looses its grip and is expelled from the host.

At the other extreme, some viruses have evolved mechanisms for evading recognition by T cells of the adaptive immune system. For example, herpes viruses can switch off expression of MHC molecules in infected cells. Because T cells use MHC molecules to detect antigen, herpes virus infection can go unrecognized. Natural killer cells have evolved to gauge the level of MHC expression on cells. If MHC expression on a cell is reduced, they are able to kill the cell. Natural killer cells thus help overcome the evasion mechanism used by herpes viruses.

Mast cells, eosinophils, and natural killer cells are all described in detail in Chapter 21.

MHC, major histocompatibility complex.

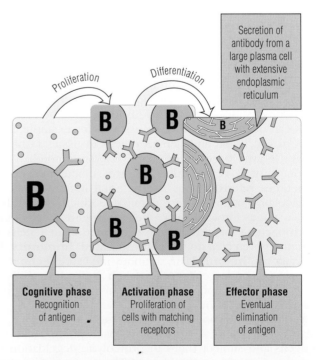

Proliferation   Differentiation

Secretion of antibody from a large plasma cell with extensive endoplasmic reticulum

Cognitive phase
Recognition of antigen

Activation phase
Proliferation of cells with matching receptors

Effector phase
Eventual elimination of antigen

Figure 2.7 Phases of an immune response illustrated for B cells and leading to antibody production.

 T cell receptor (TCR)

 Immunoglobulin (Ig)

 Antigen

 MHC I

receptor that fits the antigen. This cell is activated and proliferates (Chapter 11). Next, more and more of the same clone of cells is produced—this is the **activation phase**. The cells undergo various changes, known as differentiation, to enable a response. For example, various developmental steps occur (Chapter 14) in a B cell, leading to a whole new cell, called a plasma cell, which synthesizes and secretes large amounts of antibody molecules. At this point, the antibodies help to eliminate the antigen. This phase is a third phase, referred to as the **effector phase**. Various steps take place to downregulate the response once the antigen is eliminated. These steps are designed to regulate the response and prevent it from continuing after the antigen or microbe is neutralized or eliminated.

LEARNING POINTS Can You Now ...

1. Describe at least three characteristics of the innate and adaptive immune response systems?

2. Describe at least three ways in which the innate and adaptive systems are interrelated?

3. Explain the concept of an anticipatory immune defense system?

4. Describe the phases of an immune response and the critical role of clonal selection in achieving a specific response?

5. Describe the fundamental properties of an adaptive immune response system?

6. List the major cells involved in the innate and adaptive immune response?

 MHC II

 Cytokine, Chemokine, etc.

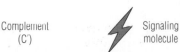 Complement (C') Signaling molecule

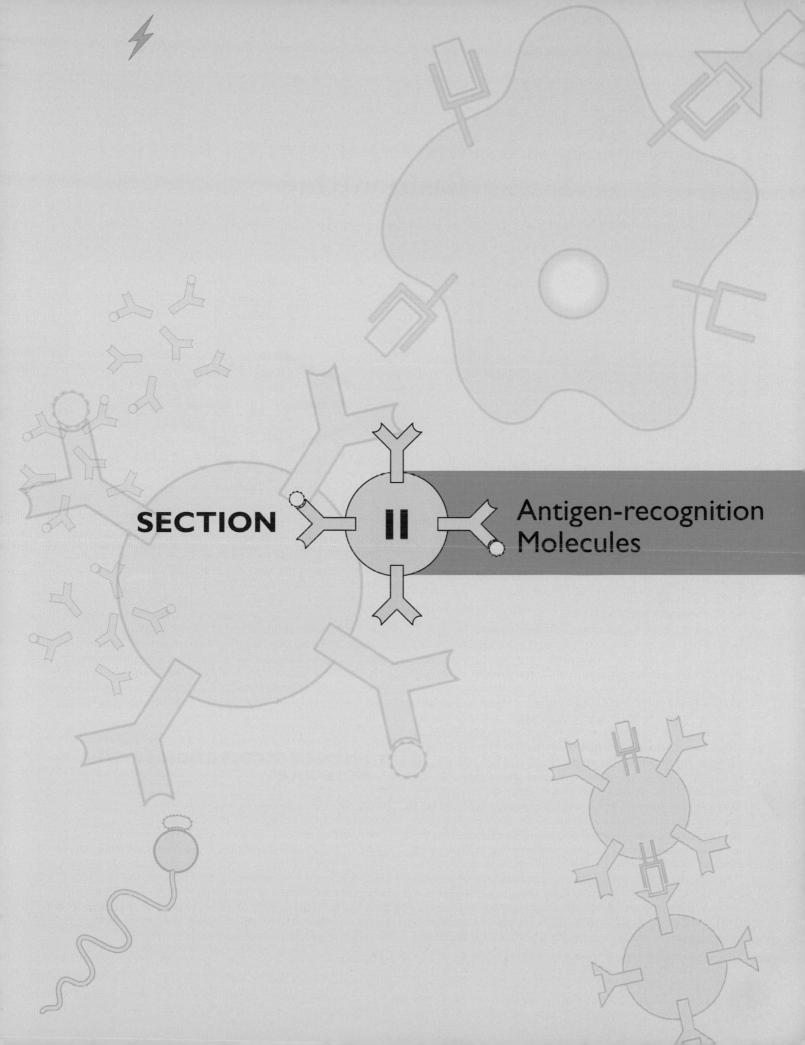

SECTION II

Antigen-recognition Molecules

3 Introduction to Antigen Recognition

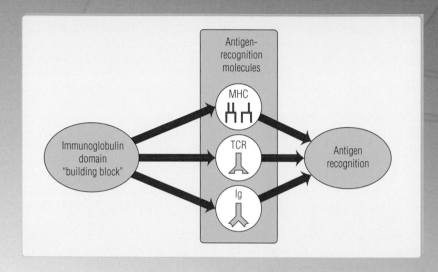

As described in Chapters 1 and 2, there are two main systems that allow humans to identify foreign (nonself) materials. These are:

- The innate immune system
- The adaptive immune system

The innate or nonadaptive immune system is characterized by the presence of phagocytic cells and blood proteins, such as the complement proteins. Complement proteins are serum proteins that form protein cascades, each activated component activating the next to generate a physiologic response. Complement can bind to bacteria, making holes in their membrane, and can also attract phagocytes to foreign material. Complement also helps to eliminate **immune complexes** (antibody-antigen) and prevent them from damaging the body. In addition to complement, pattern-recognition molecules found in the blood are also part of the innate immune system. For example, the liver makes a mannan-binding lectin (MBL) that recognizes mannose residues on glycoprotein and glycolipid molecules found in the bacterial capsule. Binding of MBLs to a bacterial capsule triggers the complement cascade and may help in direct killing of the bacterium (Chapter 19) or in the recruitment of phagocytes. In general, our own cells are not attacked by complement proteins because they possess proteins that inactivate complement.

The innate immune system relies on pre-existing molecules and cells, which nonspecifically attack invaders, and

this system protects us well against a wide range of infections. Generally, the innate system protects against infection by removing the infectious agent. However, it is unable to respond *specifically* to microbes or other foreign material (antigen). Microbes evolve much more rapidly than vertebrates, thus enabling them to evade nonadaptive defense systems by changing their structure. This is one reason that vertebrates developed an adaptive immune system. This system depends on gene rearrangement to generate a large number of pre-existing receptors (repertoire), expressed on lymphocytes, that can identify essentially any antigen.

■ ANTIGEN-RECOGNITION MOLECULES

There are three groups of molecules that specifically recognize foreign antigen for the adaptive immune system. The first two are cell-surface–located receptors found on B and T cells. The B-cell receptor is also secreted from differentiated B cells (plasma cells) to create a soluble antigen receptor, known as **antibody**. The third group of antigen receptors is encoded in the major histocompatibility complex (MHC). This cluster of genes is known as human leukocyte antigen (HLA) in humans. The MHC molecules function to present antigenic peptides to T cells.

B-Cell and T-Cell Receptors (BCR and TCR)

As described in Chapter 2, adaptive immunity depends on clonal selection for its efficient operation. Each B cell or T cell expresses a unique antigen receptor on its cell surface. On encountering foreign antigen, the cell expressing a receptor that best fits the antigen divides and produces daughter cells (**clones**) that have the same receptor. Diversity of receptors is generated by gene rearrangement (Chapters 6 and 7). This allows a vast repertoire of receptors to be made from a limited number of genes that rearrange and combine to give the diversity needed. Thus, the B-cell and T-cell antigen receptors are inherited as gene fragments. The gene fragments are joined together to form a complete antigen receptor gene only in individual lymphocytes as they develop. The process of rearranging and joining fragments of antigen receptor genes creates a diverse array of receptors. Theoretically, the number of different antibody molecules that could be made by the B lymphocytes in an individual could be as high as 10^{11}. This is why it is thought that there are sufficient B-cell and T-cell antigen receptors to identify all the antigens—for example, microbes—in our environment. Keep in mind that receptors for every antigen in a microbe need not exist as long as one or a few exist. The immune system only needs to identify one of the many potential antigens in a microbe to protect the host by interfering with the ability of the microbe to grow and divide.

The genes encoding B-cell antigen receptors also undergo a process during the immune response called **hypermutation** to create receptors that are an even better fit for the foreign antigen. This process of rapid mutation of sequences that encode the binding site for antigen creates many more unique receptors and an even more specific and diverse repertoire.

The antigen receptors of B-cells and T-cells, in addition to being generated via similar genetic mechanisms, are also similar with respect to their protein structures. They have a protein structure feature, known as the **immunoglobulin fold**, that is common to several receptor families, where parallel strands of amino acids fold into a compact globular domain, including the antigen receptors found on immune cells.

Major Histocompatibility Complex Molecules

Proteins encoded by the MHC genes represent the third group of antigen-receptor molecules. There are two main classes of molecules, which were initially named because of their role in tissue (histo-) graft rejection (compatibility). Class I MHC molecules are found essentially on all cells, and class II are found chiefly on B cells, macrophages, and dendritic cells. Their function is to present peptides to T cells. Molecules in the two MHC classes have similar structures and are also part of the family of protein molecules that uses the immunoglobulin fold (the family is known as the immunoglobulin supergene family).

The structure of the MHC molecules is described in greater detail in Chapter 8, and their function in Chapter 10. Briefly, the T-cell receptor can only recognize a foreign antigen if it is presented as a complex with an MHC molecule. The T-cell receptor contacts residues on the foreign peptide and the MHC molecule. This is a different kind of antigen recognition from that involving the B-cell antigen receptor, which binds directly to the antigen. The dual recognition requirement distinguishes T-cell receptor molecules from B-cell receptor molecules. The physiologic function of MHC molecules is to capture and display antigens from cell-associated microbes, such as viral proteins made in the host cell, for identification as foreign by T cells.

The genes that encode MHC molecules are the most variable genes we know of in the human genome. They are said to be extensively **polymorphic** (existence of multiple alleles or forms of the same gene). Their diversity, however, exists in the population as a whole, not in the individual. A comparison of MHC diversity with immunoglobulin and T-cell receptor diversity is provided in Figure 3.1. In every person, there are approximately six different class I and II MHC gene products. Given that their parents likely have completely different HLA genes, most people have 12 different class I and II MHC molecules on the surface of certain of their lymphoid cells. Unlike B-cell or T-cell receptors, which differ in every lymphocyte in an individual, all of the MHC alleles are the same in an individual, but they are different between individuals. Thus, in the population as a whole, some MHC molecules can bind antigenic peptides from a given microbe, but, potentially, any given individual may not bind a peptide from that microbe. This means that some individuals in the population may be more susceptible to a given microbe-induced disease than others. For example, if the structure of your MHC molecules makes it impossible for you to recognize and bind any peptide antigen from a given virus, you will not be able to activate a T-cell response to cells infected with that virus. Consequently, you would be susceptible to that virus-induced disease. However, the broad specificity of the peptide-binding groove in MHC molecules (described in Chapters 8 and 10) makes it unlikely that there would be no peptides from any given microbe that would fit the peptide-binding groove of an individual's MHC molecules.

 MHC II

Cytokine, Chemokine, etc.

 Complement (C')

Signaling molecule

BOX 3.1 The Advantages of HLA Diversity: HLA and HIV-1

One theory concerning the extensive polymorphism of the HLA genes is that the more different HLA class I molecules there are in the population or in an individual, the less likely it will be that a pathogen could escape the immune response by expressing no epitopes that could be bound by an MHC molecule. Therefore, by extrapolation, individuals who are heterozygous for the HLA genes should be at a survival advantage compared with homozygotes. Some evidence for this hypothesis has been obtained. A study of several hundred patients infected with HIV-1 showed that, although HIV-1-infected patients who were homozygous or heterozygous at the class I HLA loci (*HLA-A*, *HLA-B*, and *HLA-C*) could all progress to AIDS, those patients who were homozygous for the HLA class I loci progressed more quickly toward AIDS and death. In addition, it was observed that there was a faster progression to AIDS and death with an increase in the number of homozygous HLA class I loci.

This study provides some evidence for a selective advantage of MHC diversity in surviving longer with HIV/AIDS. By extension to the human population at large, it seems likely that the considerable diversity (polymorphism) of the MHC genes contributes a selective advantage for the human species (Chapter 8).

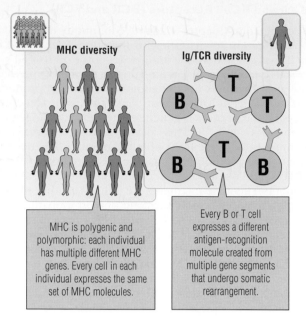

MHC is polygenic and polymorphic: each individual has multiple different MHC genes. Every cell in each individual expresses the same set of MHC molecules.

Every B or T cell expresses a different antigen-recognition molecule created from multiple gene segments that undergo somatic rearrangement.

Figure 3.1 Diversity mechanisms of major histocompatibility complexes (MHC) compared with immunoglobulin (Ig) and T-cell receptors (TCR).

LEARNING POINTS Can You Now ...

1. List the main categories of antigen-recognition molecules?

2. Explain how T-cell and B-cell receptor diversity is achieved?

3. Explain MHC polymorphism and why it is advantageous?

 T cell receptor (TCR)   Immunoglobulin (Ig)   Antigen   MHC I

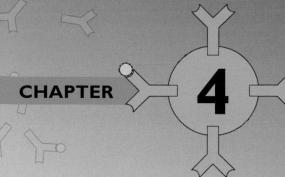

CHAPTER 4

Antigens and Antibody Structure

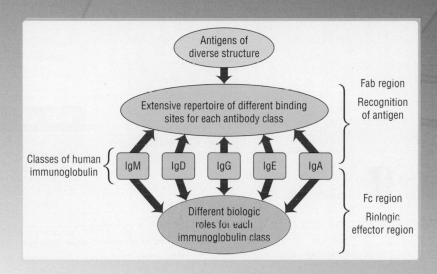

The overview figure above illustrates the topics covered in this chapter. In the first part of this chapter, we describe the various types of antigen and which antigens elicit the best immune responses. In the second part, we describe the general structure of the various classes of human **antibodies (immunoglobulins)** and selected molecular and biologic properties of antibodies. In Chapter 5 we explore in more depth the nature of antibody-antigen interaction, and in Chapter 6 we explain how antibody diversity is generated.

Antigens that cause a strong immune response can have an extensive variety of chemical structures. Antibodies are the antigen-specific proteins produced by B cells in response to contact with antigen. Antibodies circulate in the blood and lymph as plasma components. Each individual has the capacity to synthesize a vast number of different antibody molecules, each capable of specifically interacting with an antigen.

■ ANTIGENS

Antigens and Immunogens

In Chapter 1, antigens were introduced as foreign (nonself) molecules. At this point, some further definition is required to distinguish antigens, which by themselves may or may not cause an immune response, and immunogens,

which always do. An immunogen is a substance that by itself causes an immune response (e.g., production of an antibody). Effective immunogens are foreign to the host, fairly large (generally with a molecular weight greater than ≈ 6000), and chemically complex (e.g., proteins made up of 20 different amino acid residues are better immunogens than nucleic acids made up of 4 different nucleotide bases). Antigens, by comparison, are compounds capable of being bound by immunologic receptors (B-cell receptors [BCR], T-cell receptors [TCR], major histocompatibility complex [MHC]), but they do not necessarily elicit an immune response by themselves. For example, a relatively simple chemical compound, such as penicillin, cannot by itself induce an antibody response. These simple molecules are known as **haptens**. If the hapten is coupled to a macromolecule (e.g., a protein), antibodies can be generated that bind very specifically to the hapten (Fig. 4.1).

Epitopes

The terms *antigen* and *epitope* are sometimes used interchangeably. However, an **epitope** is generally used to refer to an area on a much larger molecule (e.g., a viral protein) with which an antibody can react. A viral protein may contain a large number of epitopes that are capable of interacting with many different specific antibodies. There are two different types of epitope (Fig. 4.2):

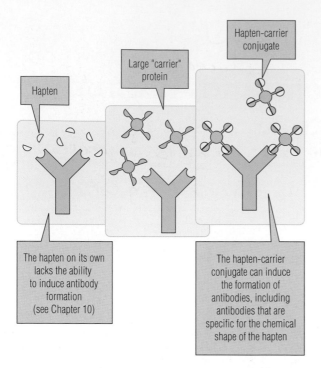

Figure 4.1 Hapten-carrier conjugate.

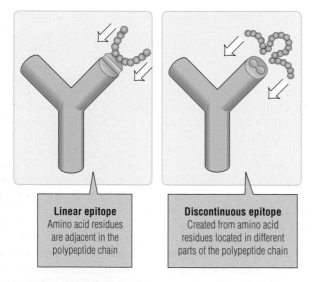

Linear epitope
Amino acid residues are adjacent in the polypeptide chain

Discontinuous epitope
Created from amino acid residues located in different parts of the polypeptide chain

Figure 4.2 Linear and discontinuous epitopes.

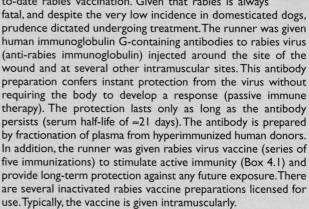
Chapter 10). Antibodies, as indicated in Figure 4.2, can recognize both types of epitope.

ANTIBODIES

Antibody Isolation and Characterization

Antibodies are immunoglobulins that react specifically with the antigen that stimulated their production. They make up approximately 20% of the plasma proteins and were initially detected by analytic techniques, such as electrophoresis, in the "gamma globulin" fraction of serum (Fig. 4.3). Serum is the liquid phase that is separated from clotted blood. It differs from plasma (the liquid phase that

- Discontinuous or conformational epitopes resulting from bringing together amino acid residues from non-contiguous areas of the polypeptide chain into a three-dimensional (3D) shape
- Continuous or linear epitopes, which are contiguous areas of sequence (e.g., amino acids 12-22 in a polypeptide chain)

Immunologic receptors on T cells recognize linear epitopes because of the way in which processed antigen is presented to them (associated with MHC molecules; see

 T cell receptor (TCR)   Immunoglobulin (Ig)   Antigen  MHC I

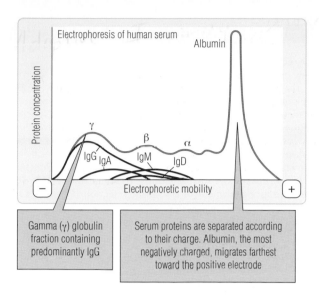

Figure 4.3 Electrophoresis of total human serum.

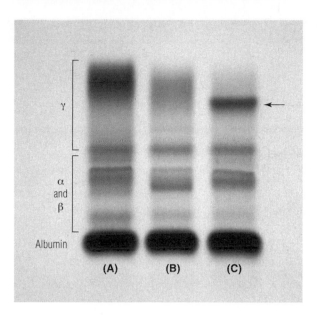

Figure 4.4 Gel electrophoresis of serum from different patients. A, Patient with polyclonal expansion of B cells and increased protein in the γ-globulin area. B, Normal serum from a control sample. C, Monoclonal expansion of B cells with an immunoglobulin spike (*arrow*) from a patient with a B-cell malignancy.

may be separated when blood is drawn and prevented from clotting) in that it is lacking the protein fibrinogen. The antibody-bearing fraction of plasma or serum is referred to as immunoglobulin. The immunoglobulins in serum constitute a highly heterogeneous spectrum of proteins, not a single molecular species (Fig. 4.3), because normal serum immunoglobulins are the heterogeneous products of many clones of B cells (polyclonal Ig). Antibodies that arise in response to a single complex antigen (e.g., a bacterial protein with multiple epitopes) are heterogeneous in chemical structure and specificity because they are formed by several different clones of B cells, each expressing an immunoglobulin capable of binding to a different epitope on the antigen (see Chapters 6 and 14). This made biochemical studies of immunoglobulins very difficult initially because pure molecules of one specificity could not easily be isolated. One finding that helped in this regard was the observation that after electrophoresis of serum, the immunoglobulin region in patients with a B-cell malignancy was often a band covering a very narrow range of electrophoretic mobility (Fig. 4.4). In this disease, a single clone of B cells may proliferate, and these multiple cells secrete a homogeneous immunoglobulin that accumulates in the serum at relatively high concentration. These immunoglobulins became a source of relatively pure protein for biochemical studies early in the investigation of their structure. Today, **monoclonal antibodies**, homogeneous antibodies from a single clone of B cells, can be prepared in virtually unlimited quantities (Box 4.3). This has been useful for studies of immunoglobulin structure and function, for clinical investigations, and for therapy.

Antibody Structure

All antibodies have the same basic molecular structure (Fig. 4.6). They are made up of light (L) and heavy (H) chains, which refer to their relative molecular weights; the light chains have a molecular weight of approximately 25,000, and the heavy chains have a molecular weight of approximately 50,000 to 70,000. In the basic immunoglobulin (Ig) molecule, there are two heavy and two light chains linked together by intermolecular disulfide bonds as shown in Figure 4.6. There are five different classes of human heavy chain with slightly different structures. These are designated by lower-case Greek letters: μ (mu) for IgM, δ (delta) for IgD, γ (gamma) for IgG, ε (epsilon) for IgE, and α (alpha) for IgA (Fig. 4.7). Light chains are divided into two types, κ (kappa) or λ (lambda). Both types of light chain are found in all five classes of immunoglobulin, but any one antibody contains only one type of light chain. Any one IgG molecule consists of identical H chains and identical L chains organized into the Y-shaped structure shown in Figure 4.6. The IgG class can be divided on the basis of physicochemical and biologic properties into subclasses. For example, human IgG molecules can be subdivided into IgG1–IgG4. The molecular structures (amino acid sequences) of members of two different subclasses (e.g., IgG_1 and IgG_3) are more similar to each other than are the structures of two immunoglobulins from different classes (e.g., IgG and IgA).

The basic immunoglobulin contains molecular parts with distinctive functions. This was shown by a number of biochemical studies. If the basic immunoglobulin molecule (IgG) is subjected to proteolytic cleavage, several fragments are produced (Fig. 4.8). For example, if the enzyme papain is used to cleave IgG, two major types of fragment are obtained. One fragment binds antigen and is referred to as Fab (fragment antigen-binding). The other fragment, known as Fc (fraction crystallizable), does not bind antigen but activates a molecular pathway known as complement

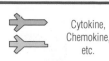 MHC II

 Cytokine, Chemokine, etc.

 Complement (C')

 Signaling molecule

BOX 4.3 Production of Monoclonal Antibodies

Monoclonal antibodies are homogeneous immunoglobulins. They can be prepared with almost any desired specificity. Hybridoma technology makes it possible to derive homogeneous immunoglobulins of any desired specificity for use in biomedical research and for therapy. The production of hybridomas is illustrated in Figure 4.5. The aim is to produce immortalized cells that only secrete immunoglobulin directed against the antigen used in immunization. It is important to be sure that myeloma cells that have not fused with immunized B cells do not survive. To do this, the myeloma cells that are used have a mutation, resulting in lack of a specific metabolic enzyme, without which they die in some culture media. After fusion, the cells are grown in these media and both nonimmortalized B cells and nonfused myeloma cells will die. Only myeloma cells that have fused with B cells and received the correct metabolic enzyme survive. Colonies of hybrid cells are grown up and screened for the production of antibody of the desired specificity. Screening for antibody-positive colonies usually involves an enzyme-linked immunosorbent assay (ELISA), described in Chapter 5. Various clinical uses have been found for monoclonal antibodies, including measurements of substances such as blood levels of hormones. In vivo, monoclonal antibody anti-CD3, which reacts with human T cells, has been used as a treatment in transplant rejection (Chapter 33). Similarly, monoclonal antibodies that react with tumor cells have been used in diagnosis and treatment of cancer (Chapter 34).

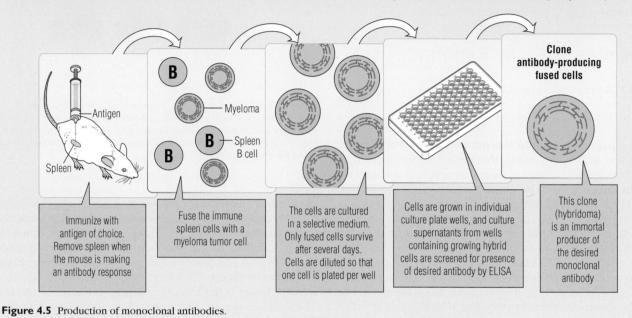

Clone antibody-producing fused cells

Immunize with antigen of choice. Remove spleen when the mouse is making an antibody response

Fuse the immune spleen cells with a myeloma tumor cell

The cells are cultured in a selective medium. Only fused cells survive after several days. Cells are diluted so that one cell is plated per well

Cells are grown in individual culture plate wells, and culture supernatants from wells containing growing hybrid cells are screened for presence of desired antibody by ELISA

This clone (hybridoma) is an immortal producer of the desired monoclonal antibody

Antigen — Spleen — Myeloma — Spleen B cell

Figure 4.5 Production of monoclonal antibodies.

Light chain

Heavy chain

Fab region binds antigen

Hinge region allows flexibility

Fc effector region binds to various cellular receptors and to complement

Carbohydrate helps protect from proteolytic degradation

Disulfide bonds

Figure 4.6 Basic antibody structure.

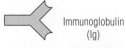 T cell receptor (TCR)

 Immunoglobulin (Ig)

Antigen

MHC I

FIG. 4.7 Selected Properties of Human Immunoglobulins

	IgM	IgD	IgG	IgE	IgA
Heavy chain symbol	μ	δ	γ	ε	α
Mean serum concentration (mg/mL)	0.4-2.5	<0.03	7-18	<0.0005	0.8-4
Serum half-life (days)	7	2	21	2	7
Activates complement	++	–	+	–	–
Placement transfer	–	–	+	–	–
Cell-binding via Fc receptors	–	–	Mononuclear cells and neutrophils	Mast cells and basophils	Mononuclear cells and neutrophils

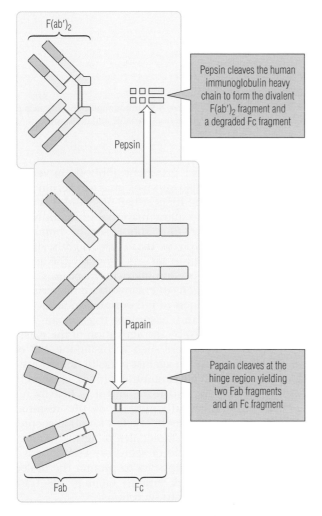

Pepsin cleaves the human immunoglobulin heavy chain to form the divalent F(ab')₂ fragment and a degraded Fc fragment

Papain cleaves at the hinge region yielding two Fab fragments and an Fc fragment

Figure 4.8. Proteolytic digestion of immunoglobulin. Fab, antigen-binding fragment; Fc, complement-fixing fragment.

(Chapter 19) and has various biologic effector functions, such as the ability to bind to receptors found on macrophages and various other cells. If the proteolytic enzyme pepsin is used, the two Fab fragments remain linked (F(ab')₂) but the Fc fragment is digested to small fragments and the effector functions are lost. These findings suggested that the different molecular parts of the Ig molecule have different functions—one for binding antigen and one responsible for other biological effector functions.

Further biochemical studies, initially involving amino acid sequencing of the L and H chains of a number of different antibody molecules, demonstrated that the L and H chains can be differentiated into regions that are highly variable in sequence (V_L and V_H) and regions that are essentially constant (C_L and C_H). If, for example, several different λ-chains from different Igs are subjected to amino acid sequencing, there will be a region of considerable similarity in sequence, but also a region of approximately 110 amino acid residues at the N-terminus of the L chain where substantial sequence differences are observed between different λ-chains (Fig. 4.9). The same is true for H chains. The C regions carry out the biologic effector functions, such as the ability to bind complement proteins, and the V regions bind antigen. The variable regions are critical for the ability to respond to a vast number of different antigen structures.

Additional 3D-structure determination has revealed that the Igs are composed of folded, repeating segments called **domains**. An L chain consists of one variable domain and one constant domain, and an H chain consists of one variable and three or more constant domains. Each domain is approximately 110 amino acid residues long and is connected to other domains by short segments of more extended polypeptide chain, as shown in Figure 4.10. Other molecules of the immune system have similar folded polypeptide domains, giving rise to the term **immunoglobulin supergene family** to describe this group of related proteins.

Selected Features and Biological Properties of the Immunoglobulin Classes

Antibodies can occur as soluble proteins in the circulation or be displayed on the surface of B cells. The primary function of all antibodies is to bind antigen. This can result in the inactivation of a pathogen—for example, by agglutinating bacteria (clumping them together) and preventing their entry to host cells. If bacteria are coated with antibody, the likelihood that they will be engulfed by phagocytic cells (opsonization) is enhanced. Antibodies can also activate complement (Chapter 19) and initiate a lytic reaction that destroys the cell to which the antibody is bound. The five classes of antibody have different functions that are a consequence of differences in structure (Fig. 4.11).

 MHC II

  Cytokine, Chemokine, etc.

 Complement (C')

 Signaling molecule

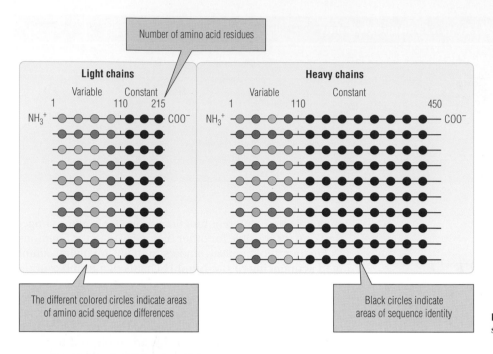

Figure 4.9. Immunoglobulin amino acid sequences: variable and constant regions.

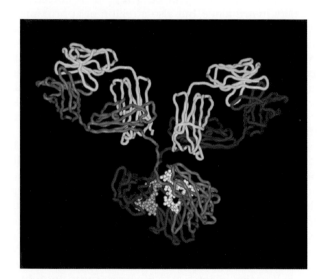

Figure 4.10. Three-dimensional domain structure of an immunoglobulin molecule. From Kumar et al: Robbins and Cotran Pathologic Basis of Disease, 7th Edition, Figure 6-5 W.B. Saunders, 2005.

- **IgM.** This is the predominant antibody early in an immune response. It has a pentameric structure, composed of five H_2L_2 units (each similar to an IgG), held together by a joining (J) chain. It has 10 potential antigen-binding sites and because of this it is the most efficient antibody at agglutinating bacteria and activating complement.
- **IgD.** IgD is chiefly found on the surface of B cells as a receptor molecule and is involved in cell activation.

- **IgG.** This is the most prevalent antibody molecule in serum (Fig. 4.7). It also survives intact in serum for the longest time (has the longest half-life), and it is able to cross the placenta to allow maternal protection of the newborn. There are four subclasses of human IgG (IgG_1–IgG_4), and each of these has slightly different properties. For example, IgG_2 is generally the antibody subclass found to predominate in responses against polysaccharide antigens of encapsulated bacteria.
- **IgE.** Binding of antigen to IgE coupled to an Fc receptor on mast cells and basophils triggers an allergic reaction (Chapter 26) by the activation of the mast cell and release of mediators such as histamine. IgE originally evolved to protect against parasitic infections.
- **IgA.** This is the main immunoglobulin in secretions such as saliva, milk, and tears, and it is heavily represented in the mucosal epithelia of the respiratory, genital, and intestinal tracts. The IgA found in secretions (sIgA) consists of two molecules of IgA, a joining (J) chain, and one molecule of secretory component. The secretory component appears to protect the molecule from proteolytic attack and to facilitate its transfer across epithelial cells into secretions.

As shown in Figure 4.7, Igs interact with a variety of cell types via the presence of receptors (Fc receptors of various kinds) on the cell. This interaction recruits the cells and their products (e.g., inflammatory macrophages and cytokines) to become a part of the protective host response to foreign antigens.

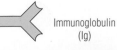 T cell receptor (TCR)   Immunoglobulin (Ig)   Antigen   MHC I

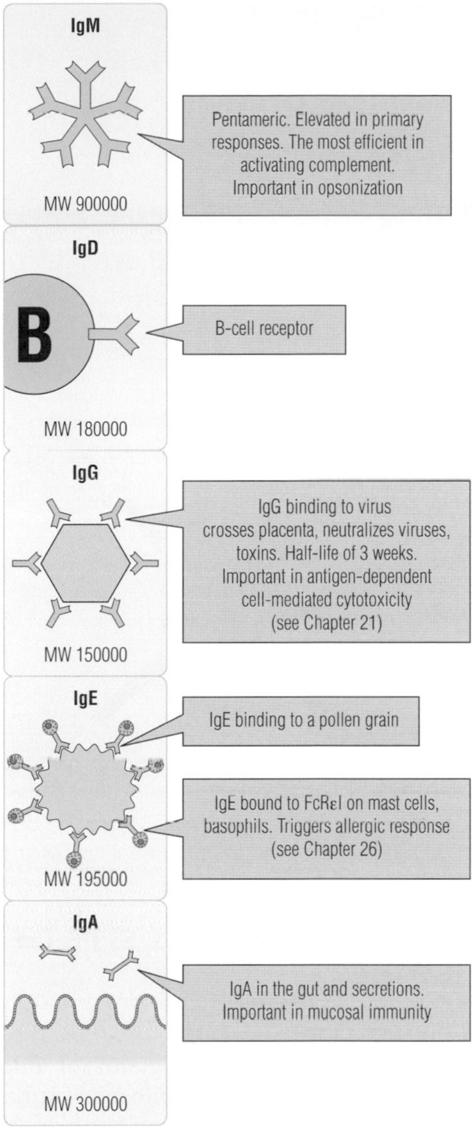
IgM
Pentameric. Elevated in primary responses. The most efficient in activating complement. Important in opsonization
MW 900000
IgD
B
B-cell receptor
MW 180000
IgG
IgG binding to virus crosses placenta, neutralizes viruses, toxins. Half-life of 3 weeks. Important in antigen-dependent cell-mediated cytotoxicity (see Chapter 21)
MW 150000
IgE
IgE binding to a pollen grain
IgE bound to FcRεI on mast cells, basophils. Triggers allergic response (see Chapter 26)
MW 195000
IgA
IgA in the gut and secretions. Important in mucosal immunity
MW 300000

Figure 4.11. Biologic properties of immunoglobulin classes.

LEARNING POINTS Can You Now ...

1. Compare antigenicity and immunogenicity?
2. Define antigen, antigenic determinant, epitope, and hapten, and give examples?
3. Draw the basic structure of the immunoglobulin molecule, indicating the location of the major structural features—for example, variable regions, hinge regions, constant domains?
4. Recall what useful fragments of immunoglobulin may be produced by proteolytic digestion—for example, the antigen-binding fragment (Fab)?
5. Recall the structural features and biologic properties of the different immunoglobulin classes and subclasses?
6. Define monoclonality and polyclonality with respect to antibodies?

MHC II
Cytokine, Chemokine, etc.
Complement (C')
Signaling molecule

5 Antibody-Antigen Interaction

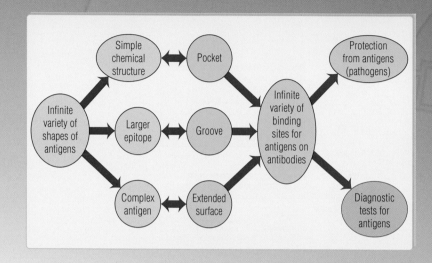

The overview figure above illustrates the topics for this chapter, which describe how antibodies interact with an almost infinite variety of shapes of antigens and how this interaction protects us from pathogens. In this chapter, we also review the development of very specific diagnostic tests for the presence of antigens or antibodies. The most striking feature of antibody–antigen interaction is its specificity. Otherwise, antibody–antigen interactions are much like other receptor-ligand interactions. Physicochemical forces are involved in the interaction between an antibody and an antigen that are similar to those between an enzyme and its substrate (or competitive inhibitor), or between a receptor (insulin receptor) and a ligand (insulin). These forces derive from:

- Electrostatic interactions between charged side-chains
- Hydrogen bonds
- van der Waals forces
- Hydrophobic interactions.

The sum of these typically weak noncovalent interactions can be a relatively strong interaction.

The extraordinary specificity of antibodies has led to their widespread use in diagnostic testing. In the latter part of this chapter, we describe several of the most important applications of antibody–antigen interaction in diagnosing disease.

■ THE ANTIGEN-BINDING SITE OF ANTIBODIES

Many experimental approaches have been used to define the structure of the antibody-binding site for antigen. By far, the most detailed and valuable information has come from x-ray crystallographic studies of antigen–antibody complexes. One conclusion from analyses of the three-dimensional (3D) structure of several antigen–antibody complexes is that the size and shape of the antigen-binding site can vary greatly. For example, the combining site can be a long, shallow crevice, or a wider, more open cleft type structure (Fig 5.1). For small chemical compounds, the site on the antibody for binding antigen is analogous to an enzyme active site. For antibodies prepared against intact larger protein molecules where the antibody will be specific for an epitope, a part of the protein antigen, namely the combining site on the antibody, may be an extended surface, rather than a cleft or crevice (Fig. 5.1). In all cases, there is chemical complementarity between the residues of the antigen and the residues of the combining site of the antibody. The walls of the combining site are formed from the amino acid residues of regions of the variable segments of the heavy and light chains (V_H and V_L), known as the hypervariable (hV) regions (Chapter 6). Antibody specificity results from the precise molecular complementarity between chemical groups in the antigen and chemical groups in the antigen-binding site of the antibody molecule.

Cross-reactivity

Occasionally an antibody binds to more than one antigen. This is referred to as cross-reactivity or multispecificity. The antibody is specific for antigen 1, but a different molecule, antigen 2, fits well enough to create a stable binding interaction (Fig. 5.2). This happens because there are a sufficient number of chemical interactions between the antigen and the antibody to create a stable structure, regardless of the total "goodness of fit." Cross-reactivity can have clinical consequences (Box 5.1).

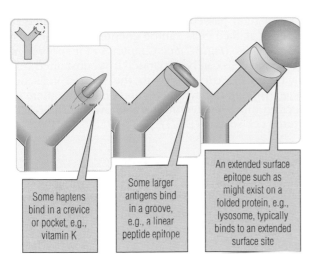

Figure 5.1 Antigen-binding sites vary in size and shape according to the type of molecule or epitope they bind.

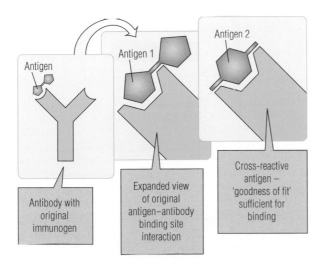

Figure 5.2 Schematic representation of antibody cross-reactivity.

BOX 5.1 Drug Allergy/IgE Cross-Reactivity

Adverse immunologic reactions to drugs, particularly antibiotics, can be a significant medical problem. For example, people die from anaphylactic reactions to penicillin (see also Chapter 26). Penicillin can form a hapten-carrier conjugate with a self-protein that can then act as an immunogen and generate an immunoglobulin (Ig)E antibody (see Fig. 4.1). Unfortunately, the anti-penicillin IgE antibodies also cross-react with a number of other antibiotics. This can complicate the treatment of bacterial infections in these patients because they are unable to take the antibiotics necessary to combat the infection.

Penicillin is a so-called β-lactam antibiotic. These antibiotics contain the four-membered β-lactam ring structure, as shown in Figure 5.3. Other antibiotics with similar chemical structures include the cephalosporins and the carbapenems.

Some anti-penicillin IgE antibodies can react with other antibiotics with similar structures. The precise specificity may vary, but there is enough "goodness of fit" (cross-reactivity) to allow significant binding to these other antibiotics and to create treatment problems.

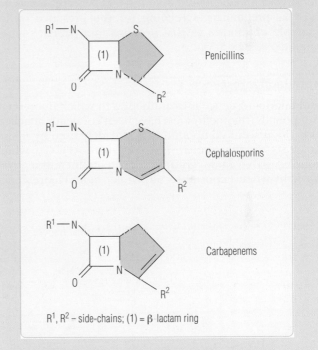

R^1, R^2 – side-chains; (1) = β lactam ring

Figure 5.3 Structures of penicillin and related antibiotics. The β-lactam ring is colored yellow.

■ DIAGNOSTIC TESTS FOR ANTIBODY OR ANTIGEN

A variety of diagnostic tests used in studying human disease are based on the specificity of antibodies. The advent of **monoclonal antibodies** has made several of these tests more reliable and useful because of the enhanced specificity and reproducibility made possible by using "tailor-

 MHC II

 Cytokine, Chemokine, etc.

 Complement (C')

 Signaling molecule

made" monoclonal antibodies. Monoclonal antibodies are derived from a single clone and all have the same specificity (see Box 4.3). The remainder of this chapter provides examples of how different tests are used and the general principle of each test. In general, these tests are used both qualitatively and quantitatively and can be used to determine the presence of either antigen or antibody.

ELISA

The enzyme-linked immunosorbent assay (ELISA) is a very sensitive and simple test for antigen that uses a covalent complex of an enzyme linked to an antibody, either to detect antigen directly or to bind to an antibody/antigen complex (Fig. 5.4). The enzyme chosen is one that is capable of catalyzing a reaction to generate a colored product from a colorless substrate (e.g., alkaline phosphatase or horseradish peroxidase) (Fig. 5.4). The amount of antibody bound to antigen is then proportional to the amount of colored end product that can be visualized (in a qualitative test) or measured in a spectrophotometer by optical density scanning (quantitative test). ELISA-type assays are used as preliminary screening for the presence of, for example, antibodies to HIV proteins in a patient's blood sample (see Box 5.3).

Immunofluorescence

Immunofluorescence uses antibodies to which fluorescent compounds (fluorochromes) have been covalently attached. One fluorescent compound that is widely used by immunologists is fluorescein isothiocyanate (FITC), which couples to free amino groups on proteins. It emits a greenish light when exposed to ultraviolet light. Fluorescence microscopes, equipped with ultraviolet (UV) sources, are used to examine specimens that have been exposed to fluorescent antibodies. This test is used extensively to detect antigens in cells or tissue sections. It is also used to screen for autoantibodies to cell or tissue antigens (Chapter 27). Either the test antibodies are directly linked to the fluorescent compound (direct test) or a ligand that can identify the antibody is linked to the fluorescent compound (indirect test) (Fig. 5.5). Often the fluorescent ligand is a second antibody that is specific for the test antibody—for example, goat anti-human immunoglobulin. An example of a clinical use of the indirect immunofluorescence assay is provided in Box 5.2.

Flow Cytometry

Flow cytometry is a technique used to enumerate live cells that express an antigen. The cells are stained with antibody that is specific for the cell-surface antigen. The antibody is coupled to specific fluorescent reagents such as FITC (several other different colored fluors are available) and then passed through the flow cytometer. The number of stained cells can be counted (e.g., the number of CD4$^+$T cells) (Fig. 5.7; see Chapter 34 for another example). Stained cells can be separated from unstained cells by applying an electric charge to the stained cells during passage through the cytometer and deflecting them into a collection tube. This technique is known as fluorescence-activated cell sorting (FACS).

Immunoblotting (Western blotting)

Immunoblotting is used to characterize antigens in complex mixtures biochemically. For example, it can be used

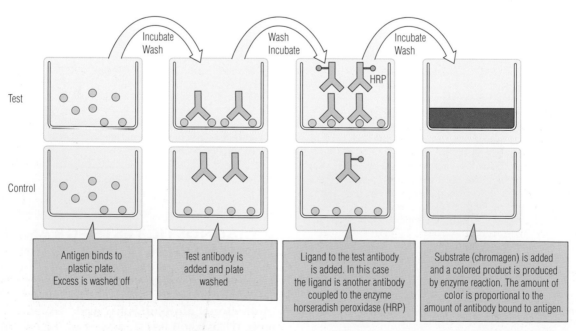

| Incubate Wash | Wash Incubate | Incubate Wash |

Test

Control

| Antigen binds to plastic plate. Excess is washed off | Test antibody is added and plate washed | Ligand to the test antibody is added. In this case the ligand is another antibody coupled to the enzyme horseradish peroxidase (HRP) | Substrate (chromagen) is added and a colored product is produced by enzyme reaction. The amount of color is proportional to the amount of antibody bound to antigen. |

Figure 5.4 Enzyme-linked immunosorbent assay (ELISA).

 T cell receptor (TCR)   Immunoglobulin (Ig)   Antigen   MHC I

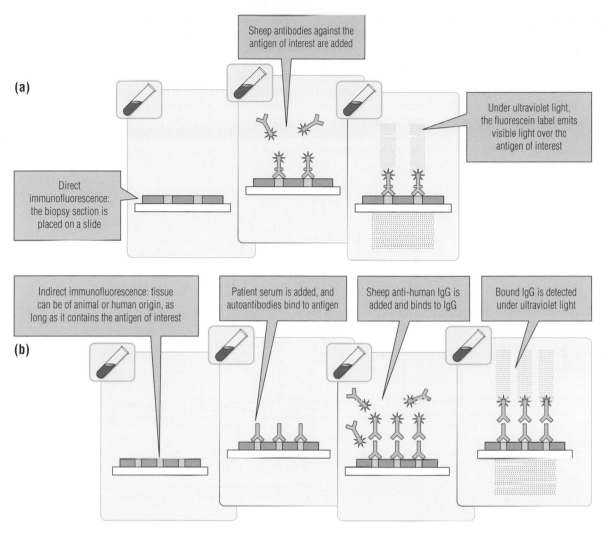

(a)

Sheep antibodies against the antigen of interest are added

Under ultraviolet light, the fluorescein label emits visible light over the antigen of interest

Direct immunofluorescence: the biopsy section is placed on a slide

(b)

Indirect immunofluorescence: tissue can be of animal or human origin, as long as it contains the antigen of interest

Patient serum is added, and autoantibodies bind to antigen

Sheep anti-human IgG is added and binds to IgG

Bound IgG is detected under ultraviolet light

Figure 5.5 Direct and indirect immunofluorescence using fluorescein isothiocyanate (FITC). Other fluorochromes can be used with different colors.

BOX 5.2 Specific Serologic Test for Syphilis

The spirochete *Treponema pallidum* causes syphilis. It can be diagnosed in the pathology laboratory using darkfield or immunofluorescence microscopy. This bacterium is a flexible, spiral rod (Fig. 5.6). To obtain the picture shown in this figure, a fluorescent treponemal antibody absorbed test (FTA-ABS) was carried out. A test serum was first absorbed with nonpathogenic treponemes to remove cross-reacting antibodies. Next, the absorbed test serum was reacted with *T. pallidum* organisms on a microscope slide. Then, as per the indirect immunofluorescence assay described in Figure 5.5, any antibodies bound to the *T. pallidum* were detected with FITC-conjugated anti-human IgG antibodies under the fluorescent microscope.

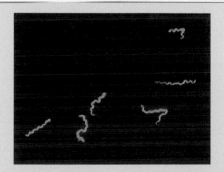

Figure 5.6 *Treponema pallidum* visualized by a fluorescent treponemal antibody absorbed test. (Illustration produced with the help of Dr. S.A. Cavalieri, Department of Pathology, and Dr. R.A. Bessen, Department of Medical Microbiology and Immunology, Creighton University School of Medicine, Omaha, Nebraska, USA.)

 MHC II

 Cytokine, Chemokine, etc.

 Complement (C')

 Signaling molecule

to detect individual antibodies to HIV proteins in serum samples to confirm an HIV-positive status indicated by an ELISA test (Box 5.3).

In Western blotting (Fig. 5.8), complex protein samples are solubilized in a strong, denaturing, charged detergent (sodium dodecyl sulfate [SDS]) and separated according to size after eletrophoresis through a polyacrylamide gel (SDS-polyacrylamide gel electrophoresis). In this example, the proteins of HIV are separated by size after electrophoresis. The larger the molecular weight of the protein, the less distance it migrates into the gel. The separated proteins are then transferred electrophoretically to a nitrocellulose membrane (blotting). Next, the blot is reacted with antibody, washed, and a ligand such as a conjugate of the enzyme horseradish peroxidase coupled to protein A (HRP-Prot A) is added to detect the bound antibody. After a substrate for HRP is added, which generates a colored insoluble product, the protein antigen can be visualized as a colored band on the nitrocellulose membrane.

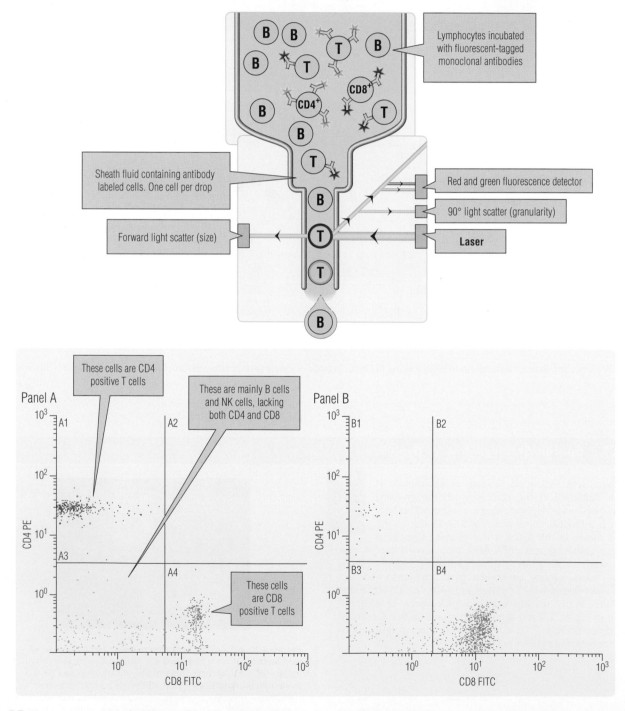

Figure 5.7 Flow-cytometry "dot plots." In panel **A**, cells stained with the red CD4 antibody account for 59% of all lymphocytes; this is a normal sample. In panel **B**, there is a reduction in the number of red-staining CD4⁺ T cells. This is a sample from a patient with HIV infection.
PE; phycoerythrin (emits red light)
FITC; fluorescent isothiocyanate (emits green light)
Flow cytometric plots courtesy of John Hewitt, Immunology, Manchester Royal Infirmary

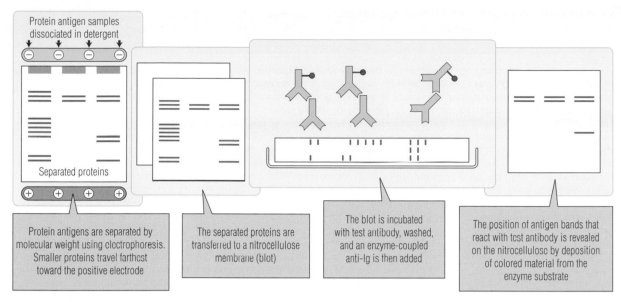

Figure 5.8 Western blotting.

BOX 5.3 Unexpected HIV-Positive Test

C.R. is a 35-year-old white woman who presents at your clinic complaining of being run down. She has had frequent low-grade fevers over the past 6 months or so, and on examination has swollen lymph nodes in her neck. She is married with two children, one 8 and the other 10 years old. None of the other members of her family has her symptoms.

On physical examination, she has white plaques (thrush) on her throat and tongue. Further examination shows that her white blood cell count and serum immunoglobulin levels are normal. An enzyme-linked immunosorbent assay (ELISA) test (see Fig. 5.4) for antibodies to HIV is positive, and this unexpected result is confirmed by the Western blot test (see Figs. 5.8 and 5.9). As shown in Figure 5.9, C.R.'s serum contains antibodies that react with some HIV proteins. Further analysis revealed that C.R.'s husband was HIV-positive, but asymptomatic, and neither of their children was found to be positive for HIV antibodies. C.R. and her husband were treated with antiretroviral therapy.

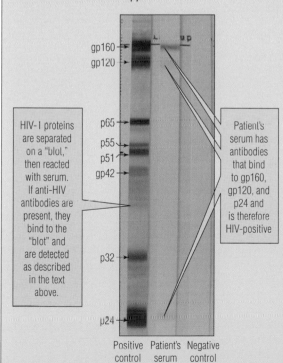

HIV-1 proteins are separated on a "blot," then reacted with serum. If anti-HIV antibodies are present, they bind to the "blot" and are detected as described in the text above.

Patient's serum has antibodies that bind to gp160, gp120, and p24 and is therefore HIV-positive

Positive control lane Patient's serum Negative control lane

Figure 5.9 A Western blot to confirm HIV-positive status. (Illustration produced with the help of Dr. S. H. Hinrichs, Department of Pathology/Microbiology, University of Nebraska Medical Center, and Dr. S.A. Cavalieri, Department of Pathology, Creighton University School of Medicine, both Omaha, Nebraska, USA.)

 MHC II   Cytokine, Chemokine, etc.   Complement (C') Signaling molecule

BOX 5.4 New Technology for the Clinical Diagnostic Laboratory—Fluorescent Microsphere-Based Immunoassay

A new approach to diagnostic testing that appears to be very valuable, especially when multiple tests must be done on a small amount of sample, is known as Luminex xMAP® technology. This technology utilizes aspects of both enzyme-linked immunosorbent assay (ELISA) and flow cytometry. In essence, polystyrene microspheres are internally color-coded with two fluorescent dyes that can be detected after laser illumination. By mixing different dyes, each bead in a set of up to 100 can be given a unique identity ("spectral signal") that can be detected in a flow cytometer (see Fig. 5.7). Each bead can also be coated with different compounds (e.g., antibodies, oligonucleotides, enzymes) that can collect molecules from a test sample. By utilizing a sandwich assay with a different-colored fluorescent reporter tag, as illustrated in Figure 5.10, the amount of a compound (e.g., antibodies to hepatitis virus) can be measured using a second laser. The microspheres are in solution in a microtiter well or test tube, and multiple beads can be present in a single container. Each bead can be derivatized with a different reactant. With a set of 100 beads, up to 100 different compounds can be assayed for. The beads are transported in fluid into the analyzer and subjected to laser illumination, much like individual cells in a flow cytometer (see Fig. 5.7). This technology can be used to carry out multiple tests (so-called multiplex testing) from a small volume of sample in a very short amount of time. The assay method has been shown to be sensitive and specific and to have some advantages over other assay formats, such as ELISA.

An example of a situation where the test could be used is as follows:

Your patient has developed jaundice shortly after a trip overseas. The patient claims no history of high-risk behavior during travel, and you request testing for antibodies to hepatitis virus. A blood sample is collected, and the serum used to assay for the presence of antibodies to hepatitis viruses A, B, or C. As shown, the patient's serum contains antibodies that bind to the Luminex beads expressing hepatitis A antigen and not to the beads that express hepatitis B or C antigens. The patient receives treatment, and the jaundice resolves.

One advantage of the microsphere bead assay is being able to test simultaneously for multiple reactants (e.g., a panel of viral antigens, a panel of cytokines).

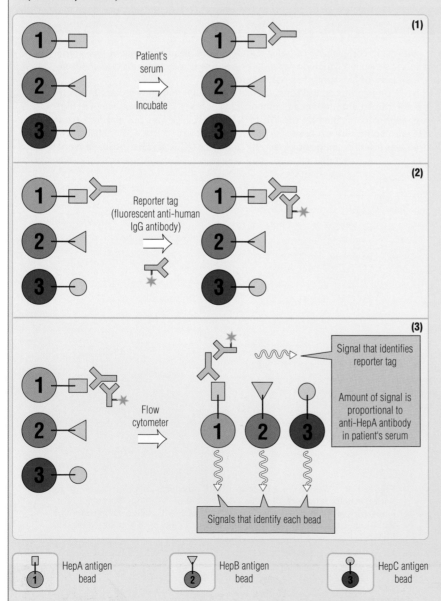

Figure 5.10 Fluorescent microsphere-based immunoassay for antibodies to hepatitis virus (Luminex xMAP® technology).

LEARNING POINTS · Can You Now ...

1. Describe antigen-antibody interaction as a subset of receptor-ligand interactions?
2. Draw the structure of the antigen binding site of antibodies for various types of antigen?
3. Explain antibody cross-reactivity in terms of "goodness of fit" of the antigen in the combining site?
4. Describe a range of diagnostic tests that are based on antigen–antibody interaction, indicating the general principle of each test?
5. List at least three examples of diseases where immunologic tests are useful in diagnosis?

  MHC II

  Cytokine, Chemokine, etc.

  Complement (C')

  Signaling molecule

6 Antibody Diversity

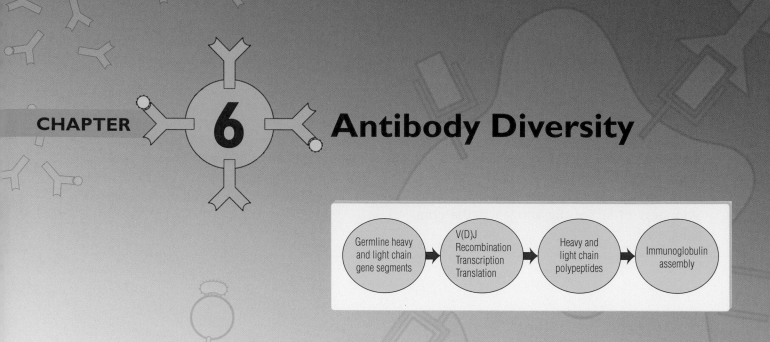

The human body appears to be capable of generating an almost infinite number of antibody (immunoglobulin [Ig]) molecules—perhaps at least one for every antigen in the universe! Some calculations suggest that there could be as many as 10^{11} different antibody molecules available in the human antibody repertoire (or collection of antibodies of different specificity). The purpose of this chapter is to describe the various mechanisms used in B cells to achieve this diversity. Similar mechanisms are used in T cells to generate T-cell receptor (TCR) diversity, but so far they have not been detected in other genes. These various mechanisms are collectively referred to as the "generation of diversity." The overview figure above illustrates the various steps on the pathway to assembling a complete Ig molecule, and this chapter provides a description of the pathway of Ig assembly in B cells.

■ IMMUNOGLOBULIN GENES

As described in Chapter 4, Igs have two kinds of polypeptide chains, heavy and light. Each chain has a variable (V) and a constant (C) region. Ig polypeptide chains are encoded by gene segments (Fig. 6.1) that are rearranged during B-cell development (Fig. 6.2) to assemble a functional gene encoding either a light or a heavy chain (Fig. 6.3). These gene segments include leader (L), joining (J), and diversity (D) gene segments in addition to the V and C gene segments. Gene segments exist in sets (or groups), which are arrays of different versions of that gene segment. For example, there are five different J_k gene segments that constitute the J_k set. Figure 6.1 illustrates the organization of the human light and heavy chain gene segments and enumerates the different gene segments for Igs.

During the development of B cells (Chapter 14), the Ig gene segments are rearranged and brought next to each other to form a contiguous functional gene (see Fig. 6.3).

The process of rearrangement is known as **somatic recombination** and occurs even in the absence of antigen to create a repertoire of potential antibody (antigen receptor) molecules. Once complete light and heavy chain genes have been assembled, the Ig light and heavy chains can be synthesized, and the polypeptide chains assembled as an Ig molecule. This molecule is either expressed at the surface of the B cell or secreted from a differentiated B cell known as a plasma cell (see Fig. 6.8 and Chapter 14).

The V regions of the chains constitute the antigen-binding site, and the C regions contribute specialized effector functions, such as binding to cellular receptors or complement proteins. Antibody diversity is created by recombining different gene segments to create different V regions. This considerably reduces the number of genes that would otherwise be needed to encode the very large number of different antibody molecules, and reduces the amount of the genome that would otherwise be given over to genes for antibody molecules.

Assembly of Variable Regions by Somatic Recombination

After the initial gene rearrangements have occurred (Fig. 6.2), the entire gene is transcribed, including the **exons** (coding sequences) and the **introns** (noncoding sequences), into a primary RNA transcript (Fig. 6.3). RNA splicing then takes place, whereby RNA processing enzymes remove the intron sequences to produce a messenger RNA (mRNA) that can be translated into protein. The leader peptide sequence (L) is then removed by proteolytic enzymes (Fig. 6.3).

The V region of light chains is composed of V and J segments, and that of heavy chains is assembled from three segments: V, D, and J (Fig. 6.2). For a complete V region to be transcribed, the V region gene segments (V and J, or V, D, and J) have to be "cut out" and then joined together by enzymes responsible for DNA recombination. For example,

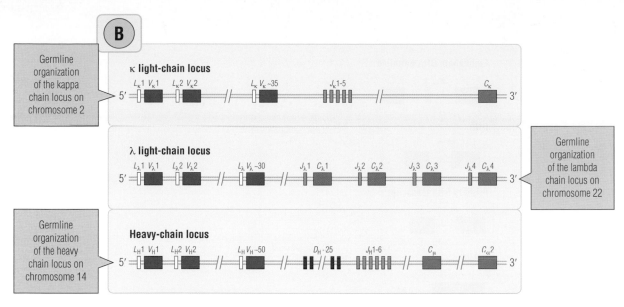

Figure 6.1 Genomic organization of the immunoglobulin loci.

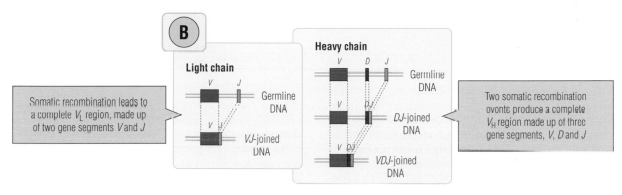

Figure 6.2 Immunoglobulin variable regions are constructed from gene segments by recombination.

one *J* segment from the array of *J* segments is combined with one *V* segment from the array of *V* segments to form a V_L region. Similarly, one *V*, one *D*, and one *J* segment are rearranged to make a V_H region. First the *D* and *J* segments are joined, then a *V* gene segment is joined to the *DJ* segment to create a complete V_H exon (Fig. 6.2). Because there are multiple *V*, *D*, and *J* gene segments (Fig. 6.1), many different complete variable regions can be created. For example, V_1 combined with J_2 forms a different V_L region with a different specificity for antigen than that formed when V_6 combines with J_2.

The complex of enzymes involved in somatic recombination in lymphocytes is known as the V(D)J recombinase. These enzymes are responsible for the cleavage and rejoining of the DNA involved in rearrangement. Two of these enzymes, RAG-1 and RAG-2 (for *r*ecombination *a*ctivating *g*enes), are responsible for the first cleavage step involved in somatic recombination of Ig genes. RAG-1 and RAG-2 are only found in lymphocytes and defects in these enzymes lead to blockage of lymphocyte development (Box 7.1).

Gene Organization and Synthesis

Human Light Chain

As described in Chapter 4, there are two types of light chain, kappa (*k*) and lambda (*l*). The events leading to synthesis of a kappa light chain are shown in Figure 6.4 and described below. The process is essentially the same for lambda light-chain synthesis.

In the germline of humans, there are approximately 35 different V_k genes found in the kappa locus on chromosome 2. Each V_k gene encodes the N-terminal 95 amino acid residues of a kappa variable region. Downstream (i.e., 3′) of the V_k region, there are five J_k exons. Each J_k segment encodes amino acids 96–108 of the kappa variable region. After a long intron, the kappa locus ends in the one C_k exon encoding the constant region of the kappa light chain.

To synthesize a kappa light chain, a cell early in the B-lymphocyte lineage (Chapter 14) selects a V_k exon (e.g., V_k3), and after a process of DNA rearrangement involving the V(D)J recombinase, joins it to a *J* segment (e.g., J_k2). The intervening DNA, in this example from approximately

 MHC II

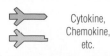 Cytokine, Chemokine, etc.

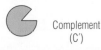 Complement (C′)

 Signaling molecule

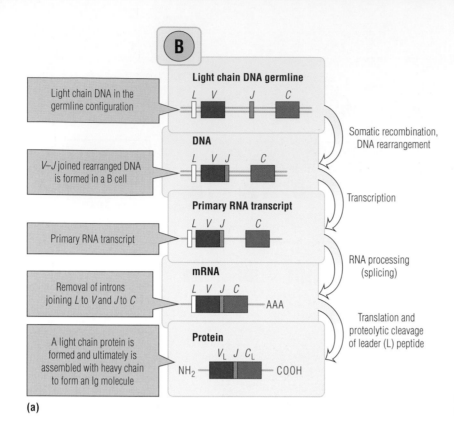

(a)

Figure 6.3 Major steps in the synthesis of (**A**) light and (**B**) heavy immunoglobulin chains.

the 3′ end of V_3 to the 5′ end of J_2, is deleted by looping it and cleaving it out for ultimate degradation. From this rearranged DNA, a primary RNA transcript is made (Fig. 6.4). This primary RNA transcript undergoes RNA splicing reactions to bring, for example, the V_k3, J_k2, and C_k exons together as a mature mRNA. Splicing removes all the intervening sequences (e.g., J_3, J_4 and J_5), thereby allowing the RNA to be translated into a kappa polypeptide chain in the endoplasmic reticulum of the cell. The process is similar for lambda chain genes, except that lambda is found on chromosome 22 in humans, and there are about 30 V_λ and four J_λ genes. Each of the J_λ genes is associated with a different C_λ gene (see Fig. 6.1). Consequently, there are four different subtypes of lambda light chain in humans.

Human Heavy Chain

In the human genome, there are approximately 50 V_H, 25 D_H, and 6 J_H gene segments in the heavy chain locus on chromosome 14 (Fig. 6.1). The D, or diversity segment, like the J segment, encodes amino acids in the third **hypervariable** (hv3) region of the heavy chain. The term *hypervariable region* is used in discussions of both Ig and T-cell receptor diversity (Chapter 7).

The mechanism of heavy chain synthesis (Fig. 6.5) is very similar to that described for kappa light chains, except that three segments, rather than two, are required for assembly of the V_H exon, and that multiple C_H exons are present in the heavy chain locus.

First the D and J segments are joined, then the V segment joins to the combined DJ segments to form the com-

plete V_H exon. C region exons are spliced to the V_H exon during processing of the heavy chain RNA transcript.

As shown in Figure 6.5, there are multiple different C_H regions. Any given V_H region may be expressed with any of the C_H regions via a process of DNA rearrangement referred to as isotype or **class switching**. The different C_H regions confer different biologic (effector) functions. This allows yet more diversity because the same antigen specificity (V region) can be associated with C_H regions that confer different effector properties—for example, ability to cross the placenta or to bind to different Fc receptors on different cell types (see Fig. 4.7).

Generation of Antibody Diversity

To generate the enormously diverse repertoire of antigen receptors that has been observed in humans, B cells use the genetic mechanisms summarized below.

1. V, D, and J gene segments are present in multiple copies; for example, there are approximately 35 V_k gene segments. This is **germline diversity**.
2. VJ and VDJ gene segments can recombine in multiple combinations (**combinatorial diversity**); for example, with 35 V_k and 5 J_k segments, there are $35 \times 5 = 175$ different human kappa light chains with different variable regions that can be formed.
3. The formation of the junction between gene segments. For example, the joining of a V gene segment to a rearranged DJ gene segment involves DNA cleavage,

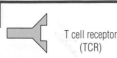 T cell receptor (TCR)

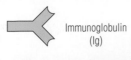 Immunoglobulin (Ig)

 Antigen

 MHC I

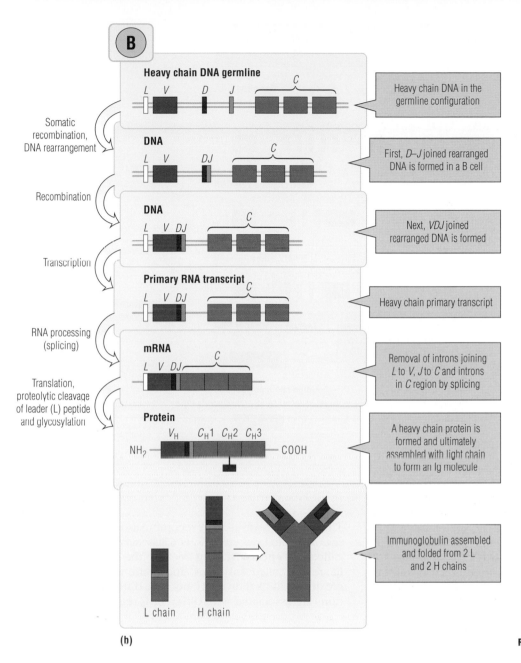

Heavy chain DNA germline

Heavy chain DNA in the germline configuration

Somatic recombination, DNA rearrangement

DNA

First, *D–J* joined rearranged DNA is formed in a B cell

Recombination

DNA

Next, *VDJ* joined rearranged DNA is formed

Transcription

Primary RNA transcript

Heavy chain primary transcript

RNA processing (splicing)

mRNA

Removal of introns joining *L* to *V*, *J* to *C* and introns in *C* region by splicing

Translation, proteolytic cleavage of leader (L) peptide and glycosylation

Protein

A heavy chain protein is formed and ultimately assembled with light chain to form an Ig molecule

Immunoglobulin assembled and folded from 2 L and 2 H chains

L chain   H chain

(h)

Figure 6.3 (cont'd)

followed by the addition and subtraction of nucleotides to create a viable joint (Fig. 6.6). The outcome of these events is that different coding sequences can be created at the joint in different B cells—for example, through the random addition of nucleotides by the enzyme terminal deoxynucleotidyl transferase (TdT). Different sequences at the joint lead to greater antibody diversity, known as **junctional diversity** (see Fig. 6.6). For example, as shown in Figure 6.6, the sequence of amino acids in a putative binding site can change from -Ala-Arg-Asn- to -Ala-Arg-Ile-, a major chemical structural change, merely by deletion of one nucleotide during joining of a V_H to a $D_H J_H$ segment.

4. Multiple combinations of light and heavy chains. In principle, any heavy chain can associate with any light chain. Because both chains contribute to the antigen-binding site, this random assortment of light and heavy chains generates different antibody specificities. For example, 200 different light chains associating in random combination with 2000 different heavy chains potentially creates 4×10^5 different antibodies.

5. Somatic hypermutation after antigenic stimulation. After a functional antibody gene has been assembled and the B cell is responding to an antigen, there is another mechanism, **somatic hypermutation**, that generates additional diversity in the V region. This mechanism operates to introduce point mutations at a very high rate into the V regions of heavy and light chains. Some of the mutations produce antibody molecules that are a better fit for antigen than the "original" antibody. These

 MHC II

 Cytokine, Chemokine, etc.

 Complement (C')

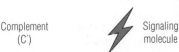 Signaling molecule

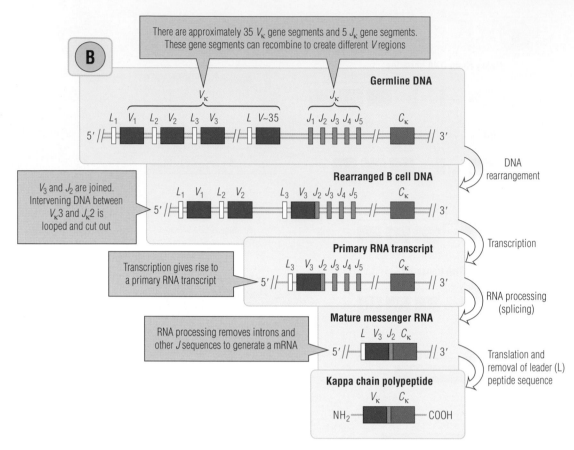

There are approximately 35 V_κ gene segments and 5 J_κ gene segments. These gene segments can recombine to create different V regions

B

Germline DNA

V_κ

J_κ

L_1 V_1 L_2 V_2 L_3 V_3 L $V\sim35$ J_1 J_2 J_3 J_4 J_5 C_κ

5′ — 3′

DNA rearrangement

V_3 and J_2 are joined. Intervening DNA between $V_\kappa3$ and $J_\kappa2$ is looped and cut out

Rearranged B cell DNA

L_1 V_1 L_2 V_2 L_3 V_3 J_2 J_3 J_4 J_5 C_κ

5′ — 3′

Transcription

Transcription gives rise to a primary RNA transcript

Primary RNA transcript

L_3 V_3 J_2 J_3 J_4 J_5 C_κ

5′ — 3′

RNA processing (splicing)

RNA processing removes introns and other J sequences to generate a mRNA

Mature messenger RNA

L V_3 J_2 C_κ

5′ — 3′

Translation and removal of leader (L) peptide sequence

Kappa chain polypeptide

V_κ C_κ

NH_2 — COOH

Figure 6.4 Kappa light chain synthesis.

new antibodies tend to bind antigen with a higher affinity, and B cells expressing them are preferentially selected for maturation into plasma cells (Chapter 14). This phenomenon is sometimes referred to as affinity maturation of the population of antibody molecules in an individual.

An example of the use of molecular genetic techniques for studies of the development of the immune response is shown in Box 6.1.

■ IMMUNOGLOBULIN CLASSES

Class Switching

As described in Chapter 4, there are five classes of human Ig: IgM, IgD, IgG, IgE, and IgA. There are also four subclasses of IgG: IgG_1, IgG_2, IgG_3, and IgG_4. There are C_H genes for each of these Igs (Fig. 6.5), and the same V_H exon can be rearranged to associate with a different C_H exon at different times in the course of an immune response. For example, early in the immune response to an antigen, a B cell will express IgM. Later, in the response to the same antigen, the assembled V region may be expressed in an IgG antibody.

This change involves DNA recombination between specific regions, called switch regions. Class switching is sometimes called **isotype switching** because the different classes of Ig are also called isotypes. Using a different constant region creates additional diversity, because different effector functions are associated with different C regions.

Expression of Both IgM and IgD on B Cells

IgD is frequently found on the surface of B cells co-expressed with IgM. These two classes are co-expressed not by class switching but by alternative processing of a primary RNA transcript (Fig. 6.7). Transcription can proceed from a VDJ region through both the C_μ and C_δ exons to yield a long primary transcript RNA. This RNA can then be differentially processed by cleavage, polyadenylation and splicing. If processing utilizes the first polyadenylation site (pA1), then a μ heavy chain mRNA is derived. If processing utilizes the second polyadenylation site (pA2), then a δ heavy chain mRNA results. The mechanisms that regulate the choice of polyadenylation site are not fully understood. The significance of co-expression of IgM and IgD for B-cell function is also not clear but may be related to B cell memory (Chapter 17).

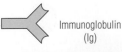

T cell receptor (TCR)   Immunoglobulin (Ig)   Antigen   MHC I

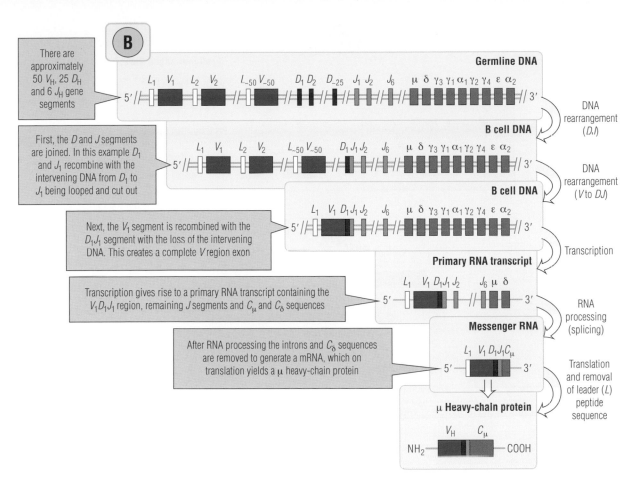

Figure 6.5 Heavy chain synthesis.

FIG. 6.6 Junctional Diversity in Joining V_H to a $D_H J_H$ Segment (V_H...A.GCG.CGA AAT.A..$D_H J_H$)

	Initial gene segments	Nuclease deletion of one nucleotide	TdT addition of one nucleotide
Germline DNA sequence ↓	V_H–A.GCG.CGA AAT.A–$D_H J_H$	V_H–A.GCG.CG ☐ AAT.A–$D_H J_H$	V_H–A.GCG.CGA⬚G⬚ AAT.A–$D_H J_H$
VDJ joined DNA ↓	V_H–A.GCG.CGA.AAT.A	V_H–A.GCG.CGA.ATA–	V_H–A.GCG.CGA.GAA.TA–
mRNA ↓	–A.GCG.CGA.AAU.A–	–A.GCG.CGA.AUA–	–A.GCG.CGA.GAA.UA–
Protein	–Ala–Arg–Asn–	–Ala–Arg–Ile–	–Ala–Arg–Glu–

Membrane-Bound AND Secreted Immunoglobulin

B cells can produce Igs as membrane-bound or secreted forms. The membrane-bound form of Ig has an additional approximately 30 amino acid residues at the C-terminus of the heavy chain. These residues include a stretch of approximately 25 hydrophobic amino acids that anchor the Ig in the cell membrane where it can act as a receptor (see Chapter 11). The two different forms are encoded in different C_H exons, and alternative RNA processing (Fig. 6.8) is used to generate either the secreted or the membrane-bound form. Again, the mechanism of regulation of this alternative RNA processing or choice of polyadenylation site is not fully understood. Presumably, signals generated by antigen binding and/or interaction with T cells are involved (see Chapter 16).

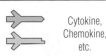 MHC II

 Cytokine, Chemokine, etc.

Complement (C')

 Signaling molecule

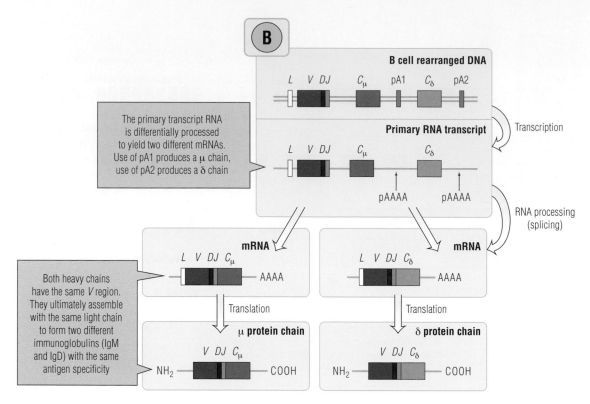

B cell rearranged DNA

L V DJ C_μ pA1 C_δ pA2

The primary transcript RNA is differentially processed to yield two different mRNAs. Use of pA1 produces a μ chain, use of pA2 produces a δ chain

Primary RNA transcript

L V DJ C_μ C_δ

Transcription

pAAAA   pAAAA

RNA processing (splicing)

mRNA

L V DJ C_μ — AAAA

Both heavy chains have the same V region. They ultimately assemble with the same light chain to form two different immunoglobulins (IgM and IgD) with the same antigen specificity

mRNA

L V DJ C_δ — AAAA

Translation

Translation

μ protein chain

V DJ C_μ

NH₂ — — COOH

δ protein chain

V DJ C_δ

NH₂ — — COOH

Figure 6.7 Alternative RNA processing to allow co-expression of IgM and IgD. pA, polyadenylation site.

■ ALLELIC EXCLUSION

There are genetic polymorphisms (numerous different alleles at a single locus) of both heavy and light chain genes; these are known as **allotypes**. In heterozygous individuals who have, for example, inherited two alternative forms of the constant region gene for IgG₁ (i.e., IgG1m(1) and IgG1m(2)), both forms will be found in the individual's total complement of Igs, but any one given B cell will express only Igs of one allotype. This phenomenon is known as **allelic exclusion**, and it indicates that only one of the two parental chromosomes expresses that gene in any given B cell (also see Chapter 14).

 T cell receptor (TCR)

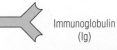 Immunoglobulin (Ig)

 Antigen

 MHC I

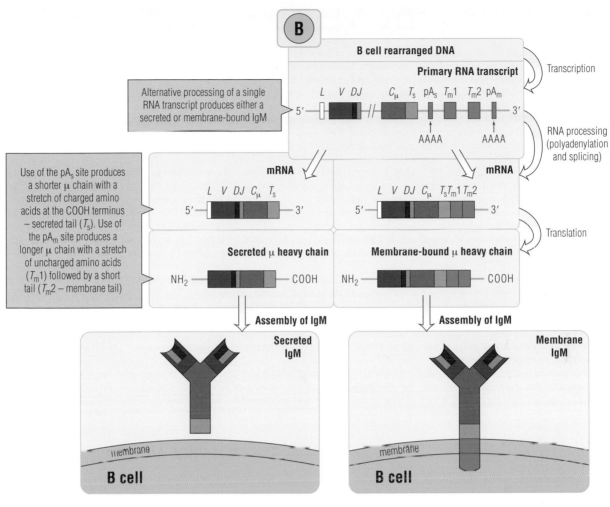

Figure 6.8 Cell surface (transmembrane) and secreted forms of immunoglobulin. pA$_s$, polyadenylation site for the secreted form; pA$_m$, polyadenylation site for the membrane-bound form.

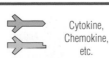

BOX 6.1 Detection of Immunoglobulin Gene Rearrangement

Ig gene rearrangement can be detected using the technique of Southern blot analysis (Fig. 6.9).

In this example, relatively intact, high molecular weight DNA was extracted from a non–B cell (e.g., skin fibroblast), a cloned B-cell line (e.g., a B-cell tumor line maintained in vitro) and polyclonal B cells purified from a normal (control) blood sample. Each of the DNA samples was then digested with the same restriction enzymes that recognize randomly distributed base pair sequences throughout the genomic DNA. The fragments of DNA obtained after enzyme digestion (the so-called restriction fragments) are of different sizes. These DNA fragments are electrophoresed through an agarose gel and separated according to size. The smaller fragments travel the farthest into the gel. The separated fragments are then "blotted" onto a membrane of nitrocellulose in a manner similar to that described for proteins in the Western blotting technique described in Chapter 5 (see Fig. 5.8). The DNA fragments remain fixed on the membrane in their gel locations.

A specific gene can then be detected by nucleic acid hybridization using a cloned piece of DNA as a probe. For example, if a cloned J_H segment from an Ig heavy chain gene is radiolabeled with radioactive phosphorus [^{32}P], this can be used to detect Ig heavy chain genes. The membrane is soaked in a solution containing the radioactive probe. The probe binds as a spot or band on the membrane where there is sequence complementarity between the DNA fragments on the filter and the probe. The "hybridized probe" is detected when the filter is exposed to photographic film. Molecular weight markers are used to determine the size of the DNA fragment containing the Ig heavy chain gene that hybridizes to the J_H probe. This technique was first used to show that Ig gene rearrangements actually do take place, and can still be used to detect Ig gene rearrangements, although it is largely being replaced by a more sensitive method involving the polymerase chain reaction (PCR).

In Figure 6.9, a Southern blot analysis of Ig gene rearrangement is diagrammed. Lane 1 shows that in DNA from a fibroblast (non–B cell), the J_H probe detects one unrearranged, so-called, germline band of approximately 4.5 kb. The DNA from a cloned (i.e., monoclonal) B-cell line (Lane 2), exhibits three bands that hybridize with the J_H DNA probe—that is, the germline band and two other bands that result from the rearrangement of both alleles of the heavy chain gene in this B-cell line. Lane 3 shows the results of hybridization of the J_H probe to DNA fragments from a polyclonal population of B cells. Because there are a very large number of B cells in a blood sample, and each exhibits a different Ig gene giving rise to DNA fragments of different sizes, there is a "smear" of DNA in the lane with no distinct bands other than the germline band.

The techniques of molecular biology/molecular genetics, such as the Southern blot technique illustrated here, have been very useful for understanding the immune system and for the detection and monitoring of lymphoid malignancies (see Chapters 14 and 34). Compare this diagram with Figure 4.4, which shows monoclonality and polyclonality of the protein product of these genes.

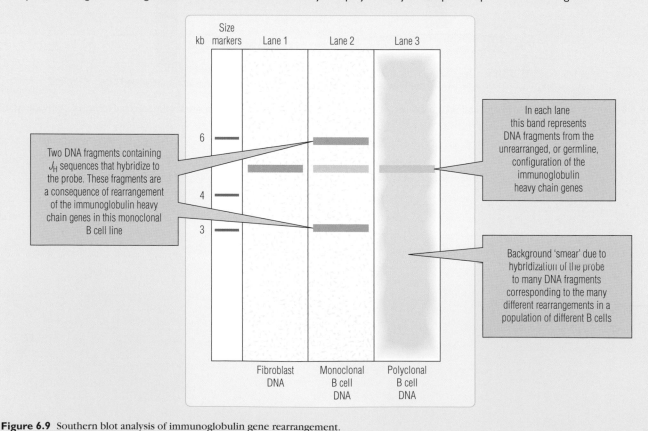

Figure 6.9 Southern blot analysis of immunoglobulin gene rearrangement.

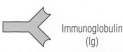 T cell receptor (TCR)

 Immunoglobulin (Ig)

Antigen

MHC I

LEARNING POINTS   Can You Now ...

1. Explain how rearrangement of gene segments generates an antibody repertoire?
2. Draw a diagram of Ig light chain gene organization and synthesis?
3. Draw a diagram of Ig heavy chain gene organization and synthesis?
4. Describe the various mechanisms that contribute to the generation of antibody diversity—for example, rearranging multiple gene segments?
5. Recall that there is allelic exclusion of Ig genes, and explain why this is functionally significant?
6. Draw a diagram of the process of class switching?
7. Draw a diagram of the process used to generate membrane-bound and secreted forms of Ig?

 MHC II  Cytokine, Chemokine, etc. Complement (C')  Signaling molecule

7 The T-Cell Receptor

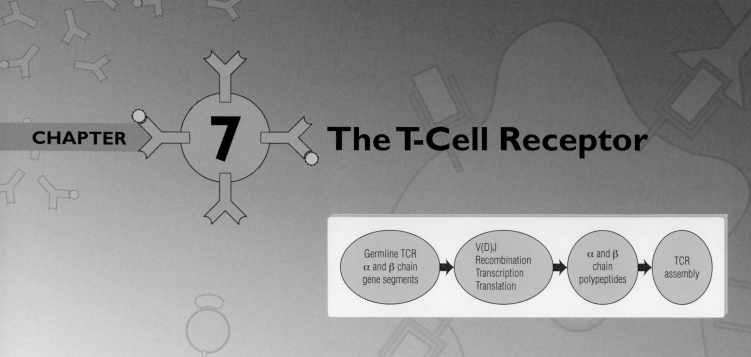

In this chapter, we describe the antigen-recognition molecule of T cells, the T-cell receptor (TCR). The overview figure above indicates the main steps on the pathway to TCR assembly that are outlined here. As described in Chapter 2, TCRs recognize peptide antigens only when they are displayed by self-MHC (major histocompatibility complex) molecules—that is, they have a dual specificity. This is quite unlike the B-cell antigen-recognition molecule (antibody), which binds various kinds of peptide and nonpeptide antigen directly. Despite the different mechanism of antigen recognition employed, the TCR is structurally similar to immunoglobulin (Ig) (Fig. 7.1). The TCR, like the B-cell antigen receptor, is clonally distributed. Every clone of T cells expresses a different antigen-receptor molecule.

■ BIOCHEMICAL CHARACTERIZATION AND RELATIONSHIP TO IMMUNOGLOBULIN

The TCR is a heterodimeric membrane protein. There are two types of receptor: receptors with αβ (alpha/beta) chains are present on approximately 95% of human T lymphocytes; receptors with γδ (gamma/delta) chains are found on approximately 5% of human T lymphocytes. Each of these chains has a molecular weight in the range of 40,000 to 60,000. The extracellular portion of each chain is composed of two domains (Fig. 7.1). The overall structure is similar to that of a membrane-bound antigen-binding fragment (Fab) of Ig. The TCR domains farthest away from the membrane are similar to Ig variable (V) region domains, and the domains closest to the membrane are similar to Ig constant (C) region domains. Antigen binds to a site created by the V domains of the αβ or γδ chains. The three-dimensional (3D) structure of the extracellular portion of

the TCR has been determined (Fig. 7.2), and this also has a great deal of similarity with that of Ig.

Protein and nucleic acid sequence data have been obtained for many TCRs with different specificities. Analyses of these sequences suggest the existence of three **hypervariable** (hv) regions in the variable region. Determination of 3D structure shows that these hypervariable regions are arranged as a relatively flat surface (Fig. 7.2) that contacts amino acid residues of both the MHC molecule and the peptide antigen.

The αβ T-Cell Receptor

The αβ TCR is the predominant (95%) human TCR found on MHC-restricted T cells. Most antigen-specific human T cells involved in host defense responses to intracellular microbes bear this form of the TCR. In general, when we refer to the TCR, we are referring to an αβ TCR. The helper T cells that collaborate with B cells are αβ T cells, as are most of the cytotoxic T cells that kill virally infected cells. The αβ TCR recognizes peptide antigens presented by MHC molecules (Chapters 2, 3, 9, and 10).

The γδ T-Cell Receptor

The γδ TCR is found on a few (5%) human T cells. These cells are derived in the thymus as a separate cell lineage from those cells expressing αβ TCR molecules (Chapter 15). γδ T cells have been found to be more frequent in some epithelial tissues, which has led to the hypothesis that they are a "first line of defense" and may initiate responses to those microbes that are frequently encountered at epithelial boundaries, such as the skin. Currently available data support the conclusion that human γδ T cells do not recognize MHC-associated peptide antigens and are not MHC-restricted. Some human γδ T cells have been shown to recognize nonpeptide phosphorylated compounds,

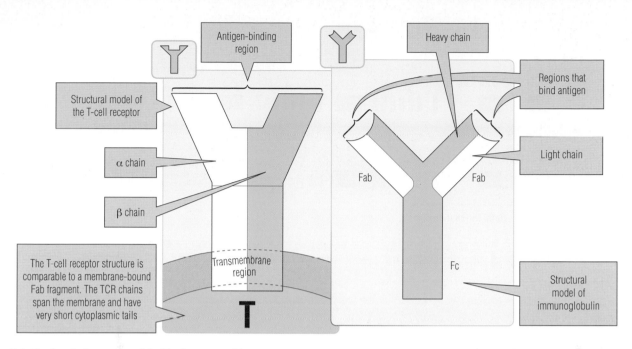

Figure 7.1 Biochemical structure of the T-cell receptor (TCR) compared to immunoglobulin. Fab, antigen-binding fragment; Fc, crystallizable fraction.

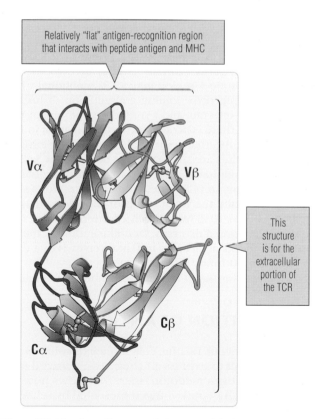

Figure 7.2 The three-dimensional structure of the T-cell receptor (TCR). MHC, major histocompatibility complex; V, Ig variable. (Adapted with permission from Garcia KC, Degano M, Stanfield RL, et al. *Science,* 274:209, 1996.)

including some lipid moieties, presented by "MHC class I–like" molecules, and others recognize protein-antigens that do not appear to undergo processing.

■ GENERATION OF DIVERSITY OF THE T-CELL-RECEPTOR GENES

The organization of the gene segments encoding the TCR chains is very like that for Ig heavy and light chain gene segments. As shown in Figure 7.3, genes for the α and γ chains are like the genes for Ig kappa and lambda light chains in that they use only *V* and *J* segments. The genes for the β and δ chains are like Ig heavy chain genes in that they utilize *V*, *D*, and *J* gene segments. An unusual feature is that the TCR δ chain gene segments are embedded in the TCR α chain locus on chromosome 14. The *V*δ genes are not shown in Figure 7.3, as they are interspersed amongst the *V*α genes. There are thought to be at least four *V*δ genes. Another difference from the Ig genes is that there are fewer TCR C-region genes. For example, there is only one *C*α gene, and although there are two *C*β genes, they appear to be functionally identical. This is in contrast to Igs in which the C regions include the μ, δ, γ, ε, and α classes; the γ1, γ2, γ3, and γ4 subclasses; and the lambda subtypes (λ1–λ4), amongst others.

The mechanisms that generate diversity before antigenic stimulation of T cells are, in essence, the same as those already described for generation of diversity in B cells (Chapter 6). After stimulation by antigen, however, the pathway in T cells is quite different from that in B cells. Whereas Ig genes continue to diversify after antigenic stimulation (e.g., by somatic hypermutation and by class

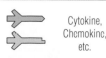 MHC II

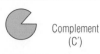 Cytokine, Chemokine, etc.

Complement (C′)

 Signaling molecule

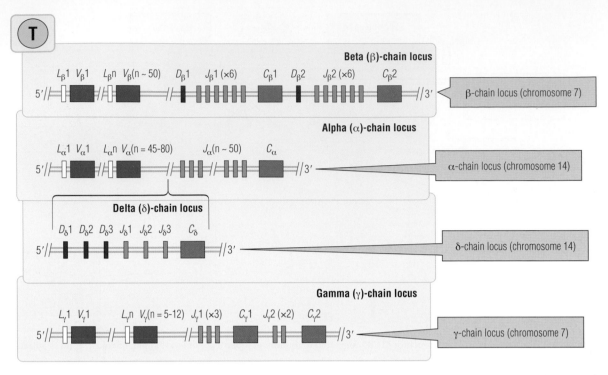

Figure 7.3 Organization of human genes for T-cell receptors. Note that the V_δ genes are not drawn because they are interspersed amongst the V_α genes.

switching, attaching a V region to a different C region), the genes for the TCRs remain unchanged. TCR genes rearrange in the thymus (Chapter 15). The basic molecular steps in synthesis of the TCR chains are very similar to those described for Ig light and heavy chains (Fig. 7.4). As for Ig genes in B lymphocytes, the V(D)J recombinase, including the RAG-1 and RAG-2 enzymes, is involved in TCR gene rearrangements (hence, defects in these functions will affect B and T cells; Box 7.1). For the α-chain, a V gene segment (e.g., $V_\alpha 2$) and a J gene segment (e.g., $J_\alpha 5$) are recombined to form a V-region exon (e.g., $V_\alpha 2 J_\alpha 5$). Transcription of the V region, along with the $C\alpha$ exon, yields a primary RNA transcript. Splicing of this RNA yields an mRNA which on translation produces a TCR α-chain protein (Fig. 7.4) in a manner similar to that described for Ig light chains in Figures 6.3A and 6.4.

Assembly of the β chain is similar to assembly of the Ig heavy chain in that first a D and a J gene segment are combined, followed by combination of this DJ unit to a V gene segment—for example, $D_\beta 1$, $J_\beta 1$, and $V_\beta 3$ as shown in Figure 7.4. The complete V-region exon is then transcribed along with $C_\beta 1$ to form a primary RNA transcript. RNA splicing yields a messenger RNA (mRNA), which, on translation, yields the β chain of the TCR (Fig. 7.4) in a manner similar to that described for Ig-heavy chains in Figures 6.3B and 6.5. The α and β chains are translated in the rough endoplasmic reticulum, and, like other membrane-bound glycoproteins, they are processed through the endoplasmic reticulum and Golgi compartments before expression at the cell-surface membrane.

As with the Igs, TCR diversity is generated by (1) the existence of multiple V-region genes, (2) junctional diversity created by imprecise joining and addition of nucleotides by the TdT enzyme, and (3) random combination of chains. Unlike Ig, there is no somatic hypermutation in TCR genes. However, the total potential B- and T-cell antigen-receptor repertoires are similar in size because the lack of somatic hypermutation is offset by a greater potential for junctional diversity in TCR genes (see Chapter 9 for a summary). Theoretically, the T-cell receptor repertoire may be as high as 10^{16} to 10^{18}, with much of the repertoire contributed by junctional diversity. One illustration of the importance of junctional diversity to TCR diversity is that there are more than 10 times as many J segments available for TCR α chains as for the Ig kappa and lambda light chains.

■ RECOGNITION OF ANTIGEN

The TCRs only occur on the cell surface; T cells do not have the potential to express an alternative secreted form like the B-cell antigen receptor. Figure 7.5 shows how the TCR interacts with peptide antigen presented by self-MHC molecules. Most peptide antigens after processing (Chapter 10) are displayed in the MHC groove (Chapters 2, 3, and 8) for binding to the TCR. A few, known as superantigens, can activate T cells independent of antigen processing and presentation. These superantigens bind simultaneously to MHC class II molecules and to certain TCRs with particular β chains. In doing so, they activate all

 T cell receptor (TCR)

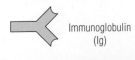 Immunoglobulin (Ig)

 Antigen

 MHC I

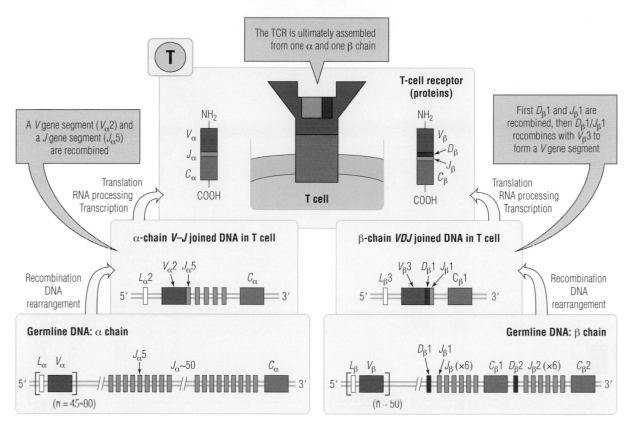

Figure 7.4 Synthesis and expression of a human αβ T-cell receptor (TCR).

BOX 7.1 Autosomal Recessive SCID Due to Defects in the Recombination Activating Gene (RAG-1, RAG-2) Products

The RAG enzymes initiate immunoglobulin gene rearrangements in B cells (see Chapters 6 and 14). As we have seen earlier in this chapter, they are also essential in T cells for T-cell receptor gene rearrangements (see also Chapter 15). Further evidence of their importance comes from the fact that deficiencies in *RAG-1* or *RAG-2* lead to autosomal-recessive severe combined immuno-deficiency disease (SCID). The form of autosomal-recessive SCID that results from *RAG-1*/*RAG-2* mutations is different from other forms of the disease in that there is a complete absence of both T and B cells. There are, however, NK cells found in the circulation. Hence, this form of the disease is known as T-B-SCID.

T-B-SCID is a rare syndrome that, without bone marrow transplantation (BMT) from a human leukocyte antigen (HLA)-compatible donor, is invariably fatal by 2 years of age. The disease presents in infants during the first few weeks of life as lymphopenia with recurrent infections. Only a very small thymus can be detected. These babies have recurrent episodes of pneumonia, otitis, and skin infections. They have persistent infections with opportunistic organisms such as *Candida albicans* and *Pneumocystis carinii*. For the parents and the pediatrician, this is an extreme emergency situation. These children are at great risk. However, if BMT is performed early enough, more than 80% of children survive. SCID as a syndrome is rare, and T-B-SCID even more rare. However, there are several hundred individuals who are alive today after BMT to correct the various forms of SCID that they suffered from. BMT is further discussed in Chapter 33.

T cells bearing this Vβ region and give rise to a massive immune response (Box 7.2).

A 3D structure analysis has been carried out on the trimolecular TCR-peptide-MHC complex and one example of this for MHC class I (HLA-A2), a viral peptide and a specific TCR is shown in Figure 7.7. This figure shows that the hypervariable sequences of this TCR V region create a "flat" surface that interacts with residues of the peptide antigen and with some of the polymorphic amino acid residues that are located in the α1 and α2 domains of the MHC molecule.

■ OTHER ACCESSORY MOLECULES INVOLVED IN T-CELL FUNCTION

As shown in Figure 7.8, there are several molecules that contribute to T-cell function; some are essential (e.g., the

 MHC II

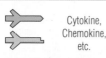 Cytokine, Chemokine, etc.

 Complement (C')

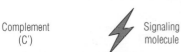 Signaling molecule

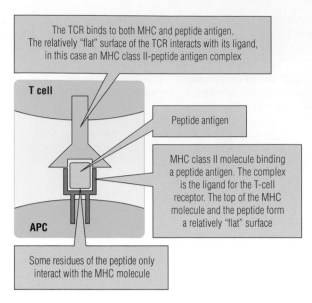

The TCR binds to both MHC and peptide antigen. The relatively "flat" surface of the TCR interacts with its ligand, in this case an MHC class II-peptide antigen complex

T cell

Peptide antigen

MHC class II molecule binding a peptide antigen. The complex is the ligand for the T-cell receptor. The top of the MHC molecule and the peptide form a relatively "flat" surface

APC

Some residues of the peptide only interact with the MHC molecule

Figure 7.5 Interaction of the T-cell receptor (TCR) with the peptide-MHC complex. APC, antigen-presenting cell; MHC, major histocompatibility complex.

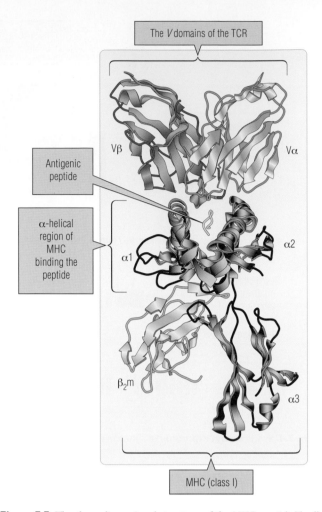

The V domains of the TCR

Vβ   Vα

Antigenic peptide

α-helical region of MHC binding the peptide

α1   α2

β₂m

α3

MHC (class I)

Figure 7.7 The three-dimensional structure of the MHC-peptide-T-cell receptor (TCR) complex. MHC, major histocompatibility complex. (Adapted with permission from Bjorkman PJ. *Cell*, 89:167, 1997.)

BOX 7.2 Superantigens

Certain proteins produced by some bacteria and viruses are recognized by αβ T-cell receptors (TCRs) expressing T cells without processing. They have been shown to bind directly (but outside the antigen recognition site) to numerous TCR Vβ sequences and to directly activate T cells. They also bind to the outside surface of major histocompatibility complex class II molecules (Fig. 7.6). The superantigens, by virtue of their binding to Vβ regions of TCRs found on many T cells, are capable of activating 1% to 20% of T cells and causing the presence of high levels of cytokines in the blood. These high levels can produce "shock-like" symptoms. Among the more common superantigens are the staphylococcal enterotoxins that cause food poisoning.

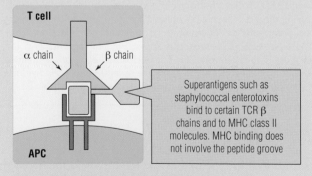

T cell

α chain   β chain

Superantigens such as staphylococcal enterotoxins bind to certain TCR β chains and to MHC class II molecules. MHC binding does not involve the peptide groove

APC

Figure 7.6 Superantigen binding to MHC class II and the T-cell receptor (TCR). APC, antigen-presenting cell; MHC, major histocompatibility complex.

CD3 complex), whereas other accessory molecules assist in T-cell function. This chapter has primarily focused on the TCR αβ and γδ chains, which bind antigen. The TCR cannot function as a receptor without the CD3 complex comprising four different transmembrane protein chains: γ, δ, ε, and ζ (zeta). CD3 molecules are necessary for a signal to be transduced to the cytoplasm after the TCR binds antigen (Chapter 11), thus allowing T-cell activation. Several additional molecules (e.g., integrins such as CD11a; also known as leukocyte function-associated antigen 1 [LFA-1]) function in adhesion of the T cell to its target cell (Fig. 7.8), and yet others function both in adhesion and signal transduction. The most important of the latter are CD4 and CD8. (The surfaces of immune cells are covered with molecules that are vital to the functions of the cells. These molecules are detected using monoclonal antibodies and are given "CD" numbers, e.g., CD4, CD8.) CD4 and

T cell receptor (TCR)

Immunoglobulin (Ig)

Antigen

MHC I

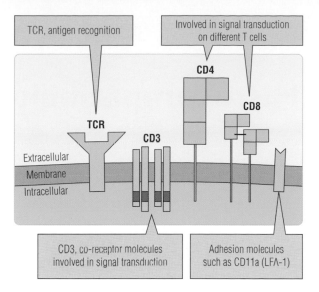

Figure 7.8 Accessory molecules involved in T-cell function. TCR, T-cell receptor.

CD8 enhance the response of specific T cells, both by stabilizing the TCR-peptide-MHC complex through binding to the class II or class I MHC molecules, respectively, and by bringing a tyrosine kinase (Lck, a member of the Src family), into the proximity of the cytoplasmic tails of the CD3 and zeta proteins, thereby facilitating signal transduction and cell activation. CD4 is the cellular receptor for HIV attachment to T cells. T cells carrying CD4 are known as T-helper cells in that they promote the responsiveness of other cells. T cells carrying CD8 have killing functions— for example, lysis of virally infected cells, and are also known as cytotoxic T lymphocytes (CTLs). The numbers of $CD4^+$ T cells and $CD8^+$ T cells are measured to assess disease progression in HIV-mediated immunodeficiency disease (see Chapter 32).

LEARNING POINTS — Can You Now ...

1. Draw the biochemical structure of the antigen-recognition proteins of the TCR?
2. Explain the roles of the various proteins in the TCR complex, and list the major accessory molecules involved in T-cell recognition?
3. Recall the structural relationship between Ig and the TCR?
4. Differentiate between the $\alpha\beta$ and $\gamma\delta$ TCRs, and recall their different functional roles?
5. Draw the TCR gene organization ($\alpha\beta$ and $\gamma\delta$)?
6. Describe the genetic mechanisms involved in the generation of TCR diversity, e.g., junctional diversity?
7. Compare the generation of diversity for Ig and the TCR?
8. Compare the recognition of antigen and superantigen by the TCR?

 MHC II

 Cytokine, Chemokine, etc.

Complement (C')

Signaling molecule

8 Major Histocompatibility Complex

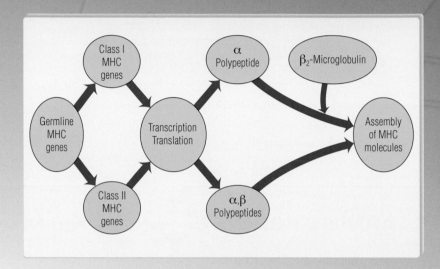

The major histocompatibility complex (MHC) is a region of DNA that encodes a group of molecules that recognize antigen. The molecules encoded by the MHC are referred to as MHC molecules and sometimes as transplantation antigens (Box 8.1). The MHCs of different organisms have specific names. The human MHC, found on human chromosome 6, is known as human leukocyte antigen (HLA). When we refer specifically to HLA, we use the terms *HLA genes* or HLA molecules (e.g., *HLA-A* genes encode HLA-A molecules). As described in Chapter 3, HLA molecules are antigen-recognition molecules, just as antibodies and T-cell receptors (TCRs) are antigen-recognition molecules. However, it was not until the three-dimensional (3D) structure of an HLA molecule was obtained that their role as antigen-recognition molecules became clear. As shown in the overview figure above, the main topics for this chapter are the genetic organization of the MHC and the structure and assembly of the MHC gene products. We also describe in more detail the role of MHC molecules in antigenic peptide "display" to T cells.

■ GENETIC ORGANIZATION

Figure 8.1 shows the organization of the genes encoded in the human MHC. Only the major loci are shown. It should be noted that, through the genome sequencing effort, some 224 loci have been identified in the HLA region. Also, note the breakdown of loci into three major classes: class I, class II, and class III. As shown in Figure 8.2, there is extensive polymorphism (existence of a large number of allelic determinants) in the MHC. Indeed, this is the most polymorphic locus known. The alleles are also unusual in that they differ in approximately 10 to 20 amino acid residues rather than just one or a few residues. Figure 8.3 shows another unusual feature of this genetic region. Blocks of alleles (**haplotypes**) are inherited together, and they are identical in families. This is largely because of a lack of genetic recombination in the MHC. Genetic recombination involves crossover, and there are relatively few crossover events that take place involving the chromosomal segment that includes the MHC.

■ REGULATION OF GENE EXPRESSION

An important difference between the *HLA class I* (A, B, and C) and *II* (DP, DQ, DR) gene products (Fig. 8.1) and the immunoglobulin and TCR gene products is that the MHC molecules are co-dominantly expressed. This means that both the maternally and the paternally derived allelic forms are expressed as cell-surface proteins. By contrast, immunoglobulin and TCR gene products exhibit allelic exclusion (only one form is expressed on each cell; see Chapters 6

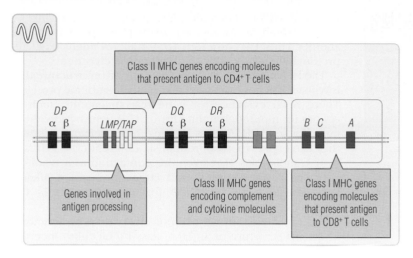

Figure 8.1 Genetic organization of major histocompatibility complex (MHC). *LMP*, large multifunctional protease; *TAP*, transporter-associated with antigen presentation.

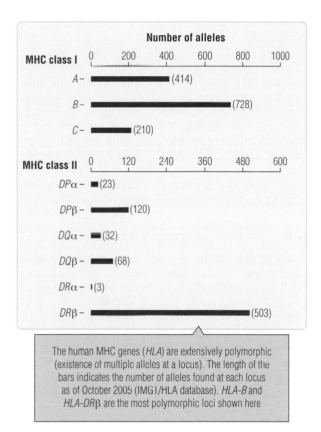

Figure 8.2 Polymorphism in the major histocompatibility complex (MHC). (Data from IMGT, The International Immunogenetics Information System®, http://imgt.cines.fr)

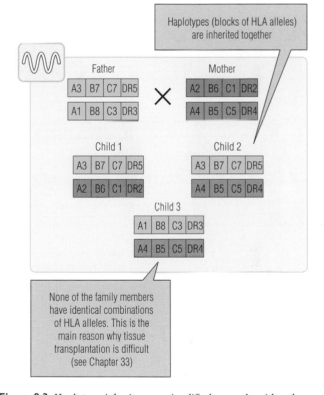

Figure 8.3 Haplotype inheritance, a simplified example with only one class II locus.

and 7). This is illustrated in Figure 8.5 for a human family. Therefore, except for the rare recombinant, children express the haplotypes they inherit from their parents. Class I molecules are found on all nucleated cells. This is in contrast to class II molecules, which are examples of differentiation antigens, and are found on only a few selected cells. Class II molecules are expressed on B cells, macrophages, and dendritic cells; they can be induced on human T cells.

STRUCTURE OF THE MAJOR HISTOCOMPATIBILITY COMPLEX GENE PRODUCTS

Class I

Figure 8.6 shows the structure of the protein products of the class I genes. The class I molecules are noncovalently

 MHC II

 Cytokine, Chemokine, etc.

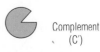 Complement (C')

 Signaling molecule

The products of major histocompatibility complex (MHC)-encoded genes were initially detected as transplantation antigens, that is, antigens recognized as non-self when tissue was exchanged between individuals as a graft (e.g., kidney transplants). Transplantation antigens are the principal cause of graft rejection between nonidentical individuals (Chapter 33). As shown in Figure 8.4, grafts between genetically identical individuals (syngeneic) succeed. All others eventually fail in the absence of other interventions—for example, immunosuppressive drugs such as cyclosporine. This is the fundamental law of transplantation. Transplantation antigens (chiefly molecules encoded in the MHC) do not exist merely to frustrate the efforts of transplant surgeons. They are important antigen-recognition molecules that "display" antigen for "review" by T cells.

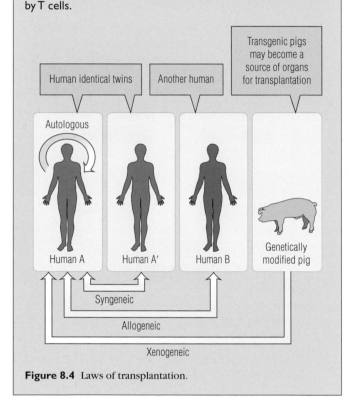

Figure 8.4 Laws of transplantation.

associated heterodimers of an approximately 45,000 molecular weight transmembrane glycoprotein (the α chain, encoded in the MHC) with an approximately 12,000 molecular weight chain (β2-microglobulin) encoded on a completely different chromosome (chromosome 15 in humans). β2-Microglobulin is a soluble protein that complexes with the α chain during synthesis and assembly in the endoplasmic reticulum. It is essential for the peptide-binding function of the MHC-encoded "heavy chain."

DNA and protein sequences obtained for a number of HLA molecules show that they are structurally homologous to one another—that is, they have very similar sequences. HLA-A molecules have very similar sequences to

HLA-B or HLA-C molecules. Alleles (alternative forms) of HLA-A, HLA-B, or HLA-C are even more similar to one another. Thus, two different *HLA-A* alleles might have approximately 90% sequence identity to each other.

The HLA class I genes have an exon/intron structure that is typical of genes encoding eukaryotic membrane proteins. There is no evidence for gene rearrangements, such as occurs in immunoglobulin (Ig) or TCR genes. Individuals inherit a set of HLA class I genes from their parents, and they can express a maximum of six different class I HLA-A, B, or C molecules. However, the population as a whole is extensively polymorphic, and large numbers of alleles, approximately 700 at *HLA-B* for example, exist in the human population.

Figure 8.6 also shows a ribbon-structure representation of the 3D structure of an HLA class I molecule. Once the structure was determined, it was clear that there was a binding groove in the molecule for peptide (antigen). This binding groove is formed entirely by the α chain in class I molecules. The amino acid residues making up the groove are the chief sites of polymorphism; that is, different *HLA-A* alleles produce different amino acids in the antigen-binding groove, and they can, therefore, bind a different range of peptide antigens. The 3D structure also shows a β-pleated sheet platform structure (with homology to Ig) supporting the α-helical binding site. The peptide antigen has been said to fit into the groove like a "hotdog in a bun." Peptides of about 8 to 11 amino acid residues fit into the class I binding site. The precise sequence of the peptide is less important than the presence of certain amino acids (referred to as anchor residues) at particular positions.

Class II

The class II MHC molecules are noncovalently associated transmembrane heterodimers, where both chains are encoded in the MHC (Fig. 8.7). The molecular weight of the α-chain is approximately 33,000, and that of the β chain approximately 29,000 (Fig. 8.7). Both are polymorphic, transmembrane glycoproteins.

As for the class I genes, there is no evidence that gene recombination is used to generate diversity (polymorphism), and the class II genes have the typical exon/intron structure of membrane proteins. There are no variable and constant region gene clusters, as there are for Ig and TCR. When collections of gene and protein sequences for the many alleles at a class II locus are compared, however, there is evidence for regions of greater and lesser diversity. These regions of diversity are called "polymorphic" regions, and they come together in the folded molecule to form the antigen-binding groove. As shown in Figure 8.7, the 3D structure of a class II molecule has a β-pleated sheet platform structure, on top of which is an α-helical binding site for peptides. The binding groove in class II molecules is created by both the α and β chains.

The overall 3D structures of the class I and II molecules differ, but there are similarities. The class II binding site for peptides is more "open" than the class I site, and longer peptides (30 amino acid residues or longer) can fit into the site and overlap at either end. Again, as is true for MHC

  T cell receptor (TCR) 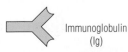 Immunoglobulin (Ig)   Antigen   MHC I

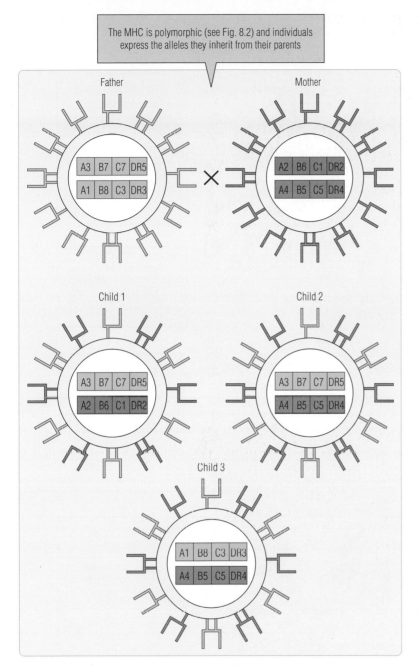

The MHC is polymorphic (see Fig. 8.2) and individuals express the alleles they inherit from their parents

Figure 8.5 Codominant expression of major histocompatibility complex (MHC) molecules, illustrated for the family combination in Figure 8.3. The MHC class I and II molecules are codominantly expressed, i.e. there is no allelic exclusion and all inherited alleles are found in all expressing cells.

class I molecules, the precise sequence of the peptide antigen is less important than that it contains particular residues at certain positions. Therefore, any given MHC molecule can accommodate a wide range of peptides (one at a time). Hence, the likelihood that any given complex antigen, such as a virus, would not contain a peptide antigen that could be efficiently recognized by, and bind to, at least one MHC molecule in an individual is very low. However, there is that possibility, and such an individual is said to be a nonresponder or low responder to that antigen. Control of immune responsiveness is, therefore, also one of the genetic traits associated with the MHC because of the role that MHC molecules have of binding antigens and

presenting them to TCRs prior to initiation of an immune response.

■ RESTRICTION OF ANTIGEN RECOGNITION

The discovery of an antigen-binding groove in MHC molecules helped to explain the concept of MHC restriction, which had been discovered earlier. It had been observed that T cells are specific for both MHC and antigen, and the MHC molecule must be self MHC. Whereas the B-cell receptor can recognize antigen directly, the TCR only

 MHC II

 Cytokine, Chemokine, etc.

 Complement (C')

 Signaling molecule

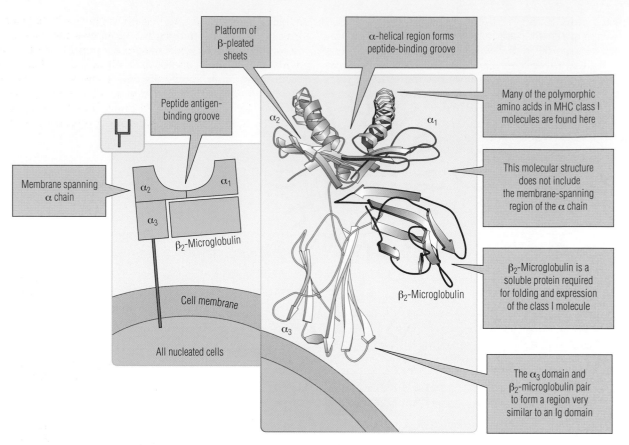

Platform of β-pleated sheets

α-helical region forms peptide-binding groove

Peptide antigen-binding groove

Membrane spanning α chain

α₂

α₁

α₃

β₂-Microglobulin

Cell membrane

All nucleated cells

α₂

α₁

β₂-Microglobulin

α₃

Many of the polymorphic amino acids in MHC class I molecules are found here

This molecular structure does not include the membrane-spanning region of the α chain

β₂-Microglobulin is a soluble protein required for folding and expression of the class I molecule

The α₃ domain and β₂-microglobulin pair to form a region very similar to an Ig domain

Figure 8.6 Structure of major histocompatibility complex (MHC) class I molecules. β₂m, β₂-microglobulin. (Adapted from Roitt I, Brostoff J, Male D. Immunology, ed 6. London: Mosby; 2001.)

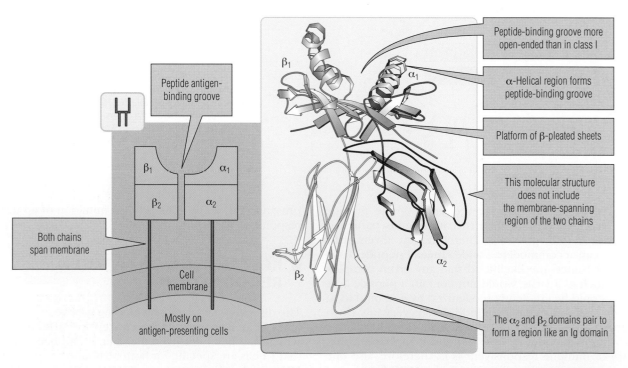

Peptide antigen-binding groove

β₁

α₁

β₂

α₂

Both chains span membrane

Cell membrane

Mostly on antigen-presenting cells

β₁

α₁

β₂

α₂

Peptide-binding groove more open-ended than in class I

α-Helical region forms peptide-binding groove

Platform of β-pleated sheets

This molecular structure does not include the membrane-spanning region of the two chains

The α₂ and β₂ domains pair to form a region like an Ig domain

Figure 8.7 Structure of major histocompatibility complex (MHC) class II molecules. (Adapted from Roitt I, Brostoff J, Male D. Immunology, ed 6. London: Mosby; 2001.)

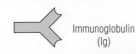 T cell receptor (TCR)

Immunoglobulin (Ig)

 Antigen

 MHC I

recognizes nonself antigen in association with self MHC, that is, there is a dual recognition process. Figure 8.8 illustrates the observations that were made. Therefore, T cells must recognize foreign antigen *and* self MHC. The function of MHC is to be both a binding site (for nonself peptides) and a ligand (for the TCR). How the peptide antigens that are recognized by TCRs are derived from complex nonself antigens, such as viruses, and how they become associated with MHC molecules is the subject of Chapter 10—Antigen Processing And Presentation.

Models of the Major Histocompatibility Complex-Antigen-T-Cell Receptor Complex

Figure 8.9 shows a schematic model of the recognition complex involving an MHC class I molecule, a nonself peptide antigen, and a TCR. The TCR contacts both amino acids from the MHC class I molecule and amino acids from the peptide antigen. Figure 8.9 also helps to illustrate how certain amino acids in the peptide antigen bind to amino acids of the MHC molecule in the peptide-binding groove, whereas other peptide antigen amino acids protrude out of the MHC groove and interact with the TCR.

The repertoire of TCRs that is selected during development in the thymus is dependent upon interaction with MHC molecules; that is, T cells "learn" self MHC in the thymus during development, and those that cannot bind appropriately to self-MHC molecules are eliminated or made anergic (nonresponsive; Chapter 15). This also helps to explain the phenomenon of MHC restriction, that is, that the T-cell receptors are specific for self MHC.

Further detailed molecular characterization of MHC-antigen-TCR interactions is relevant to various clinical situations—for example, designing peptide-based vaccines. Investigations are underway to establish the usefulness of "altered peptide ligands," where the peptide antigen amino acids that would contact the TCR are altered to create a ligand that is an antagonist and there is no T cell activation. This is being investigated as a possible approach to therapy for autoimmune diseases that have a T-cell involvement, for example, multiple sclerosis (Box 8.2).

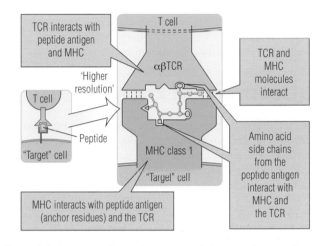

Figure 8.9 Structure of major histocompatibility complex (MHC)-antigen-T-cell receptor (TCR) complex.

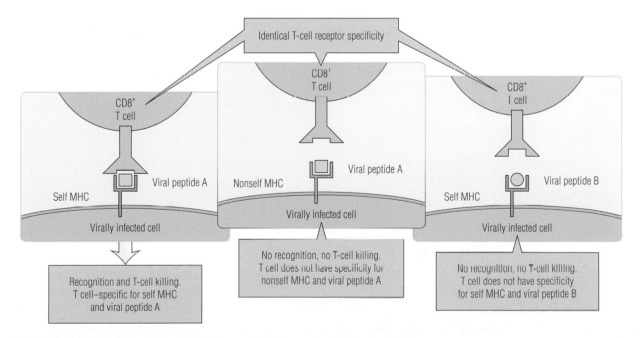

Figure 8.8 T-cell recognition of antigen is major histocompatibility complex (MHC)-restricted.

■ POPULATION ADVANTAGES OF POLYMORPHISM IN THE MAJOR HISTOCOMPATIBILITY COMPLEX ("HETEROZYGOTE ADVANTAGE")

The existence of multiple different HLA class I and II genes means that there are numerous different peptide antigen-binding molecules available for the presentation of antigen to T cells. This appears to be a selective advantage to the individual and to the population as a whole. A heterozygote can present more different pathogen-derived peptides than a homozygote. Homozygosity at HLA class I has been shown to be a disadvantage with respect to HIV/AIDS (see Box 3.1). Similarly, there is evidence that homozygosity at HLA class II increases the risk of hepatitis B virus infection persisting. Therefore, evidence is accumulating that polymorphism in the MHC may indeed confer some advantage in responding to infections by pathogens.

■ DISEASE CORRELATIONS

There are many human diseases that appear to be linked to possession of certain *HLA* alleles. These diseases are often inflammatory or autoimmune in nature. Extensive HLA typing of families has revealed correlations of varying extents with possession of certain *HLA* alleles; for example, a form of joint disease called ankylosing spondylitis is highly associated with the *HLA-B27* allele (Box 8.3). Another disease strongly correlated with HLA is insulin-dependent diabetes mellitus (IDDM). IDDM is associated with (linked to) *HLA-DQ2*. Approximately 50% to 75% of whites with IDDM have *DQ2*. Some other high correlations are listed in Figure 8.10. These observations remain to be fully explained. They could be related to the role of MHC molecules in binding peptides to present to T cells, or they could be the result of another gene linked to HLA. In the example of systemic lupus erythematosus, there is a linkage with complement genes (class III MHC)—see also Chapters 27 and 29.

FIG. 8.10 Correlations Between Various Diseases and Human Leukocyte Antigen (HLA) Alleles

Disease	HLA type
Ankylosing spondylitis	B27
Goodpasture's syndrome	DR2
Insulin-dependent diabetes mellitus	DQ2
Multiple sclerosis	DR2
Pemphigus vulgaris	DR4
Rheumatoid arthritis	DR4
Systemic lupus erythematosus	DR3

BOX 8.2 Specific Immunotherapy with Altered Peptide Ligands

The T-cell receptor (TCR) contacts amino acids of both the peptide antigen and the presenting self-MHC molecule in the trimolecular complex of TCR-peptide-MHC (Fig. 7.7). Amino acids at specific positions in the peptide antigen interact with the TCR, while others interact with the MHC molecule (Fig. 8.9). Borrowing a concept from pharmacology, and recognizing that the MHC-peptide complex is a ligand for the receptor on the T cell, some immunologists have reasoned that they could build altered peptide ligands (APLs) that are antagonists or partial agonists by substituting amino acids at certain positions in the peptide antigen. The approach has been shown to have validity in model systems and is now the subject of several clinical trials, e.g., for multiple sclerosis. Multiple sclerosis is a demyelinating disease that can involve an autoimmune T-cell response against myelin basic protein (MBP). A dominant T-cell epitope in MBP is known to be peptide MBP83-99. By substituting analogs for the amino acids at the positions in the peptide that are thought to contact the TCR, immunologists are hoping to "switch off" the T-cell response to MBP in patients with multiple sclerosis. Patients are given the APLs which should bind to MHC molecules and be presented to the MBP-specific T cells. However, instead of activating the T cells, the APLs will either prevent signal transduction and cell activation (antagonist) or activate some functions but not all (partial agonist), hopefully deflecting some of the autoimmune T cells.

 T cell receptor (TCR)   Immunoglobulin (Ig)   Antigen   MHC I

BOX 8.3 Association Between HLA-B27 and the Autoimmune Disease Ankylosing Spondylitis

Both genetic and environmental factors contribute to autoimmune disease. Among the genes associated with autoimmune disease, the strongest associations are with major histocompatibility complex (*MHC*) genes (see Fig. 8.10). One of the strongest such associations is between *HLA-B27* and the presumed autoimmune disease ankylosing spondylitis. Patients with this disease develop inflammation of the vertebral joints. For example, a patient with ankylosing spondylitis may initially present with lower back pain and stiffness that leads to difficulty in walking. Eventually the spine may become bowed. Anti-inflammatory drugs will often alleviate the symptoms of the disease.

Individuals who possess *HLA-B27* are approximately 90 times more likely to develop the disease than other individuals in the population. Neither the mechanism of the disease nor the basis for its association with *HLA-B27* is known. However, environmental factors (perhaps infection) contribute at least as much to the likelihood of contracting the disease as does HLA type. For example, only a small proportion of the people who express *HLA-B27* ever develop ankylosing spondylitis.

LEARNING POINTS Can You Now ...

1. Draw a diagram of the genetic organization of the human MHC, HLA?

2. Describe the main structural features of the *class I* and *class II MHC* gene products?

3. Recall that *MHC* gene products are co-dominantly expressed compared with the allelic exclusion demonstrated by immunoglobulin and *TCR* gene products?

4. Explain the genetic basis of MHC polymorphism and its significance for the functioning of the immune system?

5. Describe the concept of MHC restriction and draw a model of MHC-peptide-TCR interaction?

6. Compare peptide antigen binding to class I and class II molecules?

7. List some diseases associated with *HLA* alleles?

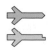 MHC II

 Cytokine, Chemokine, etc.

 Complement (C')

 Signaling molecule

9 Review of Antigen Recognition

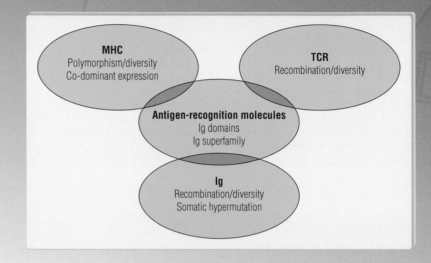

This section of the book has been focused predominantly on the process of antigen recognition and the molecules involved in this process. This is key to understanding the immune system. The genes encoding the antigen-recognition molecules influence the function of the entire adaptive immune system. In the preceding chapters, we described the structure of various antigen-recognition molecules:

- Antibodies (immunoglobulins)
- T-cell antigen receptor (TCR)
- Antigen-recognition molecules encoded in the major histocompatibility complex (MHC)

The genetic mechanisms involved in generating diversity in antibodies and TCRs were described. The generation of diversity in the genes for immunoglobulins and TCRs involves similar mechanisms, and chiefly involves somatic recombination of gene segments in each individual prior to exposure to antigen. MHC class I and II molecules are, by contrast, diverse through polymorphism. Many alternatives (alleles) exist in the human population as a whole, but the individual bears a restricted number—for example, six different *HLA-A*, *B*, and *C* (MHC class I) alleles. Chapters 3 through 8 should also have acquainted you with the various three-dimensional shapes of the antigen-recognition molecules and how they interact with antigen.

■ IMPORTANT STRUCTURAL FEATURES

The Immunoglobulin Domain Fold

As discussed in Chapter 4, the basic building block of the antibody molecule is a polypeptide chain of approximately 110 amino acid residues, folded to create an antiparallel β-pleated sheet structure and held in shape by intrachain disulfide bonds. This domain structure is shared by several other molecules, collectively referred to as the **immunoglobulin superfamily**. Most of the molecules in the superfamily are involved in recognition processes in the immune system—for example, immunoglobulin, TCR, MHC class I and II molecules, KIR, CD4, and CD8. Some representative examples of the members of this family of molecules are given in Figure 9.1.

Some essential aspects of antibody and TCR structure are listed in Figures 9.2 and 9.3; Figure 9.4 highlights some important features of MHC molecules. These should help to focus your review of these molecules.

Antigen-Recognition Sites

As we have seen earlier (Chapters 5, 6, 7, and 8), x-ray crystallographic analyses of several types of antigen-recognition

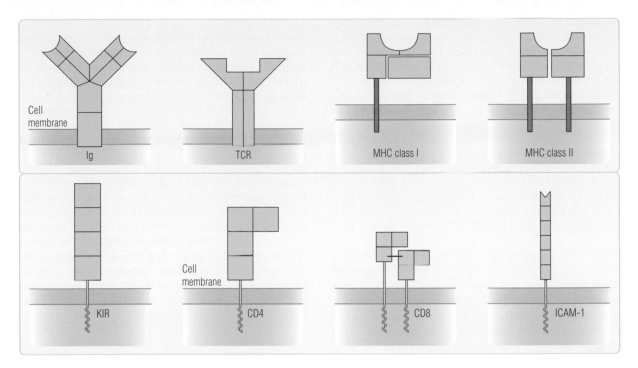

Figure 9.1 Representative members of the immunoglobulin superfamily. β_2m, β_2-microglobulin; ICAM-1, intercellular adhesion molecule 1; KIR, killer cell immunoglobulin-like receptors.

FIG. 9.2 Immunoglobulin and T-cell Receptor (TCR) Proteins and Gene Segments

Immunoglobulin Chains*	TCR Chains†	V Gene Segments Used
Heavy (γ1, μ, δ, etc.)	$\beta\delta$	V, D, J
Light (κ, λ)	$\alpha\gamma$	V, J

*May be both membrane-bound and secreted.
†Membrane-bound only.

FIG. 9.3 Immunoglobulin and T-cell Receptor (TCR) Structure-Function Relationships

Structure	Recognition of Antigen
Immunoglobulin	Directly: carbohydrate, protein, lipid, nucleic acid epitopes
TCR $\alpha\beta$	Dual recognition: self MHC + peptide antigen
TCR $\gamma\delta$	Directly: some recognize nonpeptide phosphorylated lipids and carbohydrates; others recognize protein antigens that have not been processed

FIG. 9.4 Selected Features of MHC Class I and II Molecules

	MHC Class I	MHC Class II
Genes	A, B, C	DP, DQ, DR
Cellular expression	Essentially all nucleated cells	Chiefly, antigen-presenting cells
Structure	α Chain plus β_2-microglobulin	α Chain plus β chain
Peptide binding	Peptides of 8–11 amino acid residues derived in the cytoplasm (endogenous antigen)	Peptides of 9–30 amino acid residues derived in intracellular vesicles (exogenous antigen)
Presentation to	CD8+ Tcells	CD4+ T cells

 MHC II

Cytokine, Chemokine, etc.

 Complement (C')

Signaling molecule

molecule show that the antigen-binding site in antibodies can vary considerably in shape, whereas the TCR site for interaction with peptides presented by MHC molecules tends to be a flat surface area (Fig. 7.2), at least in the TCR variable regions that have been analyzed so far. The peptide-binding grooves of MHC class I and II molecules are similar in being formed from the α-helical regions of the polymorphic domains of the MHC molecules. The groove in class II molecules is open-ended, allowing longer peptides (approximately 9–30 amino acid residues) to "hang over" the groove, whereas the class I peptide groove is closed, only allowing binding of peptides of a fixed size (approximately 8–11 residues). Knowledge accrued concerning the ways that immune molecules recognize antigens is being explored medically in immunotherapy (see Box 8.2).

Molecular analyses of the antigen-recognition molecules highlight the fundamental difference between recognition by B-cell receptors and by TCRs: immunoglobulin binds antigen directly, whereas the TCR interacts with peptide antigens presented by MHC molecules. The ligand for the B-cell receptor is antigen alone, but the ligand for the TCR is a peptide antigen-MHC molecule complex (Fig. 7.7).

■ GENERATION OF DIVERSITY

Several mechanisms have evolved to generate a wide range of antigen-recognition molecules (repertoire) capable of interacting with antigen. With respect to MHC, the MHC molecules are polygenic and polymorphic, that is, there are multiple copies of similar genes. For example, the MHC class I locus is represented by the *HLA-A*, *HLA-B*, and *HLA-C* loci in the human. In the human population, there are also a large number of alleles at these loci. This is polymorphism—existence of multiple alleles at a locus in the population. Much of the diversity in MHC (polymorphism) was created by gene conversion mechanisms, not by the somatic recombination mechanisms used by immunoglobulin and TCR genes. Gene conversion does not occur widely in the immune system, and it will not be explained further here.

The immunoglobulin and TCR genes are extremely diverse. Again, like MHC alleles, which pre-exist exposure to antigen, the repertoire of immunoglobulin and TCR genes largely precedes contact with antigen. The same enzymes, that is, the V(D)J recombinase including RAG-1/RAG-2, are involved in gene segment recombination in B and T cells. These enzymes do not appear to function in other cells. Most immunoglobulin and TCR diversity is a result of junctional diversity created during the recombination of *V* region gene segments (e.g., *D* to *J*, *V* to *DJ*, *V* to *J*). The various genetic mechanisms contributing to diversity in immunoglobulin and TCR genes are listed in Figure 9.5. Clearly junctional diversity, created by imprecise joining and by insertion and addition of nucleotides by the enzyme terminal deoxynucleotidyl transferase as gene segments are recombined, is a major contributor to this diversity (Fig. 9.6). Another point that should be highlighted is that although there is extensive "improvement" of the immunoglobulin binding site for antigen after exposure to antigen, the TCR repertoire does not continue to change after antigenic exposure (Fig. 9.5).

FIG. 9.5   Mechanisms Used to Generate Diversity in Immunoglobulin and T-cell Receptors

	Immunoglobulin	T-cell receptor
Prior to exposure to antigen		
Multiple V region gene segments	√	√
Somatic recombination of gene segments	√	√
Junctional variability	√	√
Multiple combinations of chains, e.g., light/heavy or α/β	√	√
After exposure to antigen		
Somatic hypermutation	√	−
Class switching	√	−

FIG. 9.6   Generation of Diversity: Contribution of Various Mechanisms

Mechanisms	Immunoglobulin	T-cell receptor αβ	T-cell receptor γδ
V segment recombination (*V, D, J*)	$\sim 2.5 \times 10^5$	$\sim 2 \times 10^3$	$\sim 10^2$
Estimated total repertoire	$\sim 10^{11}$	$\sim 10^{16}$	$\sim 10^{18}$

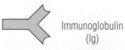 T cell receptor (TCR)   Immunoglobulin (Ig)   Antigen   MHC I

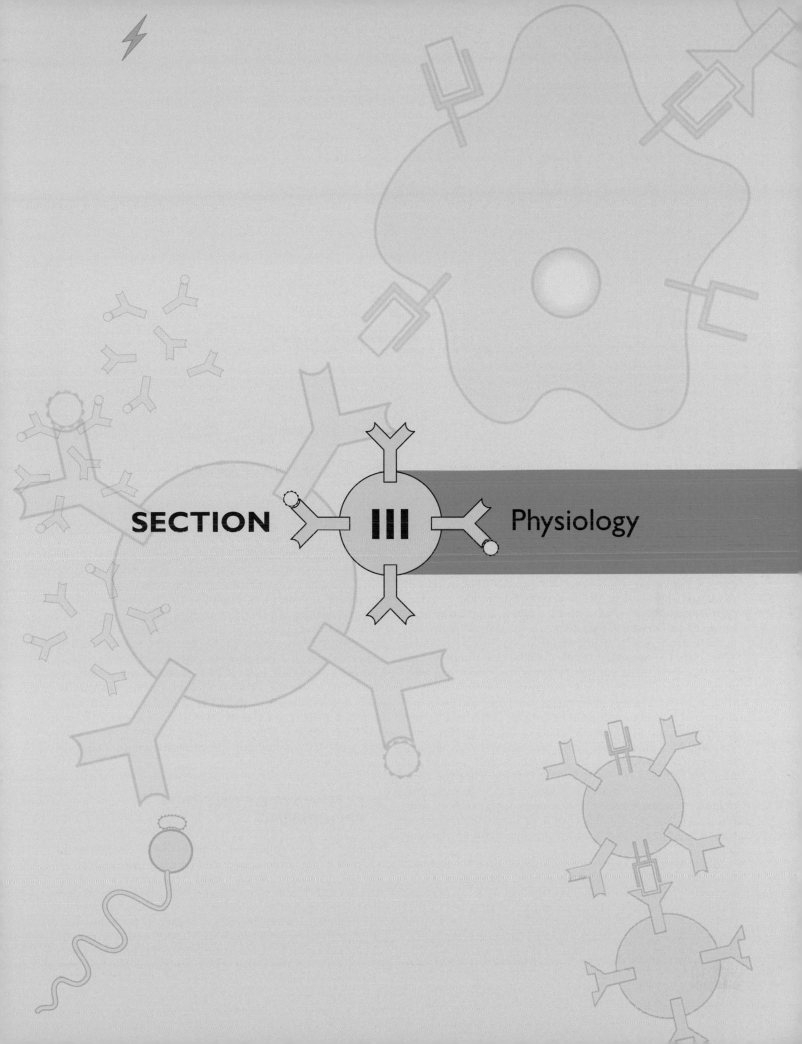

SECTION III   Physiology

Antigen Processing and Presentation

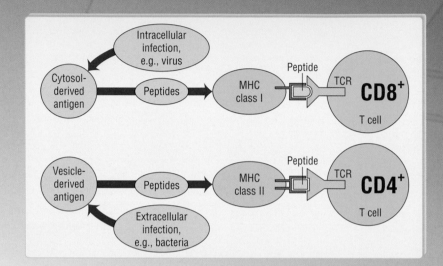

The topic for this chapter is the formation of the major histocompatibility complex (MHC)-foreign antigen complexes, which are the ligands for the αβ T-cell receptor (TCR). As depicted in the overview figure above, extracellular antigens travel in cells via a different pathway than intracellular-derived antigens. The nature of these pathways and the processes by which antigens complex with either MHC class I or class II molecules will be described.

As we have seen earlier, the body has developed barriers that are very effective in preventing foreign antigens, such as bacteria or viruses, from gaining entry and inducing disease. If a foreign organism or antigen (such as a toxin) gains entry, the protective systems of the innate immune system (e.g., phagocytic cells) may destroy the antigen before it is encountered by B or T cells and induces an adaptive immune response. Very little foreign antigen typically survives the innate immune system's various host defense systems intact, but if it does, fortunately it only requires a very small number of B- or T-cell antigen receptors to be engaged to initiate a protective adaptive immune response.

B-cell antigen receptors may interact directly with an invading microbe but αβ TCRs only recognize "processed" antigenic peptides. In addition, the αβ TCR recognizes foreign antigen only when the antigen is attached to the surface of other cells (antigen-presenting cells [APCs] or target cells; Fig. 10.1). Examples of APCs are macrophages, B cells, and the various dendritic cells (see Chapters 2, 12,

and 20). Dendritic cells, as discussed later, are APCs "par excellence" (see Box 10.1 and Chapters 12 and 20). These APCs, in addition to presenting antigen, usually provide co-stimulator activities that complete the immune activation process. Antigen is presented by APCs in association with MHC molecules (see also Chapter 8). Antigen recognition by T lymphocytes is thus said to be **MHC restricted**. The major subsets of T lymphocytes, the helper T cells (CD4+) and the cytotoxic T cells (CD8+) have different "MHC restrictions." Thus, the CD4+ T cell–APC interaction is MHC class II–restricted, and the CD8+ T cell–target cell interaction is MHC class I–restricted (see Chapters 7, 8, and 15). The process whereby antigen becomes associated with self-MHC molecules for presentation to T cells is called antigen processing.

■ PATHWAYS OF ANTIGEN PROCESSING

Peptide antigens generated in the cytosolic compartment of the cell (e.g., from viruses and bacteria that replicate in the cytosol) bind to class I MHC molecules for presentation to CD8+ T cells (see Chapter 7). Peptide antigens generated in intracellular vesicles from the endocytic uptake of extracellular antigens, such as toxins, or from microbes growing in intracellular vesicles (e.g., after the phagocytic uptake of certain bacteria by macrophages) bind to class II

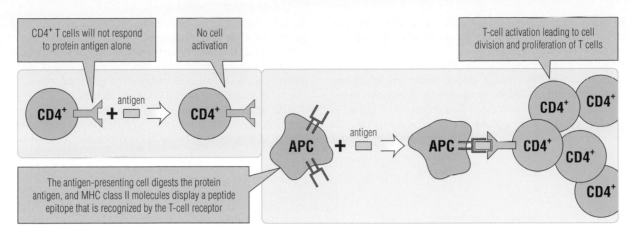

Figure 10.1 Antigen presentation to T cells by antigen-presenting cells (APCs). MHC, major histocompatibility complex.

MHC molecules for presentation to CD4$^+$ T cells. This means that CD8$^+$ T cells can monitor the intracellular environment, and CD4$^+$ T cells can monitor the extracellular environment for pathogens.

The intracellular pathway traversed by an antigen is the primary factor in determining if an antigen will be presented on class I or class II MHC molecules, not anything particular about the antigen itself. If a protein that is normally extracellular, and would therefore be processed to create an MHC class II peptide-antigen complex, is instead transfected directly into the cytoplasm using a gene expression system, the peptides that are now generated in the cytoplasm after proteolytic breakdown of the transfected protein will be presented on class I MHC molecules.

Protein antigens need to be processed by APCs to produce the antigenic peptides recognized by T cells. This processing requires time (minutes to hours) and metabolism and therefore will not occur in killed APCs, although killed cells may present preformed peptide antigens to T lymphocytes (e.g., vaccines or peptides from extracellular pathogens).

■ MECHANISMS OF ANTIGEN PROCESSING

Extracellular (or Exogenous) Antigens

Extracellular (or exogenous) antigens are either extracellular proteins (e.g., a protein vaccine) or proteins derived from a pathogen in a cytoplasmic vesicle after uptake. These antigens are processed for eventual presentation on MHC

BOX 10.1 Dendritic Cells: Antigen-Presenting Cells Par Excellence

The dendritic cells (DCs) make up a system of cells critical to the immune response, especially T cell–mediated immunity. The development of dendritic cells from progenitor cells in the bone marrow is described in Chapter 12. These cells were originally detected by their atypical cell shape (see Fig. 2.6). They have extensive "dendritic" processes that continually form and retract. Dendritic cells are found in several places in the body and are motile, migrating in the blood and lymph from peripheral organs to the lymphoid organs, particularly to T-cell areas of organs such as the lymph nodes. In essence, immature DCs function to capture antigens at sites of contact with the external environment—for example, the skin and mucosal epithelia, and then they transport and present the antigen until they encounter a T cell with specificity for that MHC-antigen complex. Dendritic cells mature in the presence of pathogens and then function to activate T cells.

Dendritic cells in different organs have been given different names (see Chapter 13). For example, epidermal DCs are known as Langerhans cells. DCs are found in virtually all the other organs and are usually known as interstitial dendritic cells because they locate in interstitial spaces. In lymphoid organs, the interstitial dendritic cells have been given the name interdigitating cells, because they are prevalent in T-cell areas and extend processes between the T cells. Another important set of DCs are the plasmacytoid-derived DCs. These cells may have a unique hematopoietic lineage (see Chapter 12). The precursors of plasmacytoid DCs are also known as type I interferon-producing cells (or IPCs). These cells have a plasma cell morphology and secrete type I interferons following viral infection. At later stages of infection, they differentiate into mature DCs that regulate the response of T cells to viral infections. Finally, DCs found in the blood and lymph are known as veiled cells. All of these dendritic cells are antigen-presenting cells, although they may have a slightly different morphology or role. Among the characteristics of DCs that contribute to their ability to present antigen effectively are: (1) they express high levels of MHC class II molecules; (2) they express high levels of costimulatory molecules, such as CD80 (B7); and (3) they retain MHC-peptide antigen complexes on their surface for long periods of time, thereby enhancing the likelihood of T-cell binding and subsequent activation. DCs initiate both CD4$^+$ and CD8$^+$ T-cell responses (see Chapter 15). Their importance as antigen-presenting cells is leading to clinical research to investigate their use in new approaches to vaccination against tumor antigens. DCs have been loaded with tumor antigens and used in clinical trials with melanoma patients, for example.

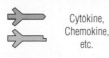 MHC II

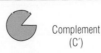 Cytokine, Chemokine, etc.

Complement (C′)

 Signaling molecule

class II molecules to CD4+ T lymphocytes (Fig. 10.2A). First, however, they must be internalized by the APC. Mostly this involves fluid phase endocytosis, but if antigen is bound by the immunoglobulin receptor, for example, internalization is via the much faster route of receptor-mediated endocytosis. Other antigens in this processing pathway are those derived from microbes that grow in intracellular vesicles after uptake by phagocytosis in cells such as macrophages. In any event, the antigen is first found inside the cell in an acidic membrane-bound compartment that can enter the endosomal pathway of the cell. Figure 10.2A illustrates only the most important stages of degradative processing, and the principal stages in the biosynthesis of integral membrane glycoproteins, such as the MHC class II α- and β-chain molecules.

The antigen derived in the intracellular vesicle moves through various acidic endosomal/lysosomal compartments where it is degraded by cellular proteases, first to peptides

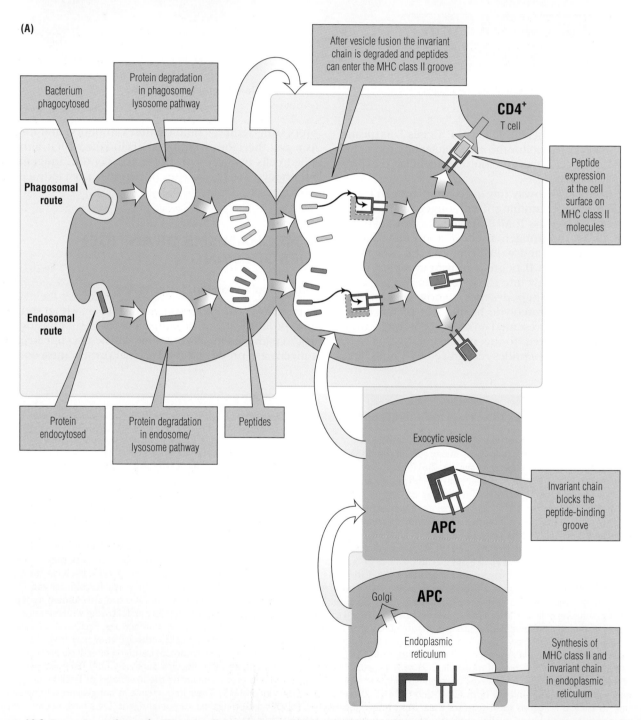

Figure 10.2 Processing pathways for **(A)** extracellular antigens and **(B)** intracellular antigens. APC, antigen-presenting cell; TAP, transporter associated with antigen presentation; TCR, T-cell receptor.

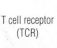 T cell receptor (TCR) 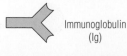 Immunoglobulin (Ig)   Antigen   MHC I

of different sizes then ultimately to amino acids. During this process, peptides are generated in the size range that can bind to class II MHC molecules (9 to 30 plus amino acid residues). The APC also synthesizes new class II MHC molecules in the endoplasmic reticulum. These molecules move out through the Golgi apparatus, where they are glycosylated, eventually becoming part of a vesicle that buds off the Golgi and may fuse with an endosomal vesicle containing peptides from an extracellular or vesicle-derived antigen. In the pathway from the endoplasmic reticulum through the Golgi and so on, the empty binding site of class II MHC is "protected" from binding other peptides (e.g., self peptides) by a molecule known as the **invariant chain** (Ii). In the acidic environment of the endosome, this protection is removed by proteolytic action, and the class II binding site is available for occupancy by any appropriate peptide available in the endosome. "Occupied" MHC class II molecules are then expressed at the cell surface when the endosomal vesicle fuses with the cell surface membrane. In this way, a foreign antigen can be presented to the repertoire of TCRs and can induce the appropriate T cell to proliferate (see Fig. 10.2A).

Intracellular (or Endogenous) Antigens

Endogenous (intracellular) antigens such as viral proteins are processed by "target cells" for eventual presentation on class I MHC molecules to CD8+ T cells (cytotoxic T lymphocytes [Fig. 10.2B]). In this case, peptides that are foreign antigens are generated in the cytoplasmic compartment. These may be derived by breakdown, via the normal cellular machinery, of viral proteins that are being synthesized and assembled in the cytoplasm of a virally infected cell (e.g., a fibroblast). In Figure 10.2B, a viral protein is being synthesized in the cytosol. The cellular degradative machinery, most importantly a complex of proteases known as the **proteasome**, may enzymatically cleave some of the viral protein molecules through various polypeptide and peptide intermediate steps until peptides of 8 to 11 residues are formed; these can bind to class I MHC molecules. Many of the peptides will undergo further degradation, making them irrelevant to the immune system. However, some will enter the endoplasmic reticulum carried by a two-chain molecule known as TAP (transporter associated with antigen presentation; see Box 10.2). TAP permits the peptides to traverse the membrane bilayer of the endoplasmic reticulum and bind in the empty peptide-binding groove of nascent MHC class I molecules being synthesized in the endoplasmic reticulum. Binding of these small peptide antigens is critical for the final stages of assembly of MHC class I molecules. In the absence of peptide, class I molecules are unable to fold correctly and are not found at the cell surface. MHC class I molecules complete their biosynthesis in the Golgi and move out to the surface membrane via the exocytic pathway. After fusion of an exocytic vesicle with the surface membrane, foreign antigenic peptides associated with MHC class I molecules may interact with T lymphocytes bearing receptors capable of binding this MHC-antigen complex (CD8+ or cytotoxic T cells).

Class I or II Association

It is important to underline that, as illustrated in Figure 10.2, the likelihood of an antigen becoming associated with class I or class II MHC is determined solely by the route of trafficking through the cell, not by some special property of the antigen. The processing of antigens in this way also explains why polysaccharides, lipids, and nucleic acids are not recognized by αβ T cells—they are not processed to fit into the binding groove of the MHC molecules.

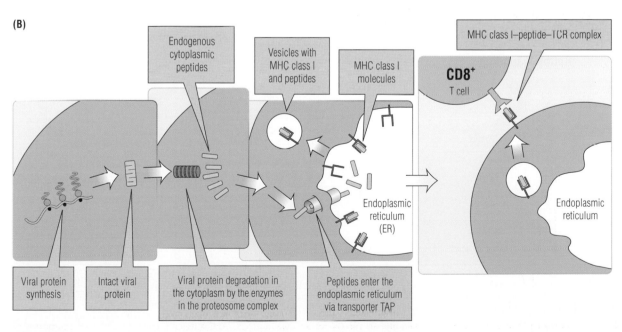

(B)

Endogenous cytoplasmic peptides

Vesicles with MHC class I and peptides

MHC class I molecules

MHC class I–peptide–TCR complex

CD8+ T cell

Endoplasmic reticulum (ER)

Endoplasmic reticulum

Viral protein synthesis

Intact viral protein

Viral protein degradation in the cytoplasm by the enzymes in the proteosome complex

Peptides enter the endoplasmic reticulum via transporter TAP

Figure 10.2, *cont'd*

 MHC II

 Cytokine, Chemokine, etc.

 Complement (C')

 Signaling molecule

Processing of cytosol- and vesicle-derived antigens to result in association with MHC class I or class II molecules, respectively, results in the activation of different subsets of T cells (Figs 10.3 and 10.4).

■ EVASION OF PROCESSING PATHWAYS BY PATHOGENS

If pathogens can avoid having their peptide antigens displayed by MHC molecules, they can avoid detection by the adaptive immune system. Consequently, numerous pathogens have developed strategies to interfere with antigen processing. For example, bacteria such as *Mycobacterium tuberculosis* have acquired the capacity to inhibit phagosome–lysosome fusion. This inhibits their exposure to lysosomal proteases and reduces the likelihood that mycobacterial peptides that will bind to MHC molecules will be generated and be expressed at the cell surface. Among the viruses, several have found ways to interfere with the processing steps leading up to binding to MHC class I molecules. For example, a protein of herpes simplex

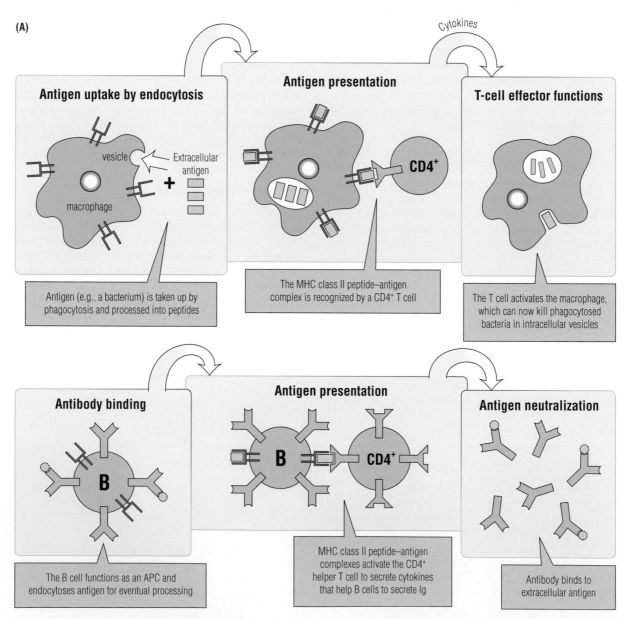

(A)

Antigen uptake by endocytosis

vesicle
Extracellular antigen
macrophage

Antigen (e.g., a bacterium) is taken up by phagocytosis and processed into peptides

Antigen presentation

CD4+

The MHC class II peptide–antigen complex is recognized by a CD4+ T cell

T-cell effector functions

The T cell activates the macrophage, which can now kill phagocytosed bacteria in intracellular vesicles

Cytokines

Antibody binding

B

The B cell functions as an APC and endocytoses antigen for eventual processing

Antigen presentation

B   CD4+

MHC class II peptide–antigen complexes activate the CD4+ helper T cell to secrete cytokines that help B cells to secrete Ig

Antigen neutralization

Antibody binds to extracellular antigen

Figure 10.3 Presentation of antigens to different subsets of T cells. (**A**) Class II MHC–associated extracellular antigen is presented to T-helper cells (CD4+ T cells) either by macrophages or by B cells. (**B**) Class I MHC–associated cytosolic antigen is presented to cytotoxic T cells (CD8+ T cells). APC, antigen-presenting cell; MHC, major histocompatibility complex.

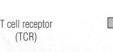 T cell receptor (TCR)

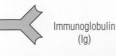 Immunoglobulin (Ig)

 Antigen

 MHC I

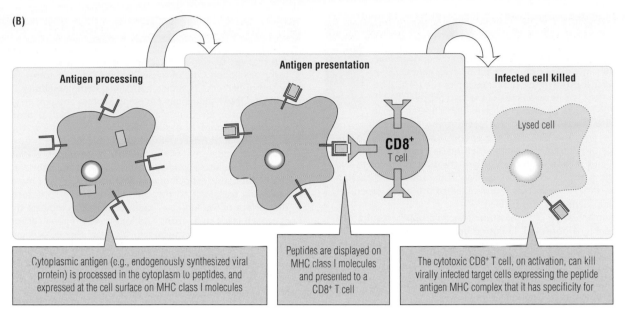

(B)

Antigen processing

Antigen presentation

Infected cell killed

Lysed cell

CD8⁺ T cell

Cytoplasmic antigen (e.g., endogenously synthesized viral protein) is processed in the cytoplasm to peptides, and expressed at the cell surface on MHC class I molecules

Peptides are displayed on MHC class I molecules and presented to a CD8⁺ T cell

The cytotoxic CD8⁺ T cell, on activation, can kill virally infected target cells expressing the peptide antigen MHC complex that it has specificity for

Figure 10.3, *cont'd*

virus (HSV) binds to TAP and inhibits peptide transport into the endoplasmic reticulum. A consequence of this is that there are fewer HSV peptides available to bind to class I MHC. Certain strains of adenovirus express a protein that inhibits the transcription of class I MHC molecules, thereby reducing the number of class I MHC molecules available to display adenoviral peptides to CD8⁺ lymphocytes.

Some of the ways pathogens have found to avoid detection by the host defense systems are a reflection of the dynamic interchange between host and microbe as both try to survive and propagate. Equally, medical research is using knowledge of the process of antigen presentation to devise new and better therapies for pathogen-mediated diseases (Box 10.3).

FIG. 10.4 Pathways of Antigen Processing

	CELL COMPARTMENT		
	Cytosol	Phagocytic vesicles	Endocytic vesicles
Source of antigen	Viruses and some bacteria	Bacteria taken up by phagocytosis, some of which are able to grow in cellular vesicles (phagosomes), e.g., the mycobacteria that cause tuberculosis	Extracellular proteins (vaccines, toxins, etc.), which are taken into the cell by endocytosis and processed in cellular vesicles (endosomes)
Molecule binding antigenic peptides	Class I MHC	Class II MHC	Class II MHC
Type of cell reacting with MHC-peptide complex	CD8⁺ T cells, which kill infected cells	CD4⁺ T cells* which activate macrophages. The activated macrophages can then destroy the intravesicular bacteria	CD4⁺ T cells* which activate B cells to make antibody

*The roles of different subsets of CD4⁺ T cells are explained further in Chapter 15

 MHC II

 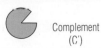 Cytokine, Chemokine, etc.

Complement (C′)

 Signaling molecule

BOX 10.2 TAP Deficiency

The peptide transporter (TAP) found in the endoplasmic reticulum membrane is encoded by two genes, *TAP-1* and *TAP-2*, located in the class II region of the MHC. The transporter is a heterodimer of the two proteins TAP-1 and TAP-2. Rare mutations exist in *TAP-1* or *TAP-2* that alter the function of TAP and prevent the efficient entry of peptides into the lumen of the endoplasmic reticulum. In the absence of peptide antigen, the MHC class I molecules are unstable, and only a small fraction are transported through the exocytic pathway to the cell surface. This reduced expression of class I MHC molecules interferes with the development of cytotoxic T lymphocytes (CTLs).

In humans with TAP mutations, chronic upper respiratory infections are observed. Humoral immunity is intact in these patients and some aspects of cellular immunity are also normal— for example, the patients' CD4$^+$ T cells can respond to antigen. However, the lack of expression of class I MHC molecules results in reduced numbers of CTL and in difficulties responding appropriately to some respiratory viruses.

BOX 10.3 DNA Vaccination

Alternatives to standard vaccination techniques are being developed. One of these involves vaccines composed of bacterial plasmids containing complementary DNA (cDNA) sequences encoding protein antigens (e.g., a viral protein or tumor antigen) against which a protective immune response is desired. Following inoculation, the bacterial plasmid transfects APCs, where the cDNA is transcribed, translated, and some of the protein molecules are eventually broken down into peptide antigens. Some of the peptides enter the endoplasmic reticulum and bind to MHC class I molecules. Following transport to the cell surface, they are detected on the surface of the APC by T cells. Early results indicate that this approach leads to a strong and long-lived immune response to certain antigens. Furthermore, because the cDNA-encoded proteins are synthesized in the cytosol, this can provide a way to introduce antigen into the intracellular processing pathway, leading to presentation on class I MHC molecules and the elicitation of a cytotoxic T-cell response. Standard vaccine approaches (e.g., protein vaccine injected intramuscularly) would result in the protein being introduced to the endocytic/class II pathway, with eventual presentation to CD4$^+$ T cells and the likelihood of stimulating an antibody response.

The relative ease of creating plasmids that include cDNAs encoding other immune system-enhancing proteins, e.g., cytokines, in conjunction with the "vaccine" protein, makes this a very attractive approach to consider adopting widely for vaccines in the future. Several DNA vaccines are entering clinical trials for breast, colon, and prostate cancer patients, and others will undoubtedly follow.

LEARNING POINTS Can You Now ...

1. List at least three examples of antigen-presenting cells (APCs; e.g., macrophages) and describe their role in antigen processing and presentation?

2. Describe how T lymphocytes recognize antigens on the *surface* of other cells associated with MHC molecules?

3. Explain why linear protein antigenic determinants are recognized by T cells and conformational determinants are recognized by B cells?

4. Draw diagrams of the different pathways of processing of an extracellular (exogenous) and an intracellular (endogenous) protein antigen (indicating the role of intracellular proteolytic compartments)?

5. Describe with a diagram the molecular interactions involved in MHC-restricted antigen presentation to CD4$^+$ and CD8$^+$ T cells?

 T cell receptor (TCR)   Immunoglobulin (Ig)   Antigen   MHC I

II Lymphocyte Activation

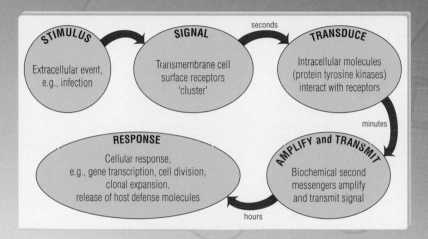

Events, such as an infection, produce a stimulus ("danger signal"), in the form of foreign antigens and inflammation (see also Chapter 20), to the immune system. As discussed earlier in Chapters 1 and 2, antigen-recognition molecules exist as cell-surface receptors on B and T lymphocytes and are able to recognize these foreign molecules. Binding to the receptors initiates a protective response. The topic for this chapter is the mechanisms involved in B and T lymphocyte activation to produce the host-defense response. The overview figure above illustrates that following antigen binding, a signal is transduced, amplified, and transmitted through the cell to the nucleus in a matter of minutes. Following a variety of biochemical changes, a cellular response is then generated. Some of the details of the events from stimulus to response will be described in this chapter.

First, an antigen must be recognized, then notice (a signal) of this recognition must be transmitted to the cellular interior, and a response is generated. The process of translating the molecular events of antigen recognition into a cellular response is known as signal transduction. Intracellular molecules are very important in **signal transduction**. They cause biochemical "second messengers" to be induced and biochemical pathways to be activated that amplify the signal throughout the cell. At the end of the biochemical pathways are transcription factors, which, on activation, initiate the new gene transcription that leads to functional changes in the cell, including proliferation, division, and differentiation.

In this overview of the activation of B and T lymphocytes, we also explain the action of some immunosuppressive drugs and indicate how enhanced knowledge of lymphocyte activation mechanisms is leading to the design of new immunomodulatory agents.

◼ ANTIGEN RECEPTORS

The B- and T-cell antigen receptors are part of multimolecular protein complexes at the cell surface (T-cell antigen receptors are described in Chapter 7 and B-cell antigen receptors in Chapters 4 and 5). Although both membrane-bound immunoglobulin and the $\alpha\beta$ (or $\gamma\delta$) T-cell receptor (TCR) have protein chains that span the cell-surface membrane and extend into the cytoplasm, they have very short cytoplasmic sequences. These short cytoplasmic "tails" are ineffective at interfacing with the intracellular molecules that activate lymphocytes. Consequently, other proteins must interact with the "receptor" proteins before there can be effective signal transduction. Functionally, both the B-cell receptor (BCR) and the TCR are multimolecular protein complexes in which several other proteins are noncovalently linked together with the antigen-receptor proteins in the cell-surface membrane. The major protein components of the BCR and the TCR complexes are illustrated in Figures 11.1 and 11.2.

The B-Cell Receptor

Functionally, the BCR is a complex of membrane-bound immunoglobulin (mIg) and two invariant proteins known

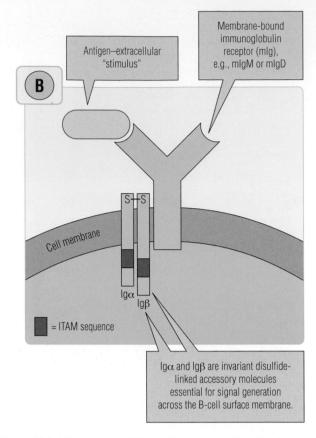

Figure 11.1 The structure of the B-cell receptor multimolecular complex. ITAM, immunoreceptor tyrosine-based activation motif.

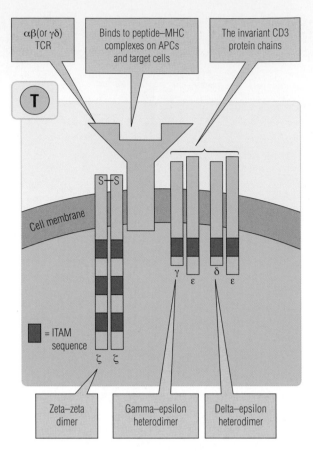

Figure 11.2 The structure of the T-cell receptor multimolecular complex. APC, antigen-presenting cell; ITAM, immunoreceptor tyrosine-based activation motif.

as Igα and Igβ. As shown in Figure 11.1, Igα and Igβ are associated with mIg as a disulfide-linked heterodimeric complex. The Igα-Igβ heterodimer is required for expression of mIg at the cell surface and for signal transduction. The intracellular regions of Igα-Igβ are large enough to interact with cellular-signaling proteins. Igα and Igβ each contain sequences found in several receptor molecules, including proteins of the TCR complex, called the immunoreceptor tyrosine-based activation motif (**ITAM**). ITAMs are essential for signal transduction in B and T cells.

The T-Cell Receptor

Functionally, the TCR complex comprises the TCR αβ (or γδ) chains and six other protein chains involved in signal transduction. The TCR αβ (or γδ) chains bind the major histocompatibility complex (MHC)-antigen complex on an antigen-presenting cell (APC), but alone cannot effectively signal to the T cell that antigen is bound. This is achieved in cooperation with the accessory protein chains, CD3 and ζ (zeta). CD3 is made of four chains, one each of γ and δ and two ε chains. There are two ζ chains in the TCR complex (see Fig. 11.2). Both the CD3 and ζ chains have substantial intracellular regions that contain ITAMs. These

sequences contain tyrosine, which becomes phosphorylated. The phosphorylated ITAMs interact with cytoplasmic signaling proteins.

Initiation of B-Cell and T-Cell Activation

There are several requirements for B- and T-cell activation. For the primary signal, the receptor complexes must be clustered. For B cells, this can occur by cross-linking of receptor molecules by multimeric antigens. This rarely occurs with soluble protein antigens, and other surface molecules become involved to enhance signaling (see later). Both B- and T-cells require a second signal for activation. The nature of the second signals, referred to as costimulatory signals, are described in Chapter 16, along with further details of the interaction of B- and T-cells. Other cell-surface molecules, referred to as coreceptor molecules, contribute to the primary signal. The role of coreceptors in B-cell and T-cell activation will be explained later.

Clustering of TCRs involves binding of the TCR to MHC-peptide antigen complexes on the APC. Immunotherapy using "altered peptide ligands" (APLs) is intended to act by modulating T-cell activation at this stage (Box 11.1 and Box 8.2). It appears that occupancy of as little as a few

 T cell receptor (TCR)   Immunoglobulin (Ig)   Antigen   MHC I

BOX 11.1 Altered Peptide Ligands and Lymphocyte Activation

Altered peptide ligands (APLs) are designed to be antagonists or partial agonists of the TCR for use in specific immunotherapy for certain diseases. Box 8.2 describes the trial of APLs in multiple sclerosis. Now that we have reviewed lymphocyte activation, we can discuss the actions of APLs on T lymphocytes in more detail. APLs that are partial agonists partially activate the cell, e.g., causing secretion of some cytokines but not cell division. T-cell recognition of APLs that are partial agonists appears to result in altered phosphorylation of receptor complex molecules, e.g., CD3 ε and the ζ chains. This partial phosphorylation reduces the ability of the receptor complex to concentrate protein tyrosine kinases (e.g., ZAP-70) on the cytoplasmic tails of the receptor proteins (see Figs 11.6 and 11.8), and impairs signal transduction. This has the ultimate effect of partially inhibiting T-lymphocyte responses.

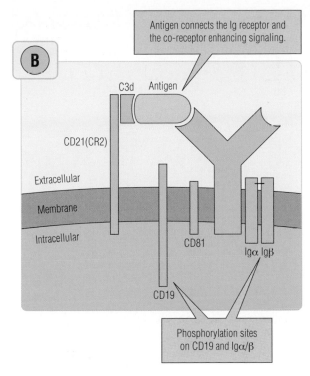

Figure 11.3 The B-cell receptor/co-receptor complex.

hundred TCRs is sufficient to initiate a primary activation signal. Again, T-cell activation requires a second costimulatory signal provided by the APC. As in B cells, co-receptor molecules contribute to the activation of T cells. CD4 and CD8 act as co-receptor molecules on T cells. Their role is also discussed further later. Finally, so-called accessory molecules facilitate T cell–APC contact and TCR–MHC-peptide binding. These accessory molecules are mostly adhesion molecules, such as CD11a or leukocyte function associated antigen 1 (LFA-1) on T cells, which binds to CD54 or intercellular adhesion molecule 1 (ICAM-1) on APCs. These adhesion molecules are discussed further in Chapter 13.

Co-Receptor Molecules in B-Cell Activation

As described earlier, the antigen-specific receptors on B and T cells are unable to transduce signals without the help of invariant proteins such as Igα/Igβ and CD3, respectively. However, optimal signaling requires even more cell-surface molecules, known as co-receptor molecules. The B-cell co-receptor (Fig. 11.3) can co-cluster with the BCR and increase the efficiency of signaling by several thousandfold. As shown in Figure 11.3, the B-cell co-receptor comprises three proteins: CD21 (also known as complement receptor 2 [CR2]), CD19, and CD81. Protein antigens bound to complement component C3d (see Chapter 19) can bind simultaneously to both CD21 and the BCR. This enables the CD21/CD19/CD81 co-receptor complex to cluster and crosslink with the BCR, and induce phosphorylation reactions on the intracellular tail of CD19. This phosphorylation allows kinases belonging to a family of similar enzymes (the Src family) to bind to the cytoplasmic tail of CD19 and to increase the concentration of signaling molecules around the BCR, thereby enhancing the efficiency of signaling.

Co-Receptor Molecules in T-Cell Activation

Optimal signaling through the TCR only occurs when co-receptor molecules are involved. The TCR co-receptor molecules are CD4 or CD8 (Fig. 11.4). As discussed in Chapters 7 and 10, CD4 binds to MHC class II molecules, and CD8 binds to MHC class I molecules. When, for example, the TCR binds to an MHC class II–peptide complex on an APC, CD4 on the T cell binds to the MHC class II molecule (see Fig. 11.6). The tyrosine kinase Lck (a Src kinase) is associated with the cytoplasmic domain of CD4 (and CD8). Consequently, Lck is localized with the TCR complex when CD4 binds to MHC class II–peptide complexes, or CD8 binds to MHC class I–peptide complexes.

Lck is integral in the signaling cascade in T cells, and, again, co-receptor molecule involvement increases the concentration of these signaling molecules in the vicinity of the TCR. The presence of the CD4 or CD8 co-receptors has been estimated to reduce the number of MHC-peptide complexes required to trigger a T-cell response by about 100-fold.

■ SIGNALING EVENTS

Intracellular molecules, chiefly protein tyrosine kinases (PTKs) and protein tyrosine phosphatases (PTPs), form the link between receptor activation and activation of biochemical pathways that amplify and transmit the signal. Within seconds of cross-linking the BCR, PTK enzymes of the Src family (Box 11.2) phosphorylate ITAMs in the re-

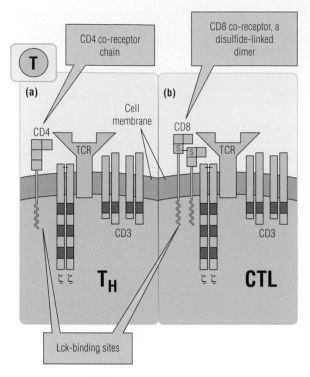

Figure 11.4 The T-cell receptor/co-receptor complex.

BOX 11.2 Intracellular Signaling: The Role of Protein Tyrosine Kinases and Protein Tyrosine Phosphatases

Phosphorylation is a common biochemical mechanism by which cells regulate the activity of proteins. Protein kinases affect protein function by adding phosphate groups to proteins. These phosphate groups are added to tyrosine residues by tyrosine kinases (e.g., ZAP-70), and to serine or threonine residues by serine/threonine kinases (e.g., protein kinase C). The phosphate groups can be removed by protein phosphatases. In general, phosphorylation activates enzymes, and dephosphorylation inactivates enzymes.

Several protein kinases are essential in signal transduction in lymphocytes, and it is important that you recognize some of the most important. For example, activation of the receptor-associated tyrosine kinases of the Src (pronounced as "Sark") family informs the interior of B and T lymphocytes that the antigen receptor is occupied. Two of the major Src family kinases in lymphocytes are known as Lyn and Lck. Another family of tyrosine kinases particularly important in lymphocytes is the Syk family. There are two members of this family: Syk and ZAP-70.

Tyrosine kinases, such as Lyn and Lck, tend to be activated early in signaling pathways, whereas serine/threonine kinases, such as protein kinase C and calcineurin, tend to be important in later stages of signaling.

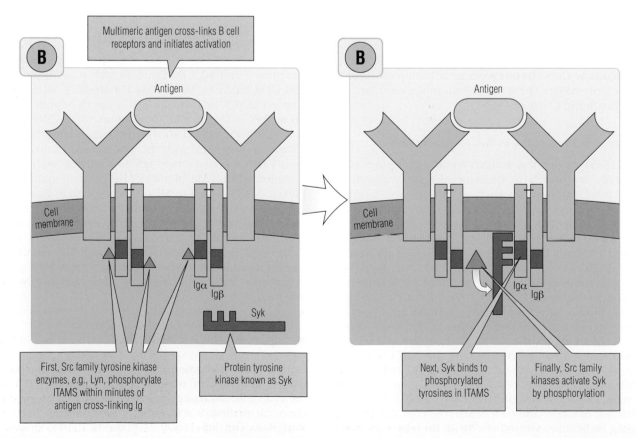

Figure 11.5 Earliest events in activation of B cells.

 T cell receptor (TCR)   Immunoglobulin (Ig)   Antigen   MHC I

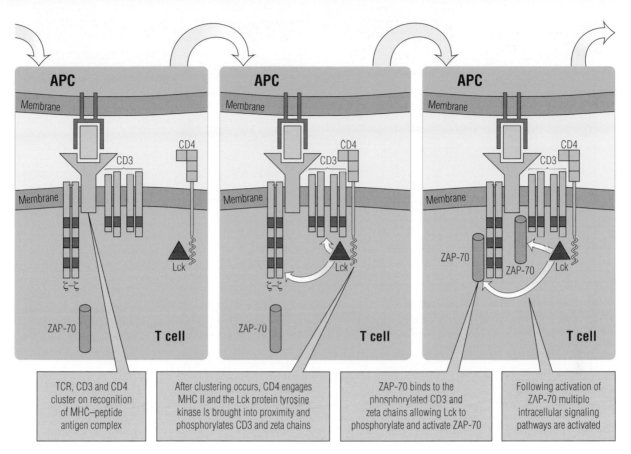

TCR, CD3 and CD4 cluster on recognition of MHC–peptide antigen complex	After clustering occurs, CD4 engages MHC II and the Lck protein tyrosine kinase is brought into proximity and phosphorylates CD3 and zeta chains	ZAP-70 binds to the phosphorylated CD3 and zeta chains allowing Lck to phosphorylate and activate ZAP-70	Following activation of ZAP-70 multiple intracellular signaling pathways are activated

Figure 11.6 Earliest events in activation of T cells.

ceptor protein cytoplasmic tails (Fig. 11.5). Phosphorylation of the receptor tails attracts other signaling molecules to the cytoplasmic side of the receptor. In B cells, the critical molecule is another PTK known as Syk. Syk is found at high levels in B cells but is also found in other cells, including some T cells. Syk binds to the phosphorylated ITAM sequences in Igα and Igβ and is then itself activated by phosphorylation. Syk may be phosphorylated by the Src family kinases associated with the BCR, as shown in Figure 11.5, or it may be phosphorylated by another Syk molecule bound to an adjacent BCR chain.

A related series of steps occurs in T cells. Clustering of the TCR, CD3, and CD4/CD8 proteins on recognition of peptides displayed by MHC molecules on APCs brings the PTK known as Lck into the receptor complex (Fig. 11.6). Lck phosphorylates the ITAMs in the cytoplasmic sequences of CD3 and ζ-chain. This attracts the PTK ZAP-70, which is unique to T cells and natural-killer cells. ZAP-70 is part of the same PTK family as Syk. ZAP-70 binds to the ITAMs of the ζ chains. More than one ZAP-70 molecule may bind to a ζ chain because of the multiple ITAMs per ζ chain (Fig. 11.6). ZAP-70 is then phosphorylated by Lck. Phosphorylation activates the PTK activity of ZAP-70.

Once a critical number of Syk or ZAP-70 kinases are activated in B or T cells, respectively, the signal is transmitted onward from the membrane, and amplified by activation of several pathways. The important role of PTKs in lymphocyte function is indicated by the occurrence of immunodeficiency in the presence of mutations affecting PTK function (Box 11.4).

■ AMPLIFICATION THROUGH SIGNALING PATHWAYS

For the signal to be propagated from the membrane to the nucleus, where it can have a major impact on a cellular response, several biochemical pathways are used that are similar in B and T cells and which amplify the signal while propagating it.

In both B and T cells, three main signaling pathways are used. The first involves phosphorylation and activation of the enzyme phospholipase Cγ (PLC-γ). This is triggered by Syk or ZAP-70 (Figs 11.7 and 11.8). Activated PLC-γ then stimulates two pathways involving (1) diacylglycerol and protein kinase C and (2) inositol 1,4,5-trisphosphate (IP_3) and the serine/threonine–specific protein phosphatase calcineurin. The third main pathway involves activation by Syk or ZAP-70 of adapter proteins that then activate single-chain guanosine trisphosphate (GTP)-binding proteins (e.g., Ras). The Ras family of proteins then activates signaling pathways leading through the mitogen-activated

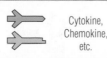 MHC II

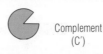 Cytokine, Chemokine, etc.

Complement (C')

 Signaling molecule

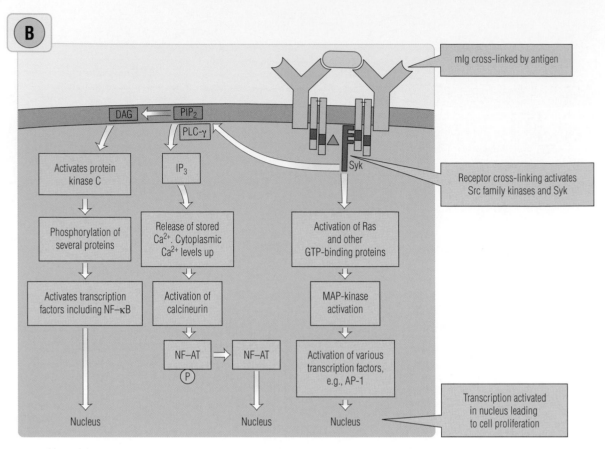

Figure 11.7   Major signaling pathways in B cells. AP-1, activation protein 1; DAG, diacylglycerol; IP$_3$, inositol 1,4,5-trisphosphate; MAP kinase, mitogen-activated protein kinase; NF-AT, nuclear factor of activated T cells; NF-κB, nuclear factor-κB; PIP2, phosphatidylinositol 4,5-bisphosphate; PLC-γ, phospholipase Cγ; .

protein kinases (MAP kinases) directly to activation of transcription factors (see Figs 11.7 and 11.8).

Phosphorylation of PLC-γ by Syk in B cells (see Fig. 11.7) and phosphorylation of PLC-γ by ZAP-70 in T cells (see Fig. 11.8) leads to migration of PLC-γ to the cell membrane where it catalyses the cleavage of phosphatidylinositol 4,5-bisphosphate to produce diacylglycerol and inositol 1,4,5-trisphosphate. The latter causes cytoplasmic calcium ion levels to increase, which, among other events, activates several calcium-dependent enzymes including a serine/threonine–specific protein phosphatase called **calcineurin**. Calcineurin is responsible for dephosphorylating the nuclear factor of activated T cells (NF-AT) family of transcription factors. NF-AT is required for expression of genes for cytokines in T cells (e.g., interleukin-2) but is also found in other cell types and is activated by BCR stimulation in B cells.

The serine/threonine kinase protein kinase C is activated by interaction with diacylglycerol and phosphorylates several cellular proteins, leading eventually to the activation of transcription factors, including nuclear factor-κB (NF-κB). The third signaling pathway involves activation of the small GTP-binding proteins of the Ras family. These

signaling molecules operate through activation of the MAP kinase family of enzymes. The MAP kinases activate several transcription factors, including one called activation protein 1 (AP-1).

■ **RESPONSE**

The various transcription factors including NF-AT, NF-κB, and AP-1 act on several lymphocyte genes to enhance their transcription. This prepares B cells for proliferation and differentiation, and in T cells leads to enhanced expression of cytokines, such as interleukin 2, which is an essential component of an effective T-cell response, being responsible for clonal expansion, among other things. Immunosuppressive drugs can modulate this response (Box 11.3).

To preserve homeostasis, a T-cell response must be regulated and eventually terminated. How this is accomplished is not fully understood. Certainly, as antigen (pathogen) is successfully eliminated, the source of the stimulus is removed, and the T-cell response will diminish. Apoptosis (programmed cell death—see also Chapter 17) is a

T cell receptor (TCR)

Immunoglobulin (Ig)

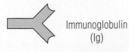
Antigen

MHC I

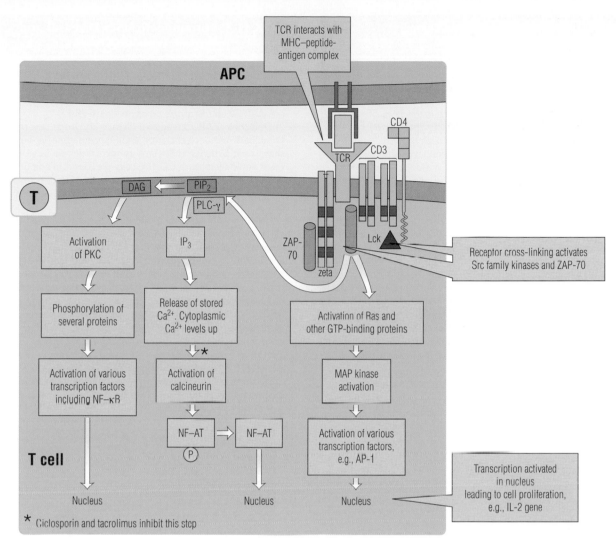

Figure 11.8 Major signaling pathways in T cells. AP-1, activation protein 1; DAG, diacylglycerol; IP$_3$, inositol 1,4,5-trisphosphate; MAP kinase, mitogen-activated protein kinase; NF-AT, nuclear factor of activated T cells; NF-kB, nuclear factor kappa B; PIP$_2$, phosphatidylinositol 4,5-bisphosphate; PLC-γ, phospholipase Cγ.

mechanism that may also contribute to termination of a T-cell response in certain circumstances. Also, if T cells fail to receive a costimulatory signal, (e.g., CD28 with CD80(B7); see Chapter 16), they enter a state of functional unresponsiveness known as anergy. How similar signals lead to different responses (i.e., activation, anergy, or apoptosis) is a topic of investigation. Presumably, different biochemical messages and pathways are induced because of the different combinations or amounts of "signal," and these generate different responses.

 MHC II

 Cytokine, Chemokine, etc.

 Complement (C')

 Signaling molecule

BOX 11.3 Immunosuppressive Drugs: Mechanism of Action

There are several immunosuppressive drugs in use to prevent allograft rejection (see Chapter 33). Two of the most useful are ciclosporin and tacrolimus. These are remarkable drugs that have revolutionized the field of transplantation surgery. Their availability has saved thousands of lives and made organ transplantation "do-able," even when there is no perfect human leukocyte antigen match available. Studies of the mechanism of action of these drugs have also helped to elucidate some of the signaling pathways in T cells.

Both ciclosporin and tacrolimus function by preventing T-cell cytokine gene transcription mediated by nuclear factor of activated T cells (NF-AT). They accomplish this by forming a complex with cytoplasmic proteins called immunophilins. The drug–immunophilin complex inhibits the action of calcineurin (Fig. 11.8). Without the dephosphorylation reaction mediated by calcineurin, NF-AT is unable to enter the nucleus and promote gene transcription—e.g., of the gene for interleukin-2 (IL-2). In the absence of this cytokine, lymphocyte proliferation is inhibited, and the immune response is suppressed. This prevents graft rejection but has the disadvantage of leaving the patient open to infectious disease because the immune response is inhibited.

BOX 11.4 Immunodeficiency Diseases and Protein Tyrosine Kinases

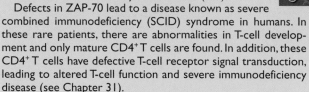

The important role of protein tyrosine kinases (PTKs) in lymphocyte function is underlined by the effects of mutations in the genes encoding two of these enzymes—i.e., ZAP-70 and Bruton's tyrosine kinase (Btk).

Defects in ZAP-70 lead to a disease known as severe combined immunodeficiency (SCID) syndrome in humans. In these rare patients, there are abnormalities in T-cell development and only mature CD4$^+$ T cells are found. In addition, these CD4$^+$ T cells have defective T-cell receptor signal transduction, leading to altered T-cell function and severe immunodeficiency disease (see Chapter 31).

Defective Btk leads to a disease known as X-linked agammaglobulinemia, in which all the classes of immunoglobulin are severely depleted, and there are no circulating B cells. Btk is involved in phosphoinositide hydrolysis during BCR signaling in pre-B cells, and defects in Btk result in impaired B-cell development and thereby prevent normal antibody production. The complications these patients experience in resisting bacterial infection are reduced by regular injections of pooled gamma-globulin preparations containing antibodies against commonly encountered pathogens (passive immunotherapy, see Chapters 2 and 31 and Box 4.2). Figure 11.9 shows a patient with Btk deficiency. He is receiving immunoglobulin replacement. This is required every 3 weeks when given i.v. The Ig replacement helps ensure a healthy life. He is attending college and has an excellent prognosis.

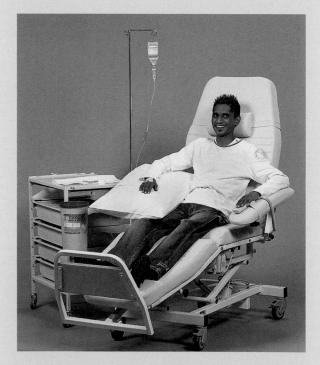

Figure 11.9 Patient with defective Btk leading to X-linked agammaglobulinemia. (From Helbert M: The Flesh and Bones of Immunology. London, Mosby, 2006.)

 T cell receptor (TCR)

 Immunoglobulin (Ig)

 Antigen

MHC I

LEARNING POINTS   Can You Now ...

1. Draw the B- and T-cell receptor complexes, and list the molecules involved?

2. Recall that B- and T-cell activation is more optimal with the aid of co-receptor complexes?

3. Describe with a diagram the earliest biochemical events in B- and T-cell activation?

4. List the major signaling pathways triggered in B and T cells by antigen recognition?

5. Recall the mechanism of inhibition of T-cell activation by immunosuppressive drugs such as ciclosporin and tacrolimus?

 MHC II

 Cytokine, Chemokine, etc.

 Complement (C')

 Signaling molecule

12 Hematopoiesis

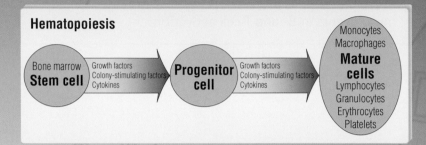

Hematopoiesis

Bone marrow **Stem cell** → Growth factors / Colony-stimulating factors / Cytokines → **Progenitor cell** → Growth factors / Colony-stimulating factors / Cytokines → Monocytes / Macrophages / **Mature cells** / Lymphocytes / Granulocytes / Erythrocytes / Platelets

Hematopoiesis is the process whereby all blood cells are formed; in adult humans, the bone marrow is the major site for hematopoiesis, and all of the differentiated blood cell types from lymphocytes to granulocytes to red blood cells are continuously generated in the adult human bone marrow. Several hundred million white blood cells (mostly neutrophils) are generated every hour in the human adult bone marrow, along with approximately 10 billion red blood cells.

The leukocytes, both lymphoid and myeloid cells, have been briefly described already in Chapter 2, and in this chapter, as illustrated in the overview figure above, their development from stem cells to progenitor cells to mature cells is explained, and some additional characterization is provided. In addition, in Chapter 13, the structure and function of the lymphoid organs where lymphocytes are generated and/or mature are described. The process by which lymphocytes move from the organs of lymphoid generation (chiefly the bone marrow and thymus in humans) to the spleen, lymph nodes, skin, mucosa, and so on, where they encounter antigen, is known as lymphocyte recirculation (or trafficking) and homing. In Chapter 13, the way that lymphocytes recirculate and home to different tissues is discussed, and the important role of cell adhesion molecules in these processes is explained.

■ THE THREE MAJOR STAGES OF HEMATOPOIESIS

Hematopoiesis can be divided into three major parts. Each part involves very different types of cells: stem cell, progenitor cell, mature cell (Fig. 12.1). **Hematopoietic stem cells** (HSCs) are pluripotential, and self-renewing. They give rise to all the blood cell types (lineages). HSCs do not express cell lineage specific marker proteins (such as CD3

on T cells or CD19 on B cells), but they do express a protein designated as CD34, which has allowed them to be enriched, by fluorescence-activated cell sorting (FACS) techniques (see Chapter 5), for further study and for use in autologous stem cell transplantation (Box 12.1).

HSCs migrate during embryonic development to the fetal liver and bone marrow. There they are induced to differentiate further by the large number of growth factors found in these tissues. Included among these growth factors are the **colony-stimulating-factors** (CSFs). Specific CSFs induce differentiation of particular cell lineages as discussed later.

In the presence of these various growth factors, including the CSFs, the HSCs become **progenitor cells** (see Fig. 12.1). Progenitor cells are less primitive than HSCs, and they have some commitment to develop along a particular cell lineage. Two separate immune system progenitor cells develop—the common lymphoid and common myeloid progenitor cells—under the influence of growth factors. These cells give rise to **mature cells**, which have fully differentiated, such as T cells (see Fig. 12.1).

■ LYMPHOID CELLS

Development

Figure 12.2 illustrates the major overall stages in the development of B and T cells from the common lymphoid progenitor (CLP). The initial stages of T-lymphocyte precursor (thymocyte) development, but not human pre–B cell development, are under the influence of the cytokine interleukin-7 (IL-7). IL-7 is produced and released from nonlymphoid stromal cells in the bone marrow. The bone marrow stromal cells include macrophages and adipocytes, and these are discussed further in Chapter 13. IL-7 is one

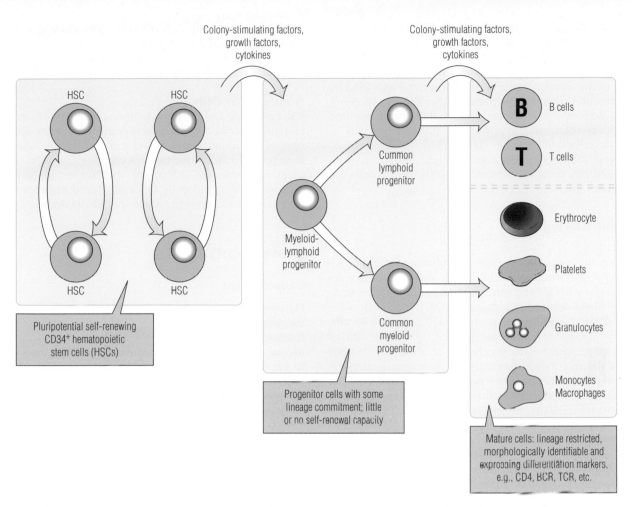

Figure 12.1 The three major stages of hematopoiesis. BCR, B-cell receptor; HSC, hematopoietic stem cell; TCR, T-cell receptor.

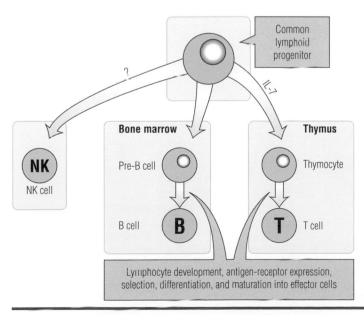

Figure 12.2 Overview of the development of the lymphoid cell lineage.

 MHC II

 Cytokine, Chemokine, etc.

 Complement (C')

Signaling molecule

of several cytokines affected by X-linked SCID (Box 12.2). Much of B-lymphocyte development takes place in the bone marrow (see Chapters 13 and 14). Most T lymphocytes develop in the thymus from thymocyte precursors derived in the bone marrow (see Chapters 13 and 15). The developmental pathway for natural-killer (NK) cells is not yet well defined. NK cells are part of the innate immune system, and their role in viral and tumor immunity is further described in Chapters 21 and 34.

X-linked SCID is discussed in Box 12.2. In this disease, T cells and NK cells are absent, and although B cells are present they are nonfunctional.

Lymphoid Cell Types

B Cells.

These are the cells that produce antibody (see Fig. 2.5). They express immunoglobulin as an antigen-specific receptor along with several other important molecules, such as major histocompatibility complex (MHC) class II molecules and the co-receptor molecule CD19. Morphologically, they have a large nucleus surrounded by a small rim of cytoplasm. In addition to producing antibody to combat extracellular infections, they can also function as antigen-presenting cells (APCs). They may be stimulated by antigen to form a larger blast cell (plasma cell; see Fig. 2.5B) with more cytoplasm, extensive endoplasmic reticulum, and secretory capacity for antibody.

T Cells.

Morphologically, T cells resemble unstimulated B cells (see Fig. 2.5)—that is, small lymphocytes with a large nucleus and small cytoplasm. They can be stimulated by antigen to become lymphoblasts with more cytoplasm and organelles. T cells consist of two major subsets: CD4+ helper cells and CD8+ cytotoxic cells (see Chapter 15). They also express an antigen-specific T-cell receptor, and they are the major source of antigen-specific protection against viral infection and other intracellular infections.

Natural Killer Cells.

NK cells (see Fig. 2.5) are lymphocytes that do not have clonally distributed antigen-specific receptors. They are part of the innate immune system and lyse certain virally infected cells and some tumor cells (see Chapter 21). They carry receptors (KIR) that are specific for molecules expressed on infected cells, or cells altered in other ways—for example, expressing tumor-specific antigens.

■ MYELOID CELLS

Development

Figure 12.3 depicts the main stages in the development of the other major white blood cells—the granulocyte and monocyte/macrophage lineages. These cells derive from the same common myeloid progenitor (CMP) that gives rise to erythrocytes and platelets. The various differentiation pathways are stimulated by the actions of different growth factor combinations—erythropoietin stimulates development of erythrocytes, and the CSFs (granulocyte-macrophage CSF [GM-CSF], granulocyte-CSF [G-CSF] and monocyte/macrophage-CSF [M-CSF]) stimulate development of the myelomonocytic progenitor cell and, ultimately, neutrophils, monocytes, macrophages, and dendritic cells (DCs) (Fig. 12.4).

Various specific CSF/cytokine combinations are necessary for the differentiation of each myeloid cell type (Figs 12.3, 12.4, and 12.5).

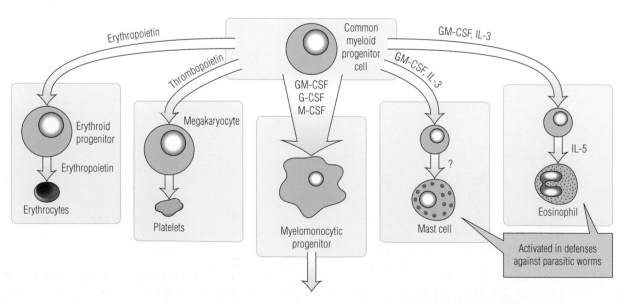

Figure 12.3 Overview of the development of the myeloid cell lineage. CSF, colony-stimulating factors; G, granulocyte; GM, granulocyte-macrophage; IL, interleukin; M, macrophage.

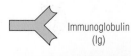 T cell receptor (TCR)

 Immunoglobulin (Ig)

 Antigen

MHC I

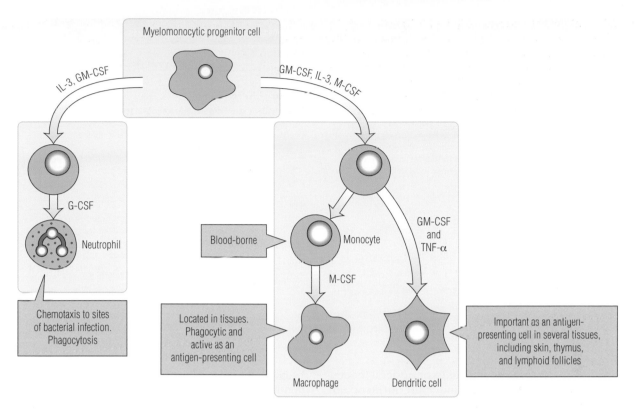

Figure 12.4 Overview of the development of the monocyte/macrophage lineage. CSF, colony-stimulating factors; G, granulocyte; GM, granulocyte-macrophage; IL, interleukin; M, macrophage; TNF, tumor necrosis factor.

Myeloid Cell Types

Neutrophils

Neutrophils (see Fig. 2.5) exhibit phagocytic and cytotoxic activities, and they migrate to sites of inflammation and infection in response to chemotactic factors. They are short-lived with a half-life of about 6 hours. Approximately 10^{11} neutrophils are estimated to be generated every day in the adult human. They contain both primary granules, loaded with lysosomal enzymes including myeloperoxidase and elastase, and secondary granules containing lysozyme, collagenase, and so on. These cells are often referred to as polymorphonuclear neutrophils (PMNs) because they have nuclei with two to five lobes. Their role as a first line of defense in the innate response to bacterial infections is discussed further in Chapter 20. Their development under the influence of G-CSF is discussed in Box 12.3.

Mast Cells

Mature mast cells (see Fig. 2.5) have large granules that can be stained purple with dyes. These granules contain heparin and histamine but do not contain hydrolytic enzymes. Mast cells express specific receptors on their surface for the Fc region of certain immunoglobulins, i.e., FcR_γ and FcR_ε. These cells have important roles in allergic responses (see Chapter 26). They are activated through their receptors for immunoglobulin E (IgE) to release the above substances.

Eosinophils

Eosinophils (see Fig. 2.5) are characterized by a nucleus with two or three lobes. They have large, specific granules, which contain heparin, as well as peroxidase and other hydrolytic enzymes. These cells have phagocytic and cytotoxic activity and express Fc receptors, specifically FcR_γ and FcR_ε. These cells also function to combat certain parasitic infections—particularly worms (see Chapter 21).

Monocytes/Macrophages

Monocytes (see Fig 2.5) are the largest blood cells. They contain many granules and have a lobular-shaped nucleus. Monocytes phagocytose, have bacteriocidal activity, and can carry out antibody-dependent cell-mediated cytotoxicity (ADCC; see Chapter 21). Monocytes migrate out of the blood into the tissues and become tissue macrophages, e.g., the Kupffer cells of the liver. They express the monocyte/macrophage marker protein designated CD14. Macrophages have a central role at the dividing line between the innate and specific immune response because of their role in antigen processing and presentation.

Dendritic Cells

Dendritic cells (DC) (see Fig. 2.6) are irregularly shaped cells with many branchlike processes. They are motile and found in the blood and lymph and in most organs. There are a variety of types of DC (see Box 10.1), and they are

 MHC II   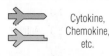 Cytokine, Chemokine, etc.   Complement (C')   Signaling molecule

FIG. 12.5 Colony-Stimulating Factors and Cytokines Important for Hematopoiesis

Molecule	Major Cellular Sources	Major Biological Activity
Colony-stimulating factors		
Granulocyte	Monocytes, macrophages, fibroblasts, endothelial cells	Stimulates neutrophil formation
Granulocyte-macrophage	T cells, monocytes, macrophages, fibroblasts, endothelial cells	Stimulates proliferation and differentiation of myeloid progenitors
Monocyte/macrophage	Monocytes, macrophages, fibroblasts, endothelial cells	Stimulates proliferation and differentiation of monocytes and macrophages
Interleukins		
3	T cells	Stimulates multiple hematopoietic cells
4	T cells, activated mast cells	Stimulates B cells (to produce IgE), T_H2 cell differentiation and mast cells
5	T cells	Stimulates differentiation and activation of eosinophils, activates B cells for immunoglobulin production
7	Stromal cells in the bone marrow	Stimulates T-cell progenitor proliferation and differentiation, and is an essential growth factor for mature T cells

critical in antigen-capture and uptake in peripheral tissues. In the presence of infection, and under the influence of cytokines, they mature and migrate to lymphoid organs where they present antigen, activate T cells, and help develop a protective adaptive immune response.

The myelomonocytic progenitor cell gives rise to various types of DC, including the interstitial DCs and Langerhans cells. The origin of the plasmacytoid-derived dendritic cells is less clear. Although these cells have certain myeloid lineage characteristics, they also have some lymphoid lineage characteristics. Their lineage is currently under active investigation. They may have a separate, unique lineage that is closer to lymphocytes than other myeloid cell types.

BOX 12.1 Autologous Hematopoietic Stem Cell Transplantation

For several weeks following chemotherapy/radiotherapy treatments for cancer, patients have severely depressed blood and immune systems. They are substantially at risk from infections. In certain circumstances, the patient's own bone marrow, which contains stem cells, is obtained prior to cancer therapy for use in treatment. This bone marrow is stored at very low temperatures in a medium that preserves the cells from destruction. It is returned to the patient (autologous bone marrow transplant) after chemotherapy/radiotherapy to help to quickly reconstitute the immune and blood cells. Because this is the patient's own marrow, there are no complications with regard to transplant rejection. However, the process of obtaining the bone marrow usually involves a relatively painful surgical procedure to aspirate cells from the pelvic bones under general anesthetic.

Large numbers of hematopoietic stem cells (HSCs) can be mobilized into the blood by giving patients granulocyte colony-stimulating factor (G-CSF). The HSCs are then identified by their expression of the CD34 molecule and harvested from the blood. Peripheral blood harvesting has been found to generate more stem cells than does bone marrow aspiration. It is also less painful for the patient, and it is becoming the approach of choice in preference to autologous bone marrow transplants in the treatment of certain patients. The general topic of transplantation is discussed in greater detail in Chapter 33.

BOX 12.2 X-linked Severe Combined Immunodeficiency Disease (XSCID)

Boys affected by XSCID are born without T and NK cells, have nonfunctional B cells, and, if untreated, will rapidly die from infection. Although there are normal numbers of B cells in these patients, the B cells are nonfunctional. This is because of both a lack of T cells to provide help and an inherent B-cell defect. Bone marrow transplant is an effective treatment for these boys, but, tragically, in many cases a human leukocyte antigen–matched donor is unavailable.

The mutation on the X chromosome responsible for XSCID has been identified. The mutation is in the gene for a subunit of several cytokine receptors, including the receptors for IL-2, IL-4, IL-7, IL-10, IL-15, and IL-21. The cytokine receptor subunit is referred to as the common cytokine receptor γ chain or γ_c chain. The B-cell defect in these boys may be related to the lack of a functioning IL-4 receptor due to the mutation in γ_c.

 T cell receptor (TCR)

 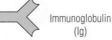 Immunoglobulin (Ig)

 Antigen

 MHC I

BOX 12.3 Administration of Granulocyte Colony-Stimulating Factor for Neutropenia

Granulocyte colony-stimulating factor (G-CSF), because of its important role in hematopoiesis, has become a well-characterized protein. The G-CSF gene has been cloned, and a recombinant form of G-CSF has been produced for use in treatment. G-CSF causes an increase in neutrophil production in the bone marrow. Apart from its role in autologous stem cell transplantation, in vivo administration of G-CSF has been approved for the treatment of neutropenias caused by several conditions, including cancer chemotherapy and acute leukemia. The enhanced neutrophil levels produced by G-CSF treatment have been shown to protect these otherwise neutropenic patients from life-threatening bacterial infections (see Box 20.1).

LEARNING POINTS Can You Now ...

1. Draw the developmental pathway from stem cell through progenitor cell to mature lymphoid and myeloid cells?

2. Describe the role of colony-stimulating factors and other growth factors in the developmental pathways to lymphoid and myeloid cells?

3. List several important morphologic features and functional activities of B and T lymphocytes, natural-killer cells, neutrophils, mast cells, eosinophils, monocytes, macrophages, and dendritic cells?

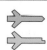 MHC II   Cytokine, Chemokine, etc.   Complement (C′)   Signaling molecule

13

The Organs and Tissues of the Immune System

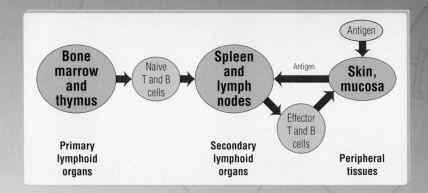

Up until this point in the book, we have primarily discussed the genes, molecules, and cells that function in the immune response. However, host defense responses take place in a whole organism, not in isolated cells or amongst subcellular components! It is now necessary to consider the immune response in the context of a physiologic system. The overview figure above depicts the main topics for this chapter, i.e., the structure and function of the primary and secondary lymphoid organs and how lymphocytes are produced, expanded, come into contact with antigen, and mature into effector cells capable of a protective immune response.

■ PRIMARY AND SECONDARY LYMPHOID ORGANS

The immune system is made up of distinct compartments, the organs and tissues, which are interconnected by the blood and lymphatic systems. In this chapter, several important features of the lymphoid organs and tissues are described, and a systems view of the immune response is introduced. In the past few years, it has become obvious that although we know much about the genes, molecules, and cells that are the basis of an immune response, there is still much more to learn about how the immune response is coordinated at a systems level, and how the complex series of physiologic events in vivo can influence the outcome of an immune response.

The immune system is comprised of those organs and tissues in which lymphocytes are produced—**the primary**

lymphoid organs—and those where they come into contact with foreign antigen, are clonally expanded, and mature into effector cells—**the secondary lymphoid organs**.

In the embryonic human (Fig. 13.1), the primary lymphoid organs (i.e., where lymphocytes are generated) are initially the yolk sac, then the fetal liver and spleen, and finally the bone marrow and thymus. In adult humans (Fig. 13.2), the primary lymphoid organs are the bone marrow and thymus. By puberty, most lymphopoiesis is B-lymphocyte production in the marrow of the flat bones, such as the sternum, vertebrae, and pelvis.

The human secondary lymphoid organs are generally considered to be the spleen, lymph nodes, and mucosa-associated lymphoid tissue (MALT) lining the respiratory, gastrointestinal, and reproductive tracts. Some consider the skin (cutaneous immune system) in this category also. These organs are distributed as shown in Figure 13.2. Lymphocytes lodge in the secondary lymphoid organs, and they expand clonally on contact with the antigen appropriate for their specific antigen receptors. They also recirculate between these organs via the blood and lymphatic systems. This lymphocyte recirculation or **trafficking** connects the various lymphoid compartments, creating one system (see later).

Lymphocytes are dispersed to almost all tissue sites, and, therefore, almost all the tissues in the human body could be thought of as "lymphoid tissues." However, some sites (e.g., eye, testis, and brain) do not have lymphoid cells, and these are said to be **immunologically privileged**. The most important sites of lymphocyte dispersal are the

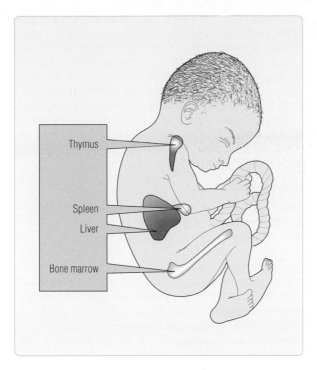

Figure 13.1 Organs of lymphocyte production in the developing human.

Figure 13.2 Major lymphoid organs in the adult human. (Adapted from Roitt I, Brostoff J, and Male D. Immunology, 6th ed. London: Mosby, 2001.)

spleen, lymph nodes, MALT, and skin. Each of these are described briefly in this chapter to create a context for understanding the physiology of the immune response.

Bone Marrow

As described in Chapter 12, the bone marrow is the major hematopoietic organ in humans. It is a richly cellular organ system. All of the blood cell types except mature T lymphocytes are generated in the extensive cavities in the bone marrow. The extensive internal cavity structures in this organ can be seen in sections (Fig. 13.3). B-cell generation takes place in these internal cavities; development

from B-cell progenitors to immature B cells occurs in a radial direction toward the center of the bone. This process will be described in more detail in Chapter 14.

Hematopoiesis is facilitated in the bone marrow by a mixture of cells and extracellular matrix components. This environment not only provides mechanical support but is also a source of the growth factors and cytokines essential for the development of the various blood cell types. The bone marrow reticular stroma, a mixture of extracellular matrix molecules, macrophages, and adipocytes, is particularly important in B-lymphocyte development, supplying cytokines and other molecules that are critical to the development of mature B cells.

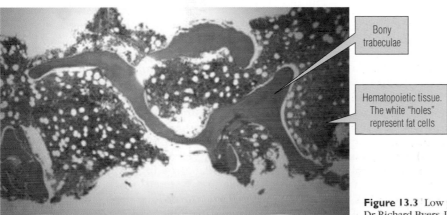

Figure 13.3 Low power view of bone marrow courtesy of Dr Richard Byers, University of Manchester, England.

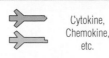 MHC II

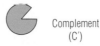 Cytokine, Chemokine, etc.

 Complement (C')

 Signaling molecule

Thymus

The thymus is a bilobed organ, found in the anterior mediastinum. The base of the thymus rests on the surface of the heart, and because of this location, the thymus is usually removed during some pediatric cardiothoracic surgical procedures, for example, surgery to repair a heart defect shortly after birth. It is notable that removing the thymus after birth seems to have little effect on the ability of these children to mount an effective T-cell–mediated immune response (see also description of DiGeorge syndrome in Box 15.1).

The thymus forms from two types of epithelial cell (endoderm and ectoderm) derived from the third pharyngeal pouch, the corresponding brachial clefts, and the pharyngeal arch. The thymus grows until puberty; it then undergoes progressive involution, and it is largely adipose tissue, with only a small amount of lymphoid tissue remaining, by late adulthood.

Each of the lobes of the thymus is divided further into lobules by connective tissue septae called trabeculae. Figure 13.4A shows a stained section, and Figure 13.4B shows a schematic drawing of the thymus. There are three main areas:

- The **subcapsular zone** containing the earliest progenitor cells
- The **cortex**, which is densely packed with developing T cells that are undergoing selection
- The **medulla** containing fewer, but more mature, T lymphocytes; these have survived the selection processes and are about to be released to the periphery (see Chapter 15).

The thymus is the primary site of T-cell development. Most T-cell progenitors (more than 95%) die in the thymus, through the process of apoptosis. There is an extensive network of epithelial cells and antigen-presenting cells that is involved in the selection process leading to the development of an appropriate T-cell receptor repertoire. An outline of some of the important cell-cell interactions in T-cell development is found in Figure 13.4B, and this topic is developed in more detail in Chapter 15.

Spleen

The spleen, a secondary lymphoid organ about the size of a clenched fist, is found in the left upper quadrant of the abdomen. It is a major "filter" for the blood, removing opsonized microbes and dead red blood cells. It is also the main site for responses to blood-borne antigens, and the source of B cells that respond in the absence of T-cell help to bacterial cell wall polysaccharide antigens (see Box 13.1). Figure 13.5A shows a stained section of a spleen. There are two main areas: the **red pulp**, containing chiefly macrophages and red blood cells in the process of disposal, and the **white pulp**, containing dense lymphoid tissue. The spleen has been estimated to lodge about 25% of the total lymphocytes in the body. The white pulp is segregated into B- and T-lymphocyte areas. The T cells are chiefly found in the **periarteriolar lymphoid sheaths** (PALS; see Fig. 13.5A and B). The PALS are concentric cuffs of lymphocytes associated with central arterioles. **Lymphoid follicles** (see Fig. 13.5A and Fig. 13.6 A and B), some with **germinal centers** (the germinal centers are lightly staining regions; see Fig. 13.5A), appear within the PALS in the spleen and in the cortex of lymph nodes. Most B cells are found in follicles. Follicles with germinal centers containing chiefly activated B cells are generally referred to as secondary follicles (see Fig. 13.6B) to distinguish them from primary follicles (no germinal center), which contain chiefly resting B cells.

Lymph Nodes

A lymph node is a bean-shaped structure (see Fig. 13.6B), usually found clustered in groups at sites where numerous blood and lymph vessels converge. For example, a large collection of nodes is found in the armpit (axillary nodes). Lymph nodes function to concentrate lymph-borne antigens for presentation to T cells. Lymph is absorbed extracellular fluid, and the lymph nodes filter (or survey) its contents for antigens before it drains into the bloodstream.

A lymph node is organized into several areas (Fig. 13.6). The cortex is predominantly the site of B cells. As for the spleen, B cells are generally found in primary or secondary follicles (Fig. 13.6A and B), depending on their state of activation. The lymph node paracortex is predominantly a CD4⁺ T-cell area. The medulla of the node contains a mixture of B cells, T cells, and macrophages.

Circulating lymphocytes enter the node via specialized high endothelial venules (HEVs) in the paracortex. The important role of HEVs in lymphocyte trafficking is discussed later.

During a response to an infection, B and T cells in the node are activated (see Box 13.2). Fluid and cells are accumulated in the node during lymphocyte activation, leading to lymph-node enlargement (the "swollen gland" typical of response to infection). After the immune system clears the infectious agent, the node returns to its normal size, and it can no longer be palpated. The location of the swollen lymph nodes reflects the site of infection. For example, an infected finger leads to swollen axillary nodes. More generalized swollen nodes (lymphadenopathy) reflect a generalized infection or tumor.

Mucosa-Associated Lymphoid Tissue

The mucosal immune system handles antigen at a contact point between the host and the environment, and it is an important first line of defense. The mucosal immune system is principally composed, in humans, of lymphoid tissue in the respiratory and gastrointestinal tracts, known as nasopharyngeal-associated lymphoid tissue (NALT; e.g., tonsils and adenoids) and gut-associated lymphoid tissue (GALT; e.g., Peyer's patches, see Fig. 13.7A), respectively. These tissues (e.g., Peyer's patch) (Fig. 13.7A) contain a specialized epithelial cell type (M cells) that takes up antigens that are inhaled or ingested (Fig. 13.7A, B, C). Antigens are taken up by M cells by the process of **pinocytosis**. Pinocytosis is the cellular intake of small vacuoles containing fluid and/or molecules. The M cells transport

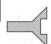

T cell receptor
(TCR)

Immunoglobulin
(Ig)

Antigen

MHC I

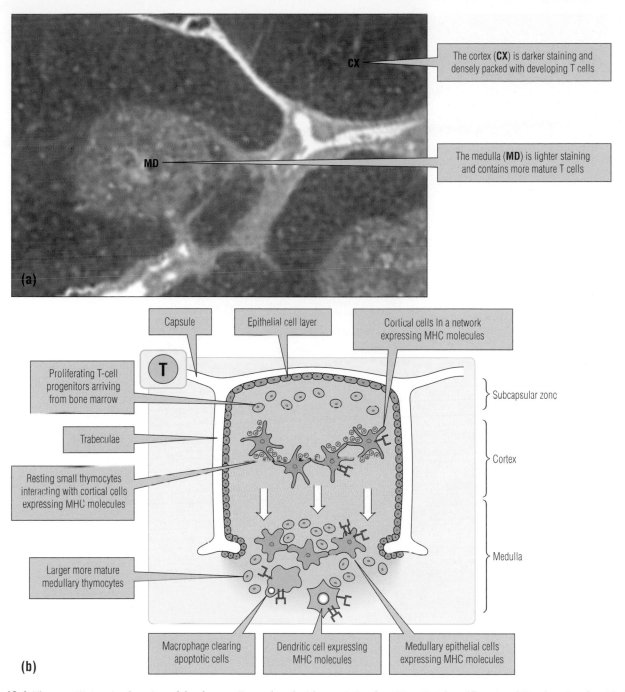

Figure 13.4 Thymus. (**A**) A stained section of the thymus. (Reproduced with permission from Kerr JB. Atlas of Functional Histology. London: Mosby, 2000.) (**B**) A simplified schematic showing the cellular organization of the thymus.

antigens by a transcellular transport process called transcytosis into the subepithelial tissues where they encounter lymphocytes. Figure 13.7D shows a section of mucosa in which the lamina propria contains T and B lymphocytes. Typically, the B cells are in follicles surrounded by a T-cell zone. The B cells secrete immunoglobulin A (IgA) across the epithelium (Fig. 13.7E). IgA is initially bound to the poly-Ig receptor (Fig. 13.7E) and, after transport across the epithelial cell membrane, it retains a piece of this

receptor (now known as secretory component), which may help protect it from degradation in the lumen.

Intraepithelial Lymphocytes
The mucosal epithelium of the gastrointestinal, respiratory, and reproductive tracts contains large numbers of lymphocytes. These lymphocytes are mostly T cells (~90%) and a greater than typical number (maybe as much as 10%–20%) are γδ T cells (Fig. 13.7D).

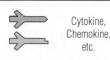 MHC II

 Cytokine, Chemokine, etc.

 Complement (C')

 Signaling molecule

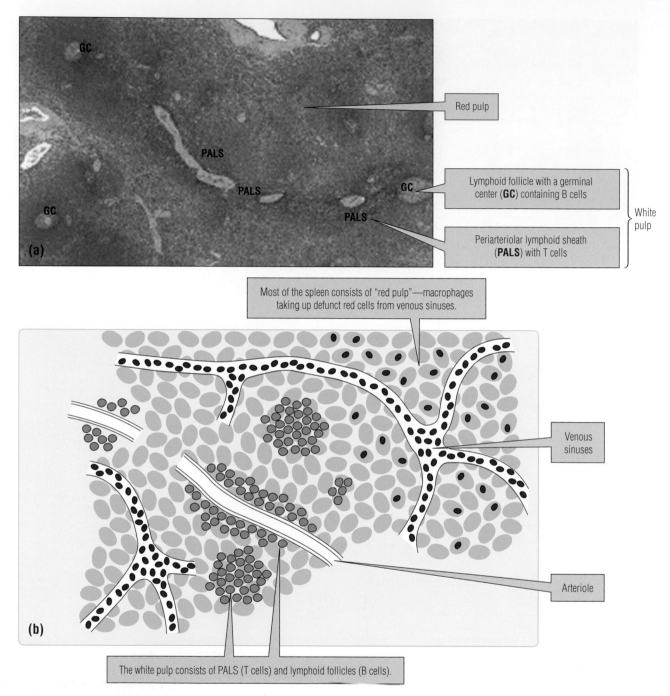

Red pulp

Lymphoid follicle with a germinal center (**GC**) containing B cells

Periarteriolar lymphoid sheath (**PALS**) with T cells

White pulp

Most of the spleen consists of "red pulp"—macrophages taking up defunct red cells from venous sinuses.

Venous sinuses

Arteriole

The white pulp consists of PALS (T cells) and lymphoid follicles (B cells).

Figure 13.5 Spleen. (**A**) Stained section of the spleen showing detail of PALS and GC (Reproduced with permission from Kerr JB. Atlas of Functional Histology. London: Mosby, 2000.) (**B**) A simplified schematic showing the organization of the spleen.

Intraepithelial T lymphocytes appear to have T-cell receptors of limited diversity. The antigens recognized by intraepithelial lymphocytes tend to be expressed as a consequence of infection. In general, intraepithelial lymphocytes act to protect the host against viral and bacterial pathogens encountered in the gut. In addition to their role as effector T cells, the intraepithelial T cells secrete cytokines that have a role in regulating immune responses in the mucosa. This regulatory role may, for example, prevent excessive responses to food antigens.

Recirculation

After exposure to antigen in the MALT, lymphocytes may leave and home to other mucosal tissues. Figure 13.7F shows this migration (recirculation or trafficking) from Peyer's patches in the gut to other mucosal surfaces—for example, the reproductive tract. This trafficking provides a potential target for vaccination, using mucosal vaccines for the initial stimulation (Box 13.3). Mucosal immune responses also occur in the lamina propria of secretory glands, such as mammary and salivary glands.

 T cell receptor (TCR)

 Immunoglobulin (Ig)

Antigen

MHC I

(a)

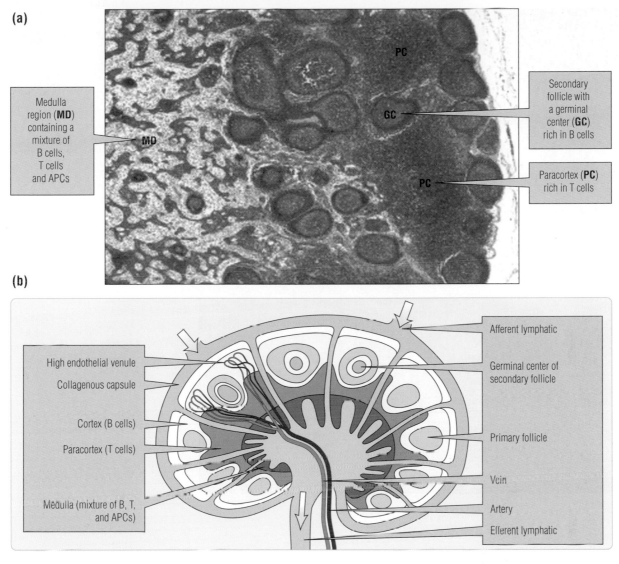

(b)

Figure 13.6 Lymph nodes. (**A**) Stained section of a node. (Reproduced with permission from Kerr JB. Atlas of Functional Histology. London: Mosby, 2000.) (**B**) A simplified schematic showing the organization of a node. APC, antigen-presenting cell.

Skin (Cutaneous Immune System)

The skin is the major physical barrier to pathogen entry, and it is a very important interface between the immune cells and the external environment. The skin has many lymphoid accessory cells (e.g., dendritic cells) that have critically important roles in handling environmental antigens that penetrate the skin. Many immune responses are initiated in the skin and, consequently, some view the skin as another peripheral organ of the immune system—the cutaneous immune tissue.

Figure 13.8A shows a photograph of inflamed skin during a delayed-type hypersensitivity (DTH) response. This type of response is described in more detail in Chapter 22. The lymphoid cells involved in immune reactions in the skin are shown in Figure 13.8B. The epidermal layer of the skin has numerous dendritic cells called Langerhans cells, which are very important in antigen processing and presentation (see also Chapter 10) in the

skin. The T cells found in the epidermal layer (intraepidermal T cells) in association with the Langerhans cells are chiefly CD8$^+$ cells. At a higher frequency than is typical, these CD8$^+$ T cells carry $\gamma\delta$T-cell receptors (Chapter 7), similar to the situation described earlier for the intraepithelial T cells of the MALT. The T-cell receptors on these intraepidermal T cells also represent a restricted set of specificities, suggesting a focus on frequently occurring pathogens that infect through the skin. The underlying dermis is rich in macrophages and T cells (Fig. 13.8B; see also Fig. 22.8).

◼ LYMPHOCYTE RECIRCULATION TRAFFICKING AND HOMING

At this point, we confine our discussion of trafficking to lymphocytes. Trafficking of other white blood cells is

 MHC II   Cytokine, Chemokine, etc.   Complement (C')   Signaling molecule

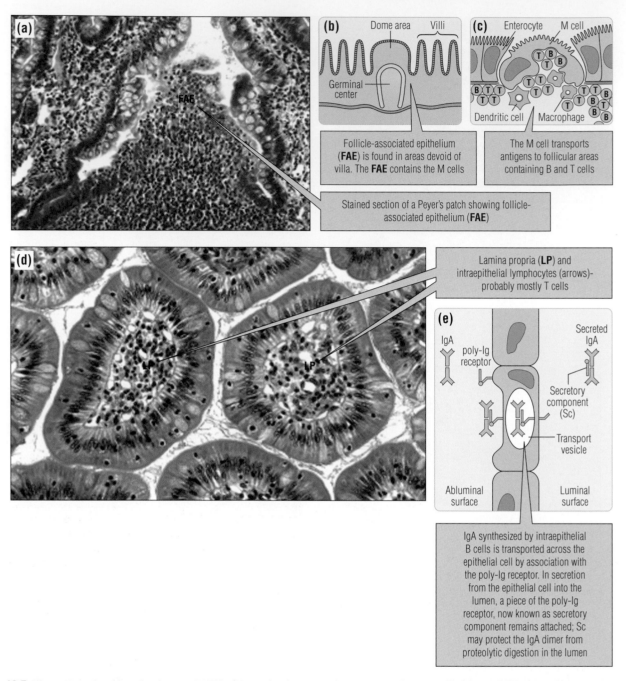

Figure 13.7 Mucosa-associated lymphoid tissue (MALT). (**A**) A stained section of a Peyer's patch (gut MALT: GALT). (**B**) The organization of GALT in Peyer's patches. (**C**) An M cell in the intestinal follicle-associated epithelium (FAE). (**D**) A section of mucosa showing T and B cells in the lamina propria (LP). (**E**) Transport of immunoglobulin A across epithelium. (**F**) Trafficking of lymphocytes from MALT. (**A** and **D**, Reproduced with permission from Kerr JB. Atlas of Functional Histology. London: Mosby, 2000; **B**, **C**, **E**, and **F**, Adapted from Roitt I, Brostoff J, Male D. Immunology, 6th ed. London: Mosby, 2001.)

discussed in Chapter 20. Most mature T lymphocytes are in constant circulation via the bloodstream and lymphatics (Fig. 13.9). They move constantly from one lymphoid tissue to another, and from lymphoid tissue to peripheral tissue. It has been estimated that a lymphocyte makes a circuit of the human body, from the blood, to the tissues, to the lymphatic system, and returns to the blood, once or twice a day. This circulation is important to ensure that the small number of lymphocytes specific for any given anti-gen has the best chance to find that antigen in any possible body site. Most of the circulating lymphocytes are T lymphocytes. B lymphocytes, because they secrete a soluble effector molecule (antibody) that interacts directly with antigen, have less requirement to recirculate, and, therefore, they spend longer time periods than T cells in the lymphoid organs.

Naive T lymphocytes—that is, T lymphocytes that have not yet encountered the antigen they have specificity for

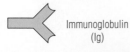 T cell receptor (TCR)

Immunoglobulin (Ig)

 Antigen

MHC I

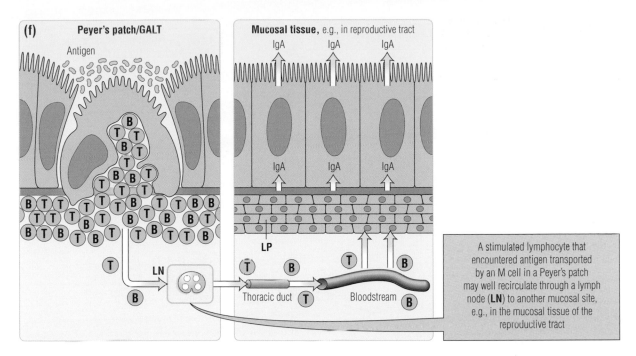

Figure 13.7, *cont'd*

(their cognate antigen; see Chapter 15), constantly circulate among the secondary lymphoid organs until they encounter antigen or die. This circulation through the lymphoid organs maximizes the chance to encounter antigen displayed on a professional antigen-presenting cell: a requirement to activate a naive T cell (see Chapter 15). Effector (or memory, i.e., long-lived cells that retain "memory" of contact with antigen and respond faster; see Chapter 17) T lymphocytes, by comparison, migrate to and lodge in selected tissue sites, where they may remain for some time. This process is referred to as **lymphocyte homing**. Positioning T cells that have already been primed by contact with antigen in peripheral sites where

they can screen for antigen enhances the likelihood of effective protection via a secondary immune response (see Chapter 17).

Lymphocyte recirculation and homing is regulated by receptor-ligand interactions between members of the different families of cell adhesion molecules (CAMs; Fig. 13.10). There are several extensive families of CAMs. The major ones are the selectins, addressins, integrins, and the CAMs that are a part of the immunoglobulin superfamily. These molecules have a variety of important roles in the immune response. Figure 13.10 illustrates some of the molecules that are most important in leukocyte recirculation and homing. The same molecules, and others in

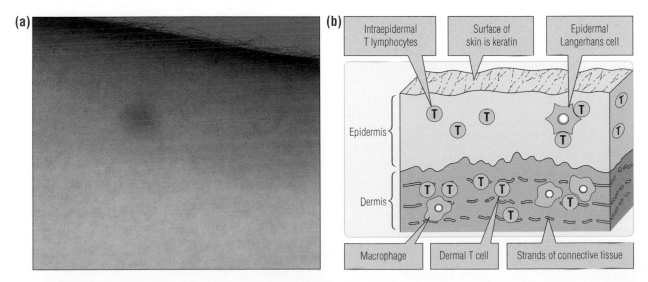

Figure 13.8 Skin: the cutaneous immune system. (**A**) A photograph of inflamed skin during a delayed type hypersensitivity test. (**B**) A simplified schematic of skin showing antigen-presenting cells (APCs) and Langerhans cells.

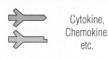 MHC II

 Cytokine, Chemokine, etc.

Complement (C')

 Signaling molecule

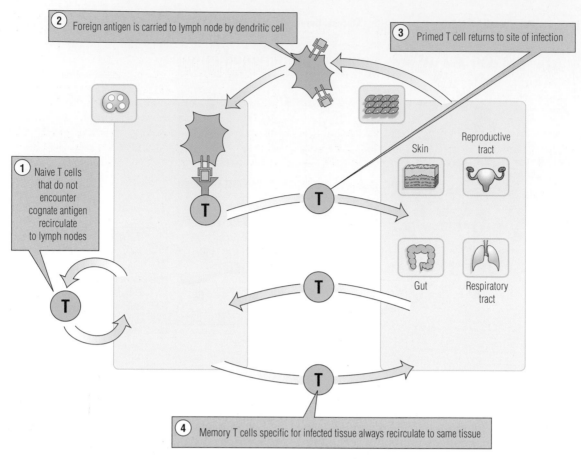

Figure 13.9 Recirculation of lymphocytes.

these families, have roles in several physiologic processes that involve cell migration, including development, tissue repair, and the adaptive and innate immune responses.

The most important of these adhesion protein interactions is between proteins on the lymphocyte surface (mostly the naive T-lymphocyte surface) and proteins on

the surface of the endothelial cells lining postcapillary venules, particularly HEVs. The HEVs have thicker than usual endothelial cell linings and are found in lymph nodes and MALT (e.g., Peyer's patches). They facilitate lymphocyte transport out of the bloodstream into the tissues, a process known as lymphocyte extravasation.

FIG. 13.10 Cell Adhesion Molecules that are Important in Lymphocyte Recirculation

Receptor	Function and Tissue Distribution	Ligand	Function and Tissue Distribution
L-selectin (CD62L) (selectin family)	Leukocyte homing receptor, binds carbohydrates	GlyCAM-1 (addressin family)	Endothelial cell adhesion molecule found on the high endothelial venules of lymph node
		MAdCAM-1 (addressin family)	Endothelial cell adhesion molecule found on the high endothelial venules of mucosal lymphoid tissue
Leukocyte function associated antigen (LFA-1; CD11a/CD18) (integrin family)	Secondary adhesion molecule found on T cells, monocytes, polymorphonuclear cells, etc.	Intercellular adhesion molecules (immunoglobulin superfamily)	Found on endothelial cells; function in secondary adhesion and transmigration
Very late antigen 4 (VLA-4; CD49d/CD29) (integrin family)	Role in primary adhesion of effector lymphocytes that are homing to sites of infection	Vascular cell adhesion molecule (CD106) (immunoglobulin superfamily)	Found on endothelial cells that have been activated by an inflammatory response

 T cell receptor (TCR)   Immunoglobulin (Ig)   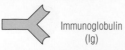 Antigen   MHC I

Lymphocyte Extravasation

Figure 13.11 is a simplified representation of the four steps in lymphocyte extravasation. The four steps are:

1. Primary adhesion to endothelium
2. Lymphocyte activation
3. Secondary adhesion (arrest)
4. Transmigration/chemotaxis.

Lymphocytes normally flow freely through the blood vessels. Analyses by videomicroscopy show that they can roll along endothelial cells, slowed down by low-affinity interactions between receptor molecules on the lymphocyte cell surface, known as homing receptors, and ligands known as addressins on the vascular endothelial cell surface (Fig. 13.10). If the lymphocyte detects signals that there is an infection in the tissue, for example, by detecting inflammatory mediators such as chemokines (see Chapter 20), the lymphocyte may be triggered, or activated, to express other adhesive molecules that can mediate strong, high-affinity, adhesive interactions. This primary adhesion, triggering, and expression of new adhesion molecules takes place in a few seconds, and lymphocyte movement is stopped even in the presence of considerable sheer forces from the ongoing blood flow.

The secondary adhesion phase is mediated by high-affinity interactions between different families of CAMs found both on the lymphocyte surface and on the endothelial cells in the tissues. Expression of different addressin molecules in different tissues allows lymphocytes to home to various tissue sites based on selective homing receptor-addressin expression and interaction (Fig. 13.10).

Lymphocyte arrest is followed by passage (**diapedesis** or transmigration) through the tight junction between adjacent endothelial cells into the tissues (Fig. 13.11). Once recruited into tissues, lymphocytes then disperse into specialized areas—for example, B lymphocytes to primary B cell follicles, T cells to PALS.

It is important to point out that the specificity of the recirculation/homing process is entirely a function of homing receptor-addressin interactions and is independent of antigen. In fact, most lymphocytes recruited to an infected tissue are not specific for the antigen causing the infection. However, an ongoing immune response influences the retention of lymphocytes at a tissue site, and it causes release of various factors that stimulate expression of adhesion proteins.

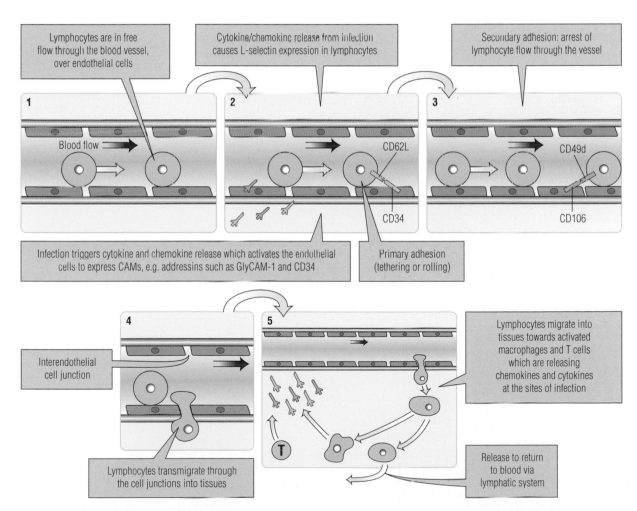

Figure 13.11 Four-step model of leukocyte extravasation. CAM, cell adhesion molecule; VCAM, vascular cell adhesion molecule; VLA, very late antigen.

 MHC II   Cytokine, Chemokine, etc.   Complement (C')   Signaling molecule

BOX 13.1 Risks of Splenectomy

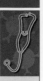

The spleen is a soft, "spongy" organ that bleeds easily following trauma. In certain situations, for example, seat-belt–mediated trauma sustained to the midsection in a car accident, the spleen can be ruptured, and it has to be surgically removed.

Splenectomized patients are more susceptible to infection by encapsulated bacteria, e.g., pneumococci, which are usually cleared by opsonization with antibody followed by phagocytosis by splenic macrophages. These patients are also less able to make antibody responses to polysaccharide antigens (T-independent (TI) responses; see Chapter 14). The marginal zone B cells in the spleen are particularly important in responses to the polysaccharide antigens found on bacterial cell walls, and splenectomy predisposes these patients to certain infections that require a TI-antibody response for protection.

Splenectomized patients are immunocompromised, and they are significantly at risk for infectious disease. They are usually maintained on life-long prophylactic antibiotics.

BOX 13.2 Lymphadenopathy

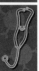

A 26-year-old man attends your clinic complaining of lumps in his throat. On further questioning, he has had a sore throat for about 4 days and is very anxious because his father was recently diagnosed with laryngeal cancer. On examination, your patient has some redness of the fauces and tonsils, which are slightly enlarged. There are also two small (approximately 1 cm diameter) lymph nodes in the right anterior triangle. You explain that the patient's symptoms are most consistent with an acute viral infection of the upper respiratory tract and that treatment is not necessary. To be safe, you take a throat swab to rule out bacterial pathogens.

Lymphadenopathy is usually the consequence of acute infection. Localized lymphadenopathy occurs as a consequence of localized infection, as is the case here, and is usually associated with a localizing sign (the inflamed throat in this case). Lymphadenopathy that persists for more than a few days or affects many different sites may indicate other disease processes, such as chronic infection (e.g., tuberculosis or HIV) or malignancy.

BOX 13.3 Mucosal Vaccines

Many pathogens, both bacterial and viral, invade the host via mucosal tissue. For example, HIV, which is primarily sexually transmitted; influenza, which invades through the respiratory mucosa; or *Shigella* and *Escherichia coli*, which cause enteric infections and diarrhea. For this reason, it would be very desirable to be able to vaccinate and induce a mucosal immune response that would prevent entry of such pathogens. Notably, vaccination at one mucosal site can confer immunity at other mucosal sites because of lymphocyte migration to other mucosal tissues (Fig. 13.7F).

Recent advances in mucosal vaccines have come from the use of mucosal adjuvants. Subunit proteins of certain bacterial enterotoxins, including the B subunit of the heat-labile toxin (LT-B) of *E. coli*, have been shown to be mucosal adjuvants when co-administered with other vaccine proteins.

One example of this is an intranasal influenza vaccine. This vaccine preparation includes the influenza virus proteins known as the neuraminidase and the hemagglutinin, which have been coupled chemically to the *E. coli* heat-labile toxin subunit as an adjuvant. When taken intranasally, this vaccine preparation produced protective levels of antibody to the influenza virus in a population studied in Switzerland.

Given that the mucosal tissues are major sites of interaction with pathogens, it is very important that we continue to learn more about mucosal immunology. It is likely that our rapidly developing understanding of the mucosal immune system will lead to effective mucosal vaccines that will confer long-term protection against pathogens such as HIV, influenza, rotaviruses, and the enteropathogenic bacteria. The impact worldwide of such mucosal vaccines would be enormous.

 T cell receptor (TCR)　　 Immunoglobulin (Ig)　　 Antigen　　 MHC I

LEARNING POINTS Can You Now ...

1. Describe the immune response in terms of a systemic physiologic response?

2. Describe the role of the bone marrow in lymphocyte generation and B-cell maturation?

3. Draw the cellular organization of the thymus, and describe the role of the thymus in T-lymphocyte generation and maturation?

4. Draw the structure of the spleen, and describe its role:
   — as a major site of responses to blood-borne antigens
   — as a "filter" for the blood
   — as a site of T-independent antibody synthesis?

5. Draw the structure of a lymph node, and describe its role as a "filter" for the lymph and as a major site for responses to lymph-borne antigens?

6. Describe the role of the various mucosa-associated lymphoid tissues (GALT, NALT, etc.) as a first line of defense, trapping environmental pathogens and presenting them to lymphocytes?

7. Describe the important role of the skin as a part of the immune system?

8. Draw the major recirculation pathways of lymphocytes around the organs and tissues of the immune system?

9. Draw the four-step model of lymphocyte extravasation?

 MHC II   Cytokine, Chemokine, etc.   Complement (C')    Signaling molecule

14

B-Cell Development

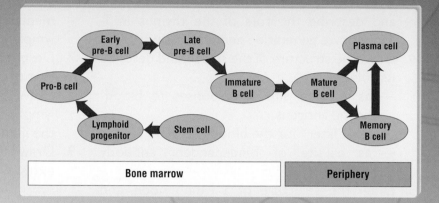

As discussed in Chapters 6 and 11, membrane-bound antibody molecules on the surface of B cells comprise a key part of the B-cell receptor (BCR) that is responsible for recognizing antigen. A series of developmental stages (defined largely by the receptor gene rearrangements that occur during these stages) results in expression of the antigen-specific BCR. B lymphocytes expressing a diverse repertoire of BCRs, as yet unselected, are generated continually in the bone marrow. Before reaching maturity, the developing B cells undergo a selection process (referred to as **negative selection**) in an attempt to ensure that their antigen receptor does not display self-reactivity. Anti-self reactivity may result in autoimmunity (Chapter 27). Those B cells surviving negative selection disperse to the peripheral lymphoid organs (Chapter 13) where they may encounter the foreign antigen they have specificity for, become activated, and, ultimately, terminally differentiate into antibody-producing cells. Those cells that do not encounter the appropriate antigen die in a matter of days or at most a few weeks. In this chapter, as illustrated in the overview figure above, the developmental stages of the B cell, from hematopoietic stem cell to mature B cell are discussed; the stages include:

- Stem cells
- Pro-B cells
- Pre-B cells
- Immature B cells

Material in this chapter contributed by Dr. Patrick Swanson, Department of Medical Microbiology and Immunology, Creighton University School of Medicine, Omaha, Nebraska, USA.

- Mature B cells
- Plasma cells
- Memory cells.

■ EARLY B LYMPHOCYTE DEVELOPMENT

Stem Cell to Immature B Cell

The B-cell lineage is derived from lymphoid progenitor cells that differentiate from hematopoietic stem cells (see Chapter 12). B cells are produced throughout life, with differentiation first occurring in the fetal liver and then shifting to the bone marrow soon after birth (see Chapters 12 and 13). In the adult bone marrow, B-cell development follows a radially organized maturation pathway, with the least developed cells close to the endosteal (inner) surface of the bone and the more mature cells concentrated in the central marrow space (Fig. 14.1). Immature B cells exit the bone marrow via the sinusoids and migrate to the periphery. Their development in the bone marrow depends on a variety of growth factors contributed by bone marrow stromal cells (see Chapter 12).

From the earliest cell progenitor, the hematopoietic stem cell, the B-cell differentiation pathway can be subdivided into several developmental stages. These stages are defined by the rearrangement status of the immunoglobulin heavy and light chain genes and the expression of differentiation-specific molecules (markers) on the cell surface (Fig. 14.2). The earliest committed B-lineage cell is called the **pro-B cell**. This cell is recognized by the appearance of surface

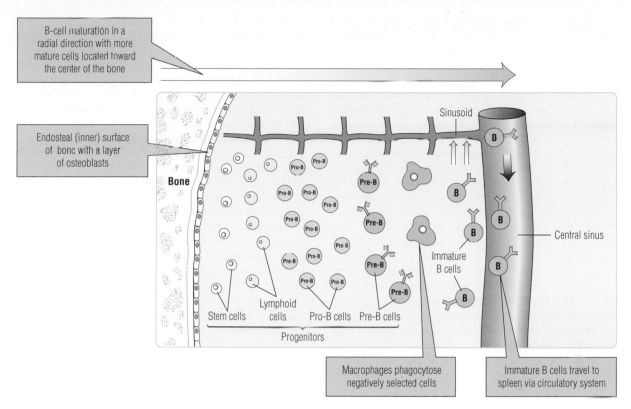

Figure 14.1 Development of B cells in bone marrow.

FIG. 14.2 Steps in B-Cell Development Pathway. Other Molecules Not Shown in this Figure Have Been Used To Define B-Cell Maturation. For Simplicity, Other Stages of Differentiation Have Also Been Omitted

	Stem cell	Pro-B cell	Early pre-B cell	Late pre-B cell	Immature cell
Surface markers					
CD34	+	+	−	−	−
CD19	−	+	+	+	+
Expression of RAG genes	−	++↑	+↓	++↑	+↓
Status of Immunoglobulin genes					
H	Germline	D_H to J_H and V_H to $D_H J_H$ rearrangement	$V_H D_H J_H$ rearrangement	$V_H D_H J_H C\mu$	$V_H D_H J_H C\mu$
L	Germline	Germline	Germline	V_L to J_L rearrangement	$V_L J_L C_L$
Expression of pre-BCR or BCR proteins					
ψL	−	+	+	−	−
μ	−	−	−	+	+
Pre-BCR	−	−	+	−	−
BCR	−	−	−	−	+

 MHC II

 Cytokine, Chemokine, etc.

 Complement (C')

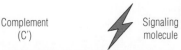 Signaling molecule

markers characterizing the B lineage (e.g., CD19, a part of the co-receptor complex; see Chapter 11). The rearrangement of immunoglobulin heavy chain diversity (D_H) and joining (J_H) gene segments (i.e., the joining of D_H to J_H) occurs during this developmental stage. Next, attempts are made to rearrange immunoglobulin heavy-chain variable region (V_H) gene segments to be adjacent to the rearranged $D_H J_H$ segments. Productive V_H to $D_H J_H$ recombination generates a contiguous variable region gene segment from which a μ heavy chain is eventually expressed (see Chapter 6). At the **early pre-B stage**, two invariant polypeptides associate noncovalently with one another to form a light chainlike structure, called the surrogate light chain (ψL), pair with the μ_H chain. The resulting complex is expressed on the cell surface in association with immunoglobulin α and β chains (see Chapter 11) to form a receptor complex called the **pre–B-cell receptor** (pre-BCR). The pre-BCR plays an important role in transducing signals leading to proliferative expansion of the pre-B cells, and thereby facilitating their further development. Proliferation promotes further development and progression toward the next main stage—the **late pre-B cell**.

Acquisition of the pre-BCR coincides with rapid cellular proliferation and downregulation of the *V(D)J* recombinase machinery: *RAG-1*, *RAG-2* (recombination activating genes 1 and 2), and terminal deoxynucleotidyl transferase (TdT) (see Chapter 6). These events have the dual effect of selecting B cells with functionally rearranged receptor genes and also preventing further V_H to $D_H J_H$ rearrangements, thereby limiting the possibility that two different antigen-binding regions are expressed on the same B cell. The recombination activating genes are essential for the immune response to function and defects can lead to deficiency diseases (see Box 7.1).

Later in the pre–B-cell stage, the *V(D)J* recombinase machinery is upregulated and light-chain gene rearrangement is initiated. The appearance of paired light- and heavy-chain polypeptides on the cell surface as a complete IgM molecule, the BCR, constitutes the transition to an immature B cell.

It is worth pointing out that until the BCR is present on the cell surface, the antigenic specificity of the receptor cannot be tested. Consequently, the recombinational processes involved in B-cell development that give rise to extensive receptor diversity necessarily generate some antigen receptors that possess self-reactivity. The next phase of B-cell development involves screening this as yet unselected receptor repertoire against self antigen, a process that occurs during the transition from the immature to mature B cell, as discussed in greater detail later.

Ordered Immunoglobulin Gene Segment Rearrangement and Allelic Exclusion

As discussed in Chapter 6, the developing B cell has an extensive array of possible *V*, *D*, and *J* gene segments from which to assemble functional Ig heavy- and light-chain genes. Moreover, each cell has two different light-chain loci (κ and λ), either of which could undergo rearrangement to generate a light chain to pair with a given heavy

chain. Finally, each cell possesses two copies of each immunoglobulin locus (one donated from each set of parental chromosomes), and both are capable of being rearranged. However, only a single parental chromosome is used to synthesize a given heavy or light chain, resulting in the expression of a single heavy- and light-chain combination (a **monospecific** BCR), a phenomenon called **allelic exclusion** (see Chapter 6). This outcome is critical because it prevents different antibodies with distinct antigenic specificities from being secreted from the same cell, a situation that is wasteful and potentially dangerous to the organism. So how is allelic exclusion achieved?

The developmentally ordered process of heavy- and light-chain gene rearrangement plays an important role in ensuring that only a single type of receptor locus is rearranged at a time—that is, first the heavy chain, then the light chain (Figs 14.3 and 14.4). But why is it that a given locus is only rearranged on one allele at a time? The answer to this question is related to how heavy- and light-chain gene rearrangements are developmentally regulated. Specifically, the general molecular processes responsible for rendering a given immunoglobulin heavy- or light-chain locus that is physically accessible to the *V(D)J* recombination machinery are also involved in keeping one allele inaccessible to the recombination machinery while the other allele undergoes *V(D)J* rearrangement. The mechanistic details underlying these processes have not been completely elucidated, but it appears that actively rearranging loci assume a less compact chromosomal organization than their quiescent counterparts. How the rearrangement status of a given allele is communicated to the other allele is also not yet clear.

■ THE TRANSITION FROM IMMATURE TO MATURE B CELL

Once the B cell completes the early maturation stages in the bone marrow, it begins to migrate to peripheral lymphoid organs to complete its development. As immature B cells mature, they pass through a transitional stage. During this stage, the *V(D)J* recombination machinery (*RAG-1* and *RAG-2*) is downregulated, surface expression of IgM is increased, and membrane-bound IgD, arising after alternative splicing of heavy-chain transcripts (see Chapter 6), begins to appear on the B-cell surface (Fig. 14.5). Once B cells progress through this stage, they become **mature B cells**, expressing surface IgM and surface IgD. B cells that have fully rearranged immunoglobulin genes but have not yet encountered nonself antigen are known as **naive B cells**. The rearrangement of Ig genes can be followed using Southern blotting or polymerase chain reaction (PCR)-based techniques (Box 14.1).

Induction of Tolerance

During the transitional phase, an important event occurs that helps to shape the final BCR repertoire. As immature B cells begin to encounter self antigens, those cells with antigen receptors that display self-reactivity are deleted or

 T cell receptor (TCR)   Immunoglobulin (Ig)   Antigen   MHC I

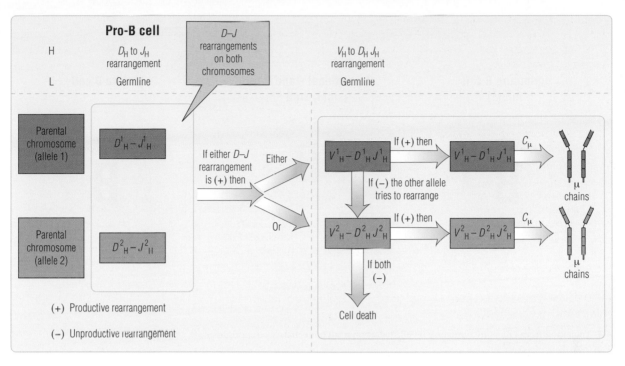

Figure 14.3 Ordered rearrangement of the immunoglobulin heavy-chain locus, enabling expression of a single heavy chain. D_H, diversity gene segment; J_H, joining gene segment; V_H, variable gene segment.

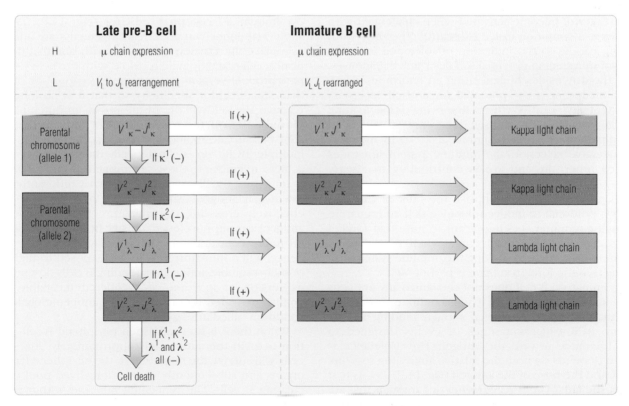

Figure 14.4 Ordered rearrangement of the immunoglobulin light-chain locus, enabling expression of a single light chain.

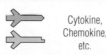 MHC II   Cytokine, Chemokine, etc.   Complement (C')   Signaling molecule

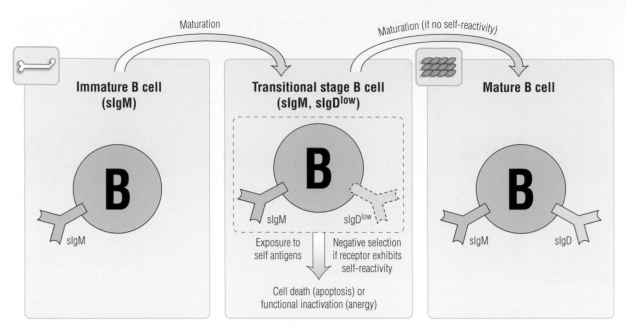

Figure 14.5 Transition from immature to mature B cell; migration from bone marrow to periphery. sIg, surface immunoglobulin.

functionally inactivated, a process called **negative selection**. This selection process results in a pool of immature B cells that do *not* become activated when challenged with self antigen, a condition called **tolerance**. The process of selection leading to the induction of tolerance to self is important in reducing potential self-destructive responses. One of the downsides of generating an enormous repertoire of receptors is the potential for antiself receptors with potentially negative effects. Removing or inactivating the cells bearing these antiself receptors is critical to avoiding pathology (i.e., autoimmune disease). By the process of negative selection, the immune system fine-tunes the B-cell repertoire and avoids contributing to disease states.

Although self antigens comprise the bulk of the antigens with potential to induce tolerance that an immature B cell will encounter, it is important to note that foreign antigens can also induce tolerance when presented to immature B cells, thereby tricking the immune system into believing that the foreign antigen is part of "self."

If the immature B cell does not recognize any antigens present in the bone marrow, it will continue to develop into a mature B cell. However, antigen binding by the immature BCR triggers a series of events designed to induce tolerance toward the antigen. How tolerance is rendered depends on both the relative ability to cross-link the BCR and the dose of the antigen (Fig. 14.7). Let us first consider the fate of cells recognizing self antigens that are abundant on the cell surface and that can extensively cross-link immature BCRs (multivalent antigens). Extensive cross-linking of the immature BCR by a multivalent self antigen induces a state of maturational arrest. During this period, the *V(D)J* recombination machinery is upregulated

to try to alter receptor specificity away from (perceived) autoreactivity by reinitiating *V(D)J* rearrangement, a process known as **receptor editing** (Fig. 14.8). Typically, additional light-chain gene rearrangements are attempted to replace the existing light chain with one that does not display self-reactivity when paired with the heavy chain. If new, productive, gene rearrangements cannot be obtained that alter receptor specificity so that it is no longer self-reactive, the cell will die by apoptosis, an outcome called **clonal deletion**. Because multivalent antigens (e.g., abundant cell-surface molecules) are capable of cross-linking multiple BCRs on a single cell, the dose required to achieve tolerance to these self antigens is quite low.

Immature B cells respond somewhat differently to univalent self antigens: small, soluble proteins that cannot effectively cross-link the immature BCR. Because these antigens can support less extensive BCR cross-linking than do multivalent antigens, they display more dose dependence. When immature B cells are exposed to high doses of such a soluble antigen, responding B cells downregulate expression of IgM and are rendered incapable of becoming activated upon subsequent antigenic challenge, a condition called **anergy** (Fig. 14.7).

When there is an established peripheral B-cell population (e.g., in the adult), only approximately 20% of new cells will survive the migration to the peripheral lymphoid organs and subsequently enter a long-lived pool of recirculating B cells. The remaining 80% die within approximately 1 week. This observation suggests that maturing B cells must compete for space in the limited sites (most likely the follicles of the lymphoid organs) that can provide a suitable environment to support their continued survival and development (see Chapter 17).

 T cell receptor (TCR) 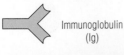 Immunoglobulin (Ig)  Antigen   MHC I

BOX 14.1 Molecular Genetic Analysis of B-Cell Tumors

Although most lymphoma cases can be diagnosed on the basis of morphologic examination coupled with what is known as "immunophenotyping"—using monoclonal antibodies and flow cytometry or fluorescence microscopy (see Chapter 5) to examine marker antigen expression, there are some difficult cases for which a molecular genetic approach will facilitate diagnosis.

As described in Chapter 6, the techniques of molecular genetics, e.g., Southern blotting, can be used to follow immunoglobulin (Ig) gene rearrangement. Ig genes rearrange in normal and neoplastic human B lymphocytes, and Southern blotting, for example, is useful in the clinical diagnosis and monitoring of lymphoma (see Chapter 6, Box 6.1). Currently, however, the methods of choice are the polymerase chain reaction (PCR)-based methods. PCR is a technique that allows DNA polymerase enzyme-based copying and amplification of DNA using short oligonucleotide primers with complementary sequences to the DNA of interest. DNA-based PCR methods are being widely utilized to examine antigen-receptor gene rearrangements in T and B cells. For example, assessing Ig heavy-chain variable gene rearrangements can aid in examining B-cell populations for the types of monoclonal expansion found in B-cell malignancies. As you will remember from Chapter 6, once a B cell begins to proliferate and expand clonally, all the progeny cells carry the same unique Ig gene rearrangements.

As a malignant B-cell population expands, the genetic features unique to this population become readily detectable over the background of diverse rearrangements present in normal B cells. Historically, Southern blotting (see Box 6.1) served as the primary means to detect "clonality" (the extent to which there is a monoclonal proliferation typical of a neoplastic cell) in B-cell populations. However, PCR-based assays are now the method of choice for molecular diagnosis of leukemia and lymphoma. To assay for clonality, PCR is used to amplify part of the hypervariable region (often the J region sequences) of the rearranged *IgH* gene. A polyclonal B-cell population will give rise to a ladder of PCR products, whereas a monoclonal B-cell population will yield a dominant PCR product with background PCR products variably present depending on the relative abundance of malignant B cells in the total B-cell population. Figure 14.6 illustrates an example of using PCR to examine patient samples for a B-cell malignancy. DNA primers were used that represented part of the hypervariable region of the Ig heavy-chain variable region exon. PCR products were amplified from various cell types and analyzed by polyacrylamide gel electrophoresis.

The monoclonal B-cell control population in lane 1 shows a single, intense, narrow band as expected because these B cells should all have hypervariable regions of the same size. Lane 2 shows PCR products from a lymph-node DNA control, where there should be a polyclonal population of B cells. A ladder of different-sized DNA products of similar intensity results from the different-sized hypervariable regions in each of the B cells represented in the lymph node. Lane 3 shows PCR products from a patient's B-cell sample. There is one intense band, no ladder, and this is representative of a high proportion of monoclonal B cells. This patient was diagnosed with a B lymphoblastic lymphoma. Lane 4 shows a different patient's sample. In this case, there is a ladder of polyclonal products but one dominant product consistent with a monoclonal expansion that has not gone quite as far as the sample in lane 3.

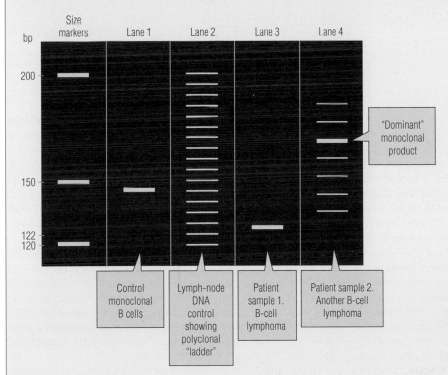

Figure 14.6 Analysis of B-cell lymphoma by PCR: polyacrylamide gel electrophoresis of PCR products from various DNA samples. PCR, polymerase chain reaction.

 MHC II

 Cytokine, Chemokine, etc.

 Complement (C')

 Signaling molecule

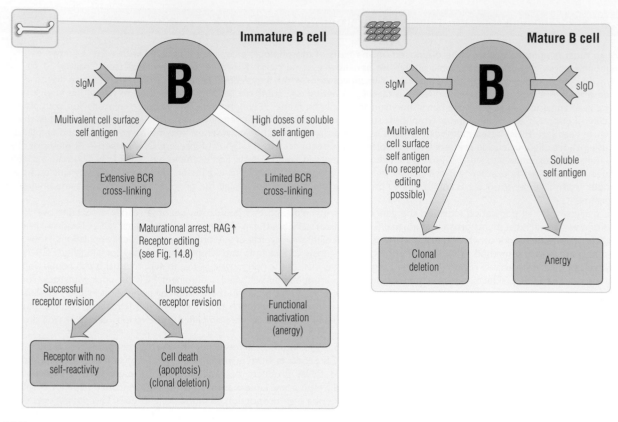

Figure 14.7 Receptor selection: generating self-tolerance. sIg, surface immunoglobulin.

■ THE MATURE B CELL

Additional Tolerance Induction

Because not all self antigens are present in the bone marrow, mechanisms have evolved to ensure that the mature B-cell pool is rendered tolerant to self antigens encountered in the periphery. As has been introduced in Chapters 10 and 11, and as discussed later in this chapter and in more detail in Chapter 16, specific T-cell help is generally required for the mature B cell to produce antibody. If the mature B cell engages an antigen and no T cell specific for the antigen responds to provide the necessary signals (see Chapters 11 and 16) for the B cell to become fully activated, the cell will undergo clonal deletion or become anergic. As with immature B cells, the outcome of receptor engagement depends on the antigen encountered. Multivalent antigens generally cause clonal deletion, and univalent antigens induce anergy (Fig. 14.7). An important difference, however, is that the *V(D)J* recombination machinery, present through most stages of B-cell development, appears to be permanently shut off when B cells acquire mature levels of surface IgM and IgD. Therefore, the option to undergo additional receptor editing in fully mature B cells is lost.

Activation and Antibody Production

Specialized anatomical structures in the secondary lymphoid organs (see Chapter 13) provide an environment in which antigen is concentrated and displayed to incoming naive B cells on specialized antigen-presenting cells (APCs) known as **follicular dendritic cells (FDCs)**, which in turn interact with localized T cells that support B-cell activation and differentiation. FDCs are an additional class of DC to those discussed in Box 10.1. The FDCs are APCs that are only found in lymphoid follicles. They do not express class II major histocompatibility complex (MHC) molecules but instead retain antigen/antibody complexes on their surface attached to Fc receptors or complement receptors. These cells are morphologically similar to other DCs, with long processes that create networks within the lymphoid follicles, but they may have a different origin from the bone marrow-derived class II–MHC-expressing DCs that we have described before.

Each type of secondary lymphoid tissue traps antigen from different sources: the spleen collects blood-borne antigens, antigens present in the afferent lymphatic system are trapped in lymph nodes, and mucosa-associated lymphoid tissues (MALT, e.g., Peyer's patches in gut and

 T cell receptor (TCR)

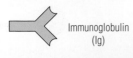 Immunoglobulin (Ig)

 Antigen

 MHC I

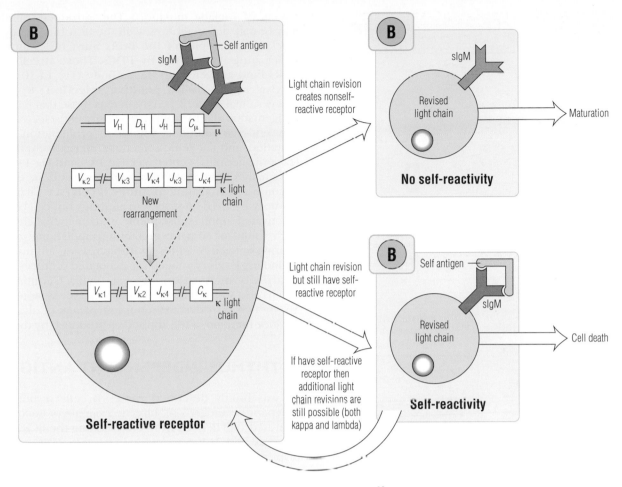

Figure 14.8 B-cell receptor editing. D_H, diversity gene segment; J_H, joining gene segment; V_H, variable gene segment.

tonsils/adenoids in nasopharynx) acquire antigen from the surrounding mucosal epithelia.

The activation of a naive B cell and its subsequent differentiation into an antibody-secreting **plasma cell** is a multistep process that usually begins when the B cell exits the bloodstream and enters a secondary lymphoid organ (Fig. 14.9). Upon entry, the B cell migrates into a region rich in T cells (called the paracortex in lymph nodes, see Fig 13.6, and the periarteriolar lymphoid sheath in spleen, see Fig 13.5; see discussion in Chapter 13). In the absence of its target antigen, the B cell traverses this region and eventually re-enters the circulation. If the B cell encounters its target antigen, antigen engagement by the BCR triggers the B cell to internalize the BCR-antigen complex. Then, the antigen is degraded and, in the case of protein antigens, processed into peptide-MHC class II complexes, which are subsequently displayed on the cell surface (see Chapter 10).

As a general rule, naive B cells cannot be activated by antigen alone. A second accessory signal is required to initiate full activation of the B cell (see Chapter 16). In the case of protein antigens, the second signal is delivered by

an activated T cell with an antigen receptor (TCR) that recognizes the peptide–MHC class II complex displayed by the B cell or by antigen presented by a neighboring APC. Antigens that require this form of B-cell–T-cell collaboration to initiate an immune response are called **thymus-dependent** (TD) antigens, because athymic animals that lack T cells are unable to mount an immune response to these antigens.

■ CONTINUED SELECTION OF B CELLS IN LYMPHOID FOLLICLES

After antigen has been administered and taken up by APCs in lymphoid organs, naive B and T cells with specificity for that antigen become activated. In a lymph node, the T cells become activated in the paracortex and the B cells in the follicles (see Fig. 13.6B). These are anatomically separate areas in the node, and on stimulation, the B cells move out of the follicles into the T-cell zone (paracortex) where they encounter activated T cells and cytokines that cause the B cells to proliferate. Some of these B cells differentiate into

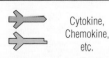 MHC II

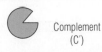 Cytokine, Chemokine, etc.

 Complement (C')

Signaling molecule

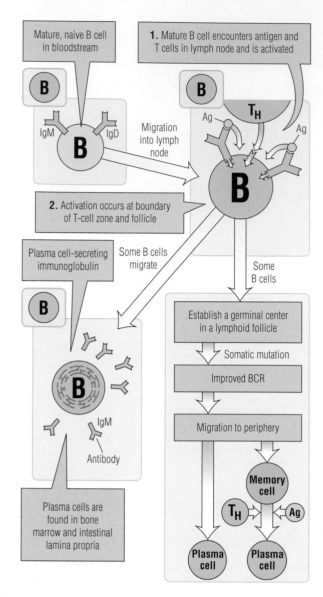

Figure 14.9 boxes text:

Mature, naive B cell in bloodstream

1. Mature B cell encounters antigen and T cells in lymph node and is activated

IgM IgD

Migration into lymph node

Ag   T_H   Ag

2. Activation occurs at boundary of T-cell zone and follicle

Plasma cell-secreting immunoglobulin

Some B cells migrate

Some B cells

Establish a germinal center in a lymphoid follicle

Somatic mutation

Improved BCR

Migration to periphery

IgM

Antibody

Plasma cells are found in bone marrow and intestinal lamina propria

Memory cell

T_H   Ag

Plasma cell   Plasma cell

Figure 14.9 Maturation of the mature B cell into an effector B cell (plasma cell). Ag, antigen; BCR, B-cell receptor; Ig, immunoglobulin.

plasma cells and home to the bone marrow or intestinal lamina propria, for example (see Fig 14.9), where they may secrete large amounts of antibody for a period of at least several weeks.

Some of the activated B cells migrate into lymphoid follicles where they proliferate rapidly (dividing about once every 6 hours) and create a germinal center (lightly stained region within the follicles; see Fig. 13.6A and B). During this period, somatic point mutations are introduced at a high rate (somatic hypermutation) into the antigen-receptor genes (see Chapter 6), resulting in the expression of BCRs that vary in their affinity toward the antigen that initiated the immune response. Somatic mutations are usually comprised of single nucleotide substitutions focused in and around the rearranged variable region exon (both heavy- and light-chain variable region exons may be

targets of somatic mutation). The introduced mutations may or may not affect how well the BCR binds antigen. As a result, the affinity of the BCRs must be evaluated on intact antigen displayed by **FDCs**. Those B cells whose BCRs bind antigen with high-affinity (Fig 14.10) receive survival signals (called **positive selection**) from FDCs and germinal center T cells, whereas those that fail to bind antigen soon die by apoptosis. Positively selected B cells may undergo additional rounds of proliferation, somatic mutation, and antigenic selection. Alternatively, they may leave the germinal center (see Fig 14.9 and Fig 14.10) and terminally differentiate into a **plasma cell**, or they may become a recirculating **memory B cell** (see Chapter 17). Memory B cells do not secrete antibody but can be rapidly reactivated upon subsequent antigenic challenge. With each round of somatic mutation, populations of B cells bearing antigen receptors with increasing affinity toward dwindling levels of antigen are generated, a process known as **affinity maturation** (see Fig. 14.10). Germinal-center T cells also support Ig class switching (see Chapters 6 and 16), which provides an important means of altering the effector function of the antibodies produced by the B cells.

■ THYMUS-INDEPENDENT ANTIGENS

As was briefly described earlier, B cells responding to polypeptide antigens require two signals to become fully activated: one derived from cross-linking the BCR, and one obtained from TCR recognition of peptide–MHC complexes displayed on the B-cell surface (see Chapter 16). However, some antigens are able to activate B cells directly in the absence of T-cell help; hence, they are called **thymus-independent** (TI) antigens. In this case, the second signal is derived from the antigen itself. Figure 14.11 illustrates how TI antigens activate B cells. TI antigens include repeating polymers, such as dextran and bacterial polysaccharides, and certain bacterial cell wall components, such as lipopolysaccharides.

It is important to consider the protective mechanism that responses to TI antigens play in host defense. As these antigens are often of bacterial origin, TI responses provide a means to generate an early and specific antibody response against bacterial pathogens that can proliferate quickly and overwhelm the immune system. However, because T cells are not usually mobilized, the antibody repertoire generated during TI responses is limited because T cell–dependent events that promote affinity maturation and class switching are not induced.

■ THE B-CELL REPERTOIRE AND HUMAN DEVELOPMENT

In adults, most peripheral B cells belong to a pool of long-lived, recirculating follicular B lymphocytes that are collectively called conventional (or B-2) B cells. However, other B-cell populations also emerge from the precursors of conventional B cells. An important subset is referred to as B-1 cells. B-1 cells appear to develop from immature B-

 T cell receptor (TCR)

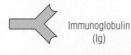 Immunoglobulin (Ig)

 Antigen

 MHC I

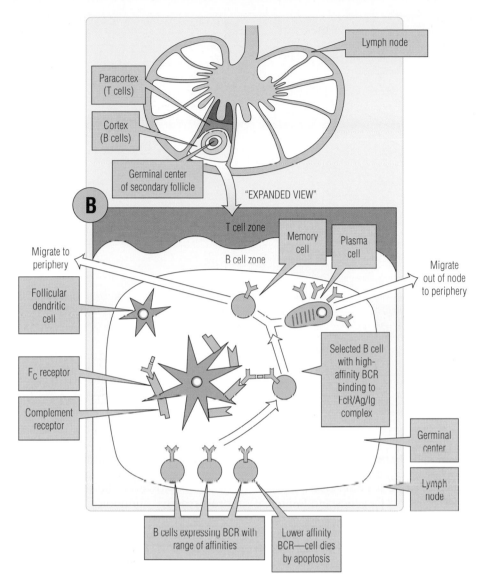

Figure 14.10 Selection of B cells expressing high-affinity receptors in lymphoid follicles.

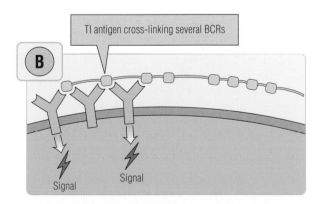

Figure 14.11 T-independent (TI) antigens. Examples of TI antigens include (1) repeating polymers, e.g., dextran and bacterial polysaccharides and (2) bacterial cell wall components, e.g., peptidoglycans and lipopolysaccharides. BCR, B-cell receptor.

cell precursors, but they are phenotypically distinct from conventional B cells, and they express different cell surface markers (Fig. 14.12). For example, many, but not all, B-1 cells express a surface marker called CD5 that is not found on conventional B cells.

B-1 cells comprise the majority of B cells found in the fetus and neonate. After birth, a developmental transition occurs during which B-cell precursors switch from being committed to the B-1 lineage to being committed to the conventional B lineage. Unlike conventional B cells, which are constantly being renewed from bone marrow precursors, B-1 cells in the adult replenish themselves by continuing division of cells carrying surface IgM (sIgM$^+$) in peripheral tissues, thereby ensuring a persistent B-1 population long after their generation has ceased. This property likely contributes to the tendency of B-1 cells (particularly the CD5$^+$ cells) to be a frequent source for a relatively

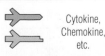 MHC II

 Cytokine, Chemokine, etc.

Complement (C')

 Signaling molecule

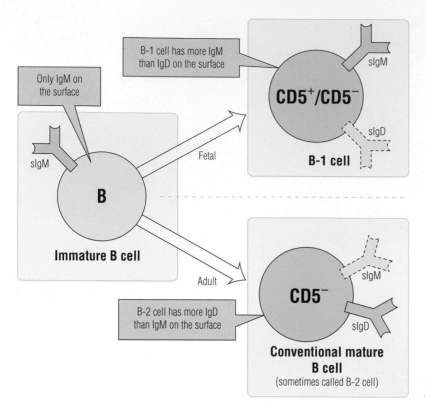

Figure 14.12 The B-cell repertoire during human development. sIg, surface immunoglobulin.

common B-cell neoplasm called chronic lymphocytic leukemia (see Box 14.2 and Chapter 34).

The B-1 cell receptor repertoire is rather restricted, as a result of preferential use of a few V_H genes and limited, if any, insertional diversity, caused by a lack of TdT expression in these cells. The BCRs expressed on B-1 cells are often reactive toward bacterial antigens (e.g., polysaccharides), and they frequently display polyspecificity—the ability to cross-react with multiple antigens. Hence, B-1 cells provide an important protective function against bacterial pathogens early in life until the adult repertoire develops. However, the tendency of B-1 cells to produce cross-reactive antibodies may partly explain the observation that B-1 cells are disproportionately represented among autoantibody-producing B cells. The antibodies produced by B-1 cells, sometimes called **natural antibodies**, are described further in Chapter 27.

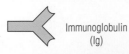 T cell receptor (TCR)

 Immunoglobulin (Ig)

Antigen

 MHC I

BOX 14.2 Microarrays or Gene Expression Profiling

The sequencing of the human genome and the availability of probes for the expressed human genes makes it possible to use a molecular technique called microarray analysis to compare qualitatively and quantitatively the expression of thousands of human genes simultaneously in, for example, normal and malignant B cells. Although this is currently largely a research tool, this gene expression profiling technique has been used to subdivide a broad class of B-cell lymphomas, called diffuse large B-cell lymphoma (DLBCL), the most frequent type of non-Hodgkin's lymphoma, into subtypes that have different patient outcomes after chemotherapy.

The basis of the microarray technique is the ability to construct an ordered array of complementary DNA (cDNA) clones on a single glass slide or microchip. Sophisticated fabrication techniques have been developed, and continue to be enhanced, that allow thousands of different gene sequences to be represented on a single chip or slide (the "microarray"). For example, there is a "lymphochip" that contains almost 20,000 cDNA clones from genes selectively enriched in lymphocytes. Next, messenger RNA (mRNA) is prepared from the cells of interest (for example, B-cell tumors of the same diagnostic category from different patients). Fluorescent cDNA probes are prepared from the total mRNA samples from each tumor cell preparation and allowed to hybridize to the microarray under conditions similar to those used for Southern blotting. Scanning devices not unlike those used in flow cytometry (see Chapter 5) are used to quantitate the amount of fluorescent cDNA probe bound to the microarray. The amount of fluorescence is proportional to the amount of probe bound, which is proportional to the amount of expression (amount of mRNA) of that gene in that cell. Thus, the genes expressed in different types of B-cell tumor can be compared.

In recent studies, most genes were found to be equivalently expressed in, for example, different B-cell lymphomas of the same clinical category, but differences were detected between lymphoma samples from certain diagnostic categories, e.g., in the category known as DLBCL. This suggested that these molecular diagnostic techniques will be very useful in establishing subtypes of tumors currently thought to be of one type, and in distinguishing them from one another, ultimately helping to better detect and monitor cancer, and raising the prospect of being able to devise targeted therapies.

LEARNING POINTS Can You Now ...

1. List the different cell types in the B-cell development pathway?

2. Recall the time-dependent changes in cell surface molecules during the B-cell development pathway?

3. Draw the order of rearrangement and expression of immunoglobulin heavy-chain and light-chain genes during B-cell development?

4. Explain with a diagram the molecular basis of allelic exclusion in B cells?

5. Compare T-dependent and T-independent B-cell activation?

6. Explain antigen-induced tolerance in immature and mature B-cell populations?

7. Describe receptor editing and affinity maturation in terms of B-cell antigen receptor improvement?

 MHC II

 Cytokine, Chemokine, etc.

 Complement (C')

 Signaling molecule

15 T-Cell Development

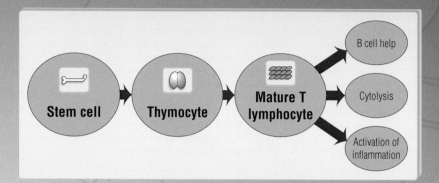

As we have already seen in Chapters 7 and 10, the highly variable T-cell receptor (TCR) recognizes foreign antigen as peptide fragments bound to self-major histocompatibility complex (MHC) molecules. To protect the host from infection, the T-cell population must contain a diverse array of antigen-specific receptors. Individual T cells express a unique receptor that is capable of recognizing foreign peptide antigen displayed by a self-MHC molecule. The main topic for this chapter, as shown in the overview figure above, is how a diverse population of mature T lymphocytes with different antigenic specificities is generated to accomplish several different protective functions for the host.

T lymphocytes are generated in the thymus. T-cell development in the thymus is a multistep process with several built-in check points to ensure that the appropriate differentiation has taken place. As a result of selection, only a small proportion of progenitor T cells, known as **thymocytes**, actually exit the thymus to the periphery as mature T cells; most ($\approx$98%) die during the selection processes that establish the T-lymphocyte repertoire. These thymic selection processes enable the host to develop a T-cell repertoire that is **self-tolerant** (mostly!), but **self-restricted** (see Chapter 8). This means that the mature T cells that are selected to develop are those most likely to be capable of recognizing nonself antigenic peptides bound to self-MHC molecules.

Different subsets of mature T cells carry out the functions of **cell-mediated immunity**, including killing virally

Material in this chapter contributed by Dr. Kristen Drescher, Department of Medical Microbiology and Immunology, Creighton University School of Medicine, Omaha, Nebraska, USA.

infected cells and tumor cells, activating the bactericidal functions of macrophages, "helping" B cells and CD8$^+$ T cells to mature into effector cells, and secreting various cytokines. This chapter, and Chapter 16, will describe how different subsets of T cells are activated to perform their effector functions.

■ THE THYMUS

The architecture of the thymus was described in Chapter 13, and its role as a primary lymphoid organ in Chapters 12 and 13. You should recall that the thymus is organized into three major areas: the subcapsular zone, the cortex, and the medulla (Fig. 15.1). Different populations of stromal cells and thymocytes are found in each of these structurally and functionally distinct regions. The critical role of the thymus in T-cell development is illustrated by the observation that individuals who never develop a thymus (complete Di George syndrome) have minimal numbers of mature peripheral T cells (Box 15.1). Despite the critical nature of the fetal thymus in establishing a peripheral T-cell population, the thymus is not necessary to maintain mature antigen-specific T cells. Thymectomy has little impact on T-cell responses in humans after birth unless the peripheral T-cell population is eliminated and needs to be reestablished, such as in the case of individuals who undergo bone marrow transplantation (see Chapter 33). Also, as was noted in Chapter 13, the thymus atrophies throughout adult life in humans. The reason for this is unknown. The production of new T cells continues throughout life, although at a declining level as the individual ages. To a great extent in later life, maintenance of

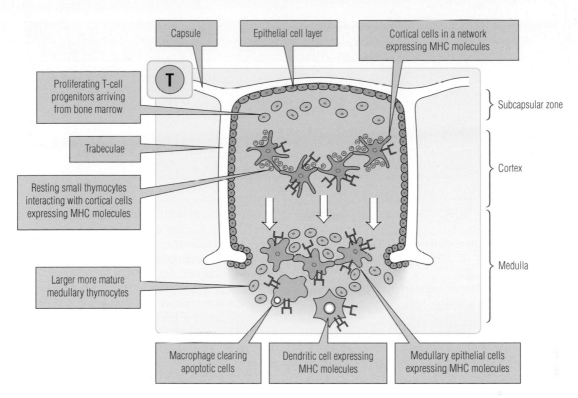

Capsule

Epithelial cell layer

Cortical cells in a network expressing MHC molecules

Proliferating T-cell progenitors arriving from bone marrow

Subcapsular zone

Trabeculae

Cortex

Resting small thymocytes interacting with cortical cells expressing MHC molecules

Medulla

Larger more mature medullary thymocytes

Macrophage clearing apoptotic cells

Dendritic cell expressing MHC molecules

Medullary epithelial cells expressing MHC molecules

Figure 15.1 Simplified schematic of thymic organization.

the pool of peripheral T cells is accomplished by mature T-cell division under the influence of interleukin-7 (IL 7).

Transition from Thymocyte to Mature T Cell

In the thymus, the different stages of thymocyte development can be identified by establishing which thymocyte cell-surface molecules are being expressed (Figs. 15.2 and 15.3). This can be done using the technique of flow cytometry (see Chapter 5) and using monoclonal antibodies that are specific for particular cell-surface molecules. Specific monoclonal antibodies that recognize T-cell surface

molecules can be used to identify different types of T cells (Fig. 15.4), establish how many of a particular subset of T cells are present in a sample, purify the subset, or block its function. These experimental approaches have been essential to understanding T-lymphocyte development in the thymus, which follows the stages:

1. Double-negative cells (DN: CD4⁻ and CD8⁻): found in the subcapsular zone
2. Commitment to αβ or γδ lineage
3. Double-positive cells (DP: CD4⁺ CD8⁺): found in the cortex

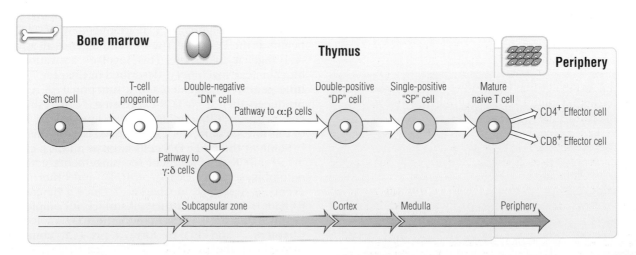

Figure 15.2 Overview of pathway of T-cell maturation.

 MHC II

 Cytokine, Chemokine, etc.

 Complement (C')

Signaling molecule

FIG. 15.3   Order of Expression of Major T-Cell Surface Molecules (e.g., CD44, CD25, CD3, CD4, CD8, TCR) During Development

Stage of Development	DN cell	CD4$^+$ CD8$^+$ DP cell	CD4$^+$ CD8$^-$ or CD4$^-$ CD8$^+$ SP cell	Mature naive T Cell
Surface Molecule				
CD44	+	−	−	−
CD25	+	−	−	−
CD4	−	+	+ or −	+ or −
CD8	−	+	+ or −	+ or −
TCR/CD3	−	+	+	+

---

4. Selection of DP cells by MHC class I or class II molecules: in the cortex
5. Selection of single-positive cells (SP: CD4$^+$ or CD8$^+$, depending on the class of MHC molecule interacted with): occurs in the medulla
6. Release of SP cells as naive mature T cells: into the periphery.

Upon migrating to the thymus and locating in the subcapsular zone, bone marrow–derived thymocytes do not express (are said to be negative for) the cell-surface molecules that are characteristic of T cells (e.g., CD3/TCR, CD4, CD8), and they are referred to as double-negative (DN) cells (see Fig. 15.3). These cells can be identified because they express cell-surface molecules such as CD44 (an adhesion molecule) and CD25 (the α chain of the IL-2 receptor). At this stage, the TCR genes are in the germline (unrearranged) configuration.

As shown in Figures 15.2 and 15.3, the DN thymocyte subpopulation undergoes several important differentiation events. The DN cells become committed to the T-cell lineage as TCR gene rearrangements begin to occur (described later). Another important choice that is made at this stage is commitment to either the αβ or γδ T-cell lineage. As mentioned earlier (see Chapter 7), there are two major lineages of T cells expressing different types of TCR. The γδ T cells are a minor population in terms of numbers, and they are most often found in the skin and in mucosal tissue, especially the gut. The major T-cell population is represented by αβ TCR-expressing T lymphocytes. Notably, both these T-cell lineages derive from a common progenitor cell, with commitment to one lineage or the other being a competitive process based on which TCR genes productively rearrange first (compare with the process of immunoglobulin light-chain gene expression in B cells; see Chapter 14).

The next major step in the T-cell development pathway is the double-positive (DP) stage (see Figs 15.2 and 15.3). DP cells express both CD4 and CD8. DP cells are rarely found in normal blood; they are essentially always found in the thymic cortex. The DP stage is the point at which cells are positively selected (retained) if they express a TCR that can recognize self-MHC and negatively selected (deleted) if they express receptors that recognize self-peptide antigens with self-MHC molecules. These selection processes are critical in reaching the developmental goal of establishing a T-lymphocyte population that is **self-tolerant** and **self-restricted**. Most (≈95%) DP cells never mature because they lack TCRs that can appropriately recognize self-MHC.

At the next step in the T-cell development pathway (see Figs. 15.2 and 15.3), the cells migrate to the thymic medulla. At this point, depending on whether or not the TCR interacts appropriately with a class I or class II MHC molecule, the cells become single positive (SP): either CD4$^-$ CD8$^+$ or CD4$^+$ CD8$^-$. This is known as **lineage commitment**. SP cells undergo further selection, and they are then released into the periphery as naive mature T cells (see Figs. 15.2 and 15.3).

Order of T-Cell Receptor Gene Rearrangements

As shown in Figure 15.5, rearrangement of TCR genes begins at the DN stage. The β, γ, and δ genes all attempt to rearrange at this stage. This involves activation of the biochemical "machinery" described in Chapter 7, and multiple gene rearrangements. If a functional γδ receptor is produced then a γδ TCR-expressing T-cell results. Those cells with γδ TCRs establish the γδ lineage. The functions of this lineage of T cells are discussed later in this chapter.

Some of the other DN cells express a TCR β-chain. This involves TCR gene segment rearrangements, activation of recombinase genes (*RAG-1*, *RAG-2*), and other molecular events as described in Chapter 7. Once a functional TCR β-chain is expressed at the cell surface, it complexes with an invariant pre-T α-chain, and the CD3 molecule (see Chapters 7 and 11) to form a pre-TCR complex. Expression of the pre-TCR allows signal transduction (see Chapter 11), and, in some fashion that is not yet entirely

---

FIG. 15.4   T-Cell Surface Molecules and Cyctokines Used in Identifying T-Cell Subsets

T-cell Subset	CTL	T$_H$1	T$_H$2
Surface Molecule			
CD3/TCR	√	√	√
CD4	−	√	√
CD8	√	−	−
Cytokine			
IL-2	√	√	√
IL-4	−	−	√
IFN-γ	−	√	−

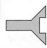   T cell receptor (TCR)

   Immunoglobulin (Ig)

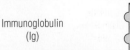   Antigen

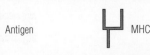   MHC I

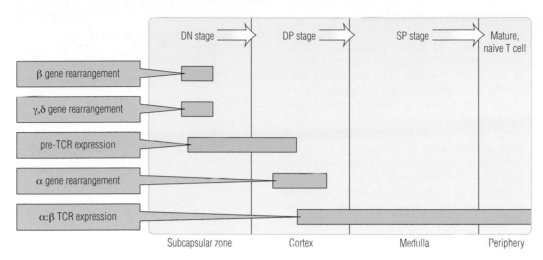

Figure 15.5 Order of T-cell receptor gene rearrangements. TCR, T-cell receptor.

clear, signals from the pre-TCR halt further β-chain rearrangements and allow proliferation of the DP-T cells. Proliferation promotes TCR α-chain rearrangement after recombinase expression. Therefore, similar to the role of the pre-BCR (see Chapter 14), expression of the pre-TCR is a critical step in the pathway to assembly of an αβ TCR and formation of the αβ T-cell population.

Positive Selection: Establishment of Self-Restriction

The DP cell, based on interaction with MHC molecules, may mature into an SP cell. However, most DP cells die in the cortex because they lack receptors capable of interacting with self-MHC. Cortical epithelial cells play an important role in positive selection by displaying MHC–self-peptide antigen complexes to the TCRs expressed on the DP cells. Survival (**positive selection**) of any given DP thymocyte is dependent on the ability of the TCR expressed on that cell to interact with the MHC–self-peptide antigen complex on the cortical epithelial cell and transduce a signal

that triggers differentiation into an SP cell. The TCR may interact with either an MHC class I or MHC class II molecule depending on its particular structure and recognition capability. Positive selection depends on the intensity of the signal generated by the TCR during the interaction. In ways that are not entirely understood, this signal influences the expression of either the CD4 or CD8 molecule on the cell surface. In a second step in the process, the combination of TCR and co-receptor (CD4 or CD8) is "double-checked." This step involves ensuring that a T cell that is CD8+, for example, expresses a TCR that preferentially recognizes peptides displayed by MHC class I molecules. Only those cells with a co-receptor that matches the specificity of that cell's TCR (i.e., CD4 with a TCR that is specific for [restricted to] MHC class II molecules, and CD8 with a TCR that is specific for [restricted to] MHC class I molecules) are able to complete the maturation process and move out into the periphery. Figure 15.6 illustrates some of the steps in this positive selection process.

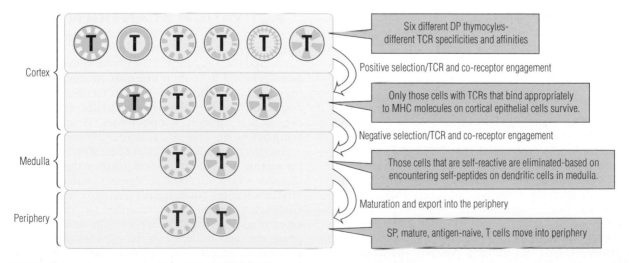

Figure 15.6 Positive and negative selection processes. TCR, T-cell receptor.

 MHC II   Cytokine, Chemokine, etc.   Complement (C')   Signaling molecule

Negative Selection: Establishment of Central Self-Tolerance

The pool of cells generated by positive selection in the thymus is self-MHC restricted, but it also includes some self-reactive cells. These self-reactive cells must be eliminated or the host risks autoimmune disease. Elimination of self-reactive cells involves a process called **negative selection** (Fig. 15.6). During negative selection, clones that are strongly reactive (have high-affinity) with self-peptides are eliminated, and a state of self-tolerance is (largely) established. The process of negative selection involves encountering self-peptides displayed on MHC molecules on the surface of dendritic cells in the medulla of the thymus. Many, but not all, tissue and soluble self antigens are encountered in the thymus. Therefore, negative selection is not a perfect way to eliminate self-reactivity—some cells with receptors reactive with self-peptides will survive. Mutations in a gene known as the autoimmune regulator (AIRE) gene illustrate this concept well. The AIRE gene is thought to be involved in regulating expression of a variety of self-peptides derived from endocrine organ proteins in thymic epithelial and nonepithelial cells. Mutations in this gene in humans result in destruction of several endocrine organs, including the adrenals and pancreatic islets (an autosomal recessive disorder known as autoimmune polyendocrine syndrome I [APS-I]). Mutations in the AIRE gene prevent expression of the endocrine organ peptides in the thymus. Consequently, developing T cells do not encounter these self-antigens in the thymus. This results in T cells that are specific for these endocrine organ antigens escaping negative selection and deletion and being available to attack the endocrine organs, through recognition of self-endocrine proteins, after they emerge from the thymus into the periphery.

Negative selection is mediated by signal transduction through the TCR, leading to induction of apoptosis and eventual clonal deletion. Apoptosis is the mechanism responsible for cell death induced by negative selection in the thymus. Apoptotic cells are disposed of by thymic macrophages.

It has been estimated that two thirds of the cells that survive positive selection in the cortex are subsequently deleted by negative selection in the medulla. Consequently, a very small number of the original thymocytes emerge into the periphery as mature, but still antigen-naive, T cells. **Naive** refers to the fact that these cells have not yet encountered the foreign, nonself antigen that specifically "fits" their TCR.

T-Cell Receptor Signaling in Positive and Negative Selection

The same molecular interaction (i.e., TCR binding to MHC-peptide antigen complex) mediates both positive and negative selection (Fig. 15.7). How can very different outcomes result from the same type of receptor-ligand interaction? It has been suggested that different affinities of interaction between TCRs and MHC-peptide complexes generate different intracellular signals. These signals might be quantitatively or qualitatively different. Investigations are underway to determine the nature of these signals and

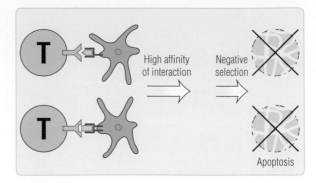
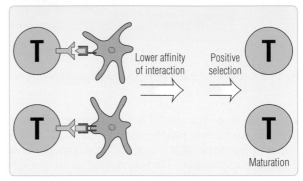

Figure 15.7 T-cell receptor signaling in positive and negative selection.

to establish an answer to this paradox. Currently, one simplified interpretation of the available data would be that high-affinity interactions between the TCR and the appropriate MHC molecule lead to negative selection (deletion) of the cell expressing that TCR, whereas lower (but not too low!) affinity interactions, perhaps best described as "intermediate affinity" interactions, between the TCR and the MHC molecule lead to positive selection and continued maturation.

■ THE PERIPHERY: NAIVE T-CELL ACTIVATION BY ANTIGEN

The mature T cells that leave the thymus have not yet encountered the antigen that they have specificity for (sometimes referred to as their **cognate antigen**). At this stage, they are said to be naive, mature T cells. These cells may circulate from the bloodstream to the central lymphoid organs (e.g., spleen, lymph nodes, Peyer's patches) for years before they die or encounter antigen.

Antigen is usually encountered on a professional antigen-presenting cell (APC) in a secondary lymphoid organ (see Chapter 13). If the TCR recognizes antigen displayed on MHC molecules (first signal) and also receives a second costimulatory signal (see Chapter 16), the T cell is activated (Fig. 15.8; see Chapter 11). The activated cells then proliferate and undergo clonal expansion and differentiation into effector cells, most of which are short-lived. These effector cells are often said to be "antigen primed,"

 T cell receptor (TCR)   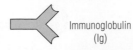 Immunoglobulin (Ig)   Antigen   MHC I

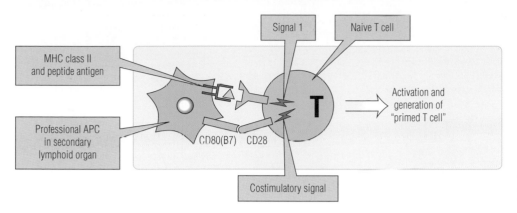

Figure 15.8 Activation of naive T cells. APC, antigen-presenting cell; MHC, major histocompatibility complex.

and this process is referred to as "priming" the T cells. These primed or effector cells undergo several changes, e.g., expression of new cell surface molecules such as CD154 (CD40 ligand) and various adhesion molecules (see Chapters 13 and 16). The effector T cells can move into peripheral tissues and other organs to handle pathogen infection directly, or they can migrate to germinal centers to help to activate B cells with specificity for the same antigen to secrete antibody.

The end result is a vigorous T-cell response and destruction of the pathogen. Most of the activated T cells then die by apoptosis, restoring homeostasis to the T-cell pool. A few effector cells mature into memory T cells, which can respond faster and more effectively on re encountering antigen (see Chapter 17).

Peripheral T-Cell Tolerance

As described earlier, negative selection is used to help generate a self-tolerant, mature, T-cell population. However, because not all self antigens are encountered in the thymus, some self-reactive cells may "escape" from the thymus and appear in the periphery. There are several mechanisms that act in the periphery to ensure that potentially self-reactive T-cell clones that have "escaped" into the periphery are controlled and rendered harmless. For example,

1. If a T cell is specific for a common peripheral antigen, and the T cell is repeatedly stimulated by encountering this antigen, the T cell will undergo apoptosis and be deleted. This mechanism is known as deletion-induced tolerance.
2. If a T-cell encounters the antigen it has specificity for in the absence of a costimulatory signal (CD80/CD28; see Fig. 15.8), the T cell will be rendered functionally inactive. This mechanism is known as clonal anergy.
3. A population of regulatory T cells with apparent specificity for self antigen has been described. These T cells express high amounts of CD25 and appear to be generated both in the periphery and in the thymus. They are capable of suppressing T-cell effector functions via expression of inhibitory cytokines such as IL-10 and transforming growth factor-β (TGF-β). By suppressing

the function of helper T cells recognizing a self-antigen, they effectively induce tolerance for that antigen.

The development of regulatory T cells (T reg) is dependent on a transcription factor, Foxp3. Mutations in Foxp3 result in a multisystem autoimmune disease in humans that is thought to be caused by a reduction in regulatory T-cell numbers.

Mature T-Cell Responses and Functions

After the naive, mature T cell has encountered its cognate antigen-MHC complex and received either a costimulatory signal from a professional APC or stimulation by an appropriate cytokine, it proliferates and differentiates into an effector cell. Cytokines such as IL-2 are also released from the T cell and contribute to the clonal expansion. The CD8+ and CD4+ T-cell subsets can then develop with different effector functions.

By virtue of the different specificities of CD4+ and CD8+ effector T cells, the immune response can monitor extracellular pathogens (e.g., bacteria and parasites; Fig. 15.9 and see Fig. 15.11) and intracellular pathogens (e.g., viruses; Fig. 15.10), respectively. CD4+ T cells monitor MHC class II molecules, which display peptides generated in vesicles (e.g., from extracellular pathogens taken up by phagocytosis), and CD8+ T cells monitor MHC class I molecules, which display peptides generated in the cytoplasm (e.g., from intracellular pathogens such as viruses replicating in the cytoplasm). Nonpeptide antigens can be recognized by γδ T cells. The clinical consequence of a failure to express MHC molecules in the thymus is illustrated in Box 15.2.

CD4+ T Cells

CD4+ T cells recognize antigen displayed on MHC class II molecules (see Chapters 8 and 10). As is discussed in more detail in Chapter 16, CD4+ T cells may differentiate into one of two helper cell subsets (T_H1 or T_H2), depending on the type of immune response taking place and in particular the cytokines present in the environment of the T cell (Fig. 15.11). If the response involves the innate immune system and, for example, macrophages are stimulated by IFN-γ released from NK cells to produce large

 MHC II

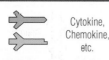 Cytokine, Chemokine, etc.

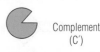 Complement (C')

 Signaling molecule

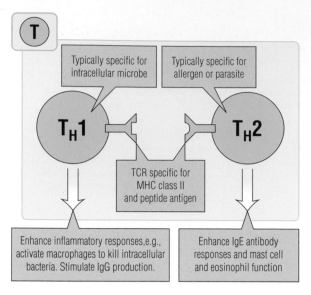

Figure 15.9 The CD4⁺ T cells as effectors in extracellular infections. MHC, major histocompatibility complex; TCR, T-cell receptor.

amounts of IL-12, the environment favors the production of the T_H1 population of CD4⁺ T cells. IL-12 stimulates primed CD4⁺ T cells to differentiate into T_H1 cells. These cells mainly have the role of activating the bactericidal function of macrophages. This is largely accomplished by the release of interferon IFN-γ from T_H1 cells. This cytokine is a potent activator of macrophage phagocytic activity

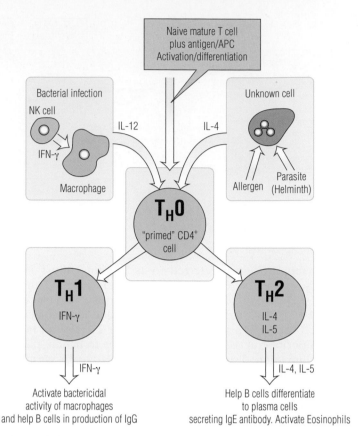

Figure 15.11 The function of the T-helper subsets T_H0, T_H1 and T_H2. APC, antigen-presenting cell; IFN, interferon; IL, interleukin; NK, natural killer.

and thereby helps to enhance the destruction of bacteria and viruses present in the macrophages. In addition, T_H1 cells stimulate B cells to undergo class switching to production of IgG. This antibody has excellent opsonizing properties and therefore also helps to promote microbial clearance through phagocytosis. T_H1 responses may be involved in exacerbations of multiple sclerosis (Box 15.3).

In contrast, an immune response that has little, if any, involvement of innate system—for example, macrophage or NK cell activation—and instead mostly involves lymphocyte activation, can create an environment enriched in IL-4 (e.g., IL-4 released when the host encounters a parasitic worm or allergen), which preferentially stimulates the production of CD4⁺ T-helper cells of the T_H2 subset. These cells are characterized by the release of IL-4 and IL-5, cytokines that stimulate B cells, and enhance antibody class switching toward the production of IgE. These conditions also favor production of eosinophils and mast cells, which can help eliminate parasitic infections.

Chapter 16 provides more information on the T_H1 and T_H2 subsets of CD4⁺ T-helper cells (see Fig. 16.6).

CD8⁺ T Cells (Cytotoxic T Lymphocytes)

Naive CD8⁺ T cells emerge from the thymus. They require further activation and differentiation to become the effector T cells that lyse virally infected target cells and tumor

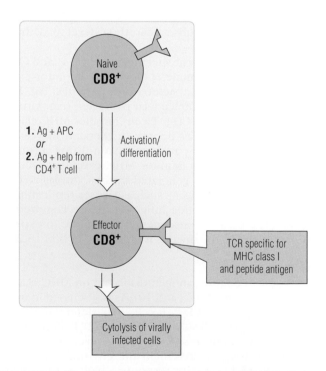

Figure 15.10 The CD8⁺ T cells as effectors in intracellular infections. APC, antigen-presenting cell; MHC, major histocompatibility complex; TCR, T-cell receptor.

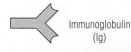 T cell receptor (TCR)   Immunoglobulin (Ig) 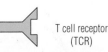 Antigen   MHC I

cells (see Box 15.4). CD8$^+$ T cells recognize antigen displayed on MHC class I molecules. Because MHC class I molecules are found on essentially all nucleated cells of the body, CD8$^+$ T cells can monitor all cells for signs of infection, but they may encounter antigen on a nonprofessional APC. CD8$^+$ T cells are activated to become effector T cells either by encountering antigen on a professional APC and receiving activation signals from both MHC class I and costimulatory molecules (e.g., CD80 (B7)), or by encountering antigen on a non-APC target cell and receiving a "second signal" from cytokines released by CD4$^+$ T-helper cells.

In any event, CD8$^+$ T cells require activation signals from antigen and either costimulatory molecules or cytokines to differentiate into effector CTLs with the function to lyse other cells. The cellular machinery required for cell killing and the mechanisms employed by CTLs to lyse target cells are described in Chapter 21.

The γδ T-Cell Subset

As described earlier in this chapter, γδ TCR-expressing T cells are a minor population (<5%) of all T cells and represent a separate lineage from the αβ T cell. The γδ TCR recognizes antigen very differently from the αβ TCR in that it recognizes certain peptide and nonpeptide antigens without processing and in the absence of MHC class I or II molecules.

The γδ T cell acts as a part of the first line of defense, recognizing microbial invaders in the skin and gut mucosa predominantly. They appear to recognize commonly occurring microbial pathogens.

Their unique ability to recognize some common microbial protein and nonprotein antigens (such as bacterial cell wall phospholipids; see Chapter 7) without processing and presentation distinguishes them from αβ T cells, and this enables them to have a unique protective role in the first line of defense against invading microbes.

 MHC II
  Cytokine, Chemokine, etc.
 Complement (C')
 Signaling molecule

BOX 15.1 Partial Di George Syndrome

As a neonatologist, you are called to the pediatric surgical unit to see an infant who has been diagnosed as having a fistula between the esophagus and trachea and who is having a series of convulsions due to low calcium levels. An incidental finding is the subtly unusual facial appearance, and on chest radiograph, it has been noted that the thymus is absent. This combination is seen in Di George syndrome, where structures derived from the third and fourth pharyngeal pouches do not develop, including the thymus and parathyroid glands (which control blood calcium levels). The infant fortunately does not have any cardiac defects, the other major anomaly associated with Di George syndrome. Further testing shows part of chromosome 22 has been deleted, confirming the diagnosis.

This female infant continues to develop fairly normally. She is observed to have a decreased number of CD3⁺T cells (see flow cytometry figure—Fig 15.12). However, her immunoglobulin levels are normal. She handles normal childhood infections well, and she is not provided any special immunologic treatment. By early adulthood, she is leading a normal life (see clinical photo, Fig. 15.13).

Children with partial Di George syndrome, as in our example, tend to develop fairly normally, provided they do not have other associated problems, such as heart defects. However, patients with complete Di George syndrome suffer from opportunistic infections (e.g., from fungi and viruses) in much the same way as do those with severe combined immunodeficiency disease (SCID; see Chapter 31).

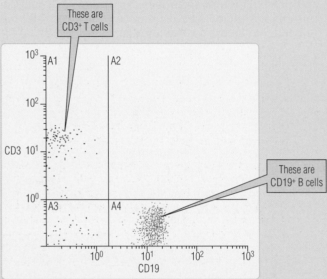

Figure 15.12 Flow cytometric analysis, courtesy of John Hewitt, Immunology, Manchester Royal Infirmary, England. Lymphocytes from a female infant with Di George syndrome. Despite low T-cell numbers this infant survived, as shown in Figure 15.13

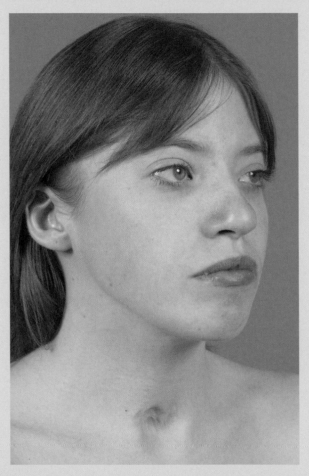

Figure 15.13 Patient with Di George syndrome. Courtesy of Medical Illustration, Manchester Royal Infirmary, England. The picture indicates the subtle "elfin-like" appearance of individuals with this syndrome. The scar is from surgery on the trachea.

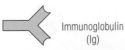 T cell receptor (TCR)

 Immunoglobulin (Ig)

 Antigen

MHC I

BOX 15.2 MHC Class II Antigen Deficiency

The clinical consequences of a lack of major histocompatibility complex (MHC) molecule expression in the thymus can be illustrated by the human immunodeficiency disease known as MHC class II antigen deficiency. Many patients with this autosomal-recessive condition are of North African descent. The patients' B cells (and blood monocytes) lack MHC class II molecules on the cell surface. Those affected by this syndrome exhibit persistent problems with viral and bacterial infections. These patients also exhibit thymic hypoplasia. The lack of MHC class II molecules results in abnormal thymic selection processes and a block in CD4$^+$ T-cell development.

Laboratory analyses show that there are normal numbers of CD8$^+$ T cells but very low levels of CD4$^+$ T cells. The low level of CD4$^+$ T cells creates difficulties in providing T-helper function and this probably explains the hypogammaglobulinemia in these patients, which is present despite normal numbers of B cells.

Detailed molecular genetic analyses have pinpointed the genetic alterations in these patients. The mutations determined so far lie in regulatory genes that affect the expression of MHC class II genes and not in the MHC class II genes themselves.

BOX 15.3 Influence of the Pregnancy-induced Reduction in T-Cell Immune Responses on Multiple Sclerosis

Multiple sclerosis (MS) is an inflammatory demyelinating disease of the central nervous system (CNS). Most patients experience relapsing-remitting disease characterized by periods of disability followed by periods of disease resolution. T-cell-mediated autoimmune responses to CNS components are involved in the development of symptoms, and, while the disease is heterogeneous, the CNS lesions of many patients are infiltrated by macrophages and T cells. The T cells in the MS lesions are primarily of the CD4$^+$ T$_H$1 phenotype, and investigators have postulated that downregulation of the T$_H$1 response may alleviate exacerbations. A recent study of pregnant patients with MS supports this hypothesis.

A prospective study was performed to determine the effects of pregnancy on MS. It was found that MS relapse rates were significantly decreased during the third trimester, then significantly increased at 3 months postpartum. Pregnancy is associated with a reduction in cellular immunity, that is, a reduction in T$_H$1 type responses. Following childbirth, there is a return toward T$_H$1 type responses. Therefore, the changes in immune response during pregnancy correlate with the changes observed in disease symptoms, and support the hypothesis that modulating T$_H$1 type responses in MS patients would improve their lives. These changes in the immune response during pregnancy, when other profound endocrinologic changes also take place, indicate the interrelationship between the immune system and other physiologic systems.

 MHC II

 Cytokine, Chemokine, etc.

  Complement (C')

 Signaling molecule

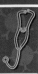

BOX 15.4 Acute Epstein-Barr Virus Infection

Most people have been infected with Epstein-Barr virus (EBV). In the developing world, infection takes place in early childhood, and it is usually asymptomatic. In the developed world, infection is usually delayed until adulthood, and it causes infectious mononucleosis (also known as glandular fever). Symptoms of infectious mononucleosis (IM) include a sore throat, malaise, lymphadenopathy, and, possibly, an enlarged spleen. There may also be malignancy associated with EBV infection, and this complication is discussed in Chapter 34.

From the point of view of the host response, acute EBV is characterized by a massive increase in the number of CD8⁺ T cells in the peripheral blood. The increase appears to be of EBV antigen-specific T cells (Fig. 15.14). Based on studies using a technique for enumerating virus-specific T cells, known as tetramer analysis (see Box 17.1), it has been suggested that the enormous expansion of T cells during acute EBV infection may be a result of the expansion of a few dominant clones of CD8⁺ T cells with specificity for EBV antigens—a so-called oligoclonal expansion.

The original EBV-specific CD8⁺ T cells are generated in the thymus and clonally expanded on contact with EBV antigens in the periphery. EBV infects its target cell, the B cell, for life. Thus, EBV establishes a latent infection. Infected B cells proliferate, although very little free virus is produced. CD4⁺ T cells also respond to acute EBV infection and produce interleukin-6, interferon-γ, and tumor necrosis factor. These cytokines contribute to the fever and fatigue observed in these patients.

An antibody response, mostly immunoglobulin M, is also mounted during acute EBV. The antibody response is not as useful in limiting this infection as the CTL response. The combination of antibody and CD8⁺ CTL, however, reduces, but does not eliminate the infection. Finally, some of the CD4⁺ T and CD8⁺ T cells become memory cells and help in a future response to the virus (Fig. 15.14). This infection is a good example of how the immune system may not always be able to accomplish "sterilizing immunity," but sometimes has to settle for limiting the infection.

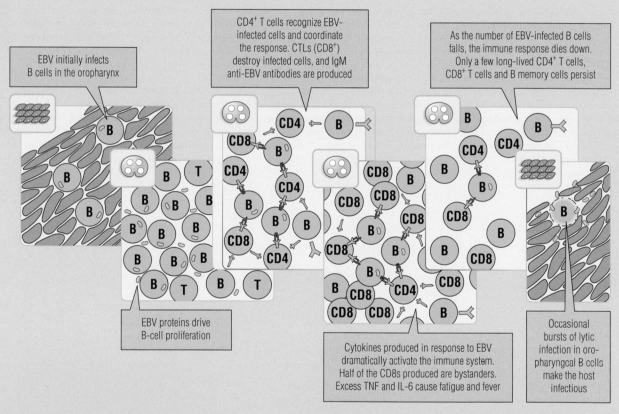

Figure 15.14 Infection with Epstein-Barr virus (EBV) and immune responses. IL, interleukin; TNF, tumor necrosis factor.

 T cell receptor (TCR)   Immunoglobulin (Ig)   Antigen   MHC I

LEARNING POINTS Can You Now ...

1. Recall the role of the thymus in establishing the T-cell repertoire?

2. Draw the major steps in the pathway of T-cell development and indicate the cell surface molecules that are expressed at different stages?

3. List the major cell surface molecules expressed on thymocytes at different stages of development and indicate their function?

4. Compare positive and negative selection?

5. Draw the events involved in naive T-cell activation?

6. Recall the mechanisms used to generate central and peripheral tolerance in T cells?

7. List the functional properties of different T-cell subsets?

8. Compare and contrast the roles of $\gamma\delta$ and $\alpha\beta$ T cells?

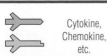 MHC II

 Cytokine, Chemokine, etc.

Complement (C')

Signaling molecule

16 Cell-Cell Interaction in Generating Effector Lymphocytes

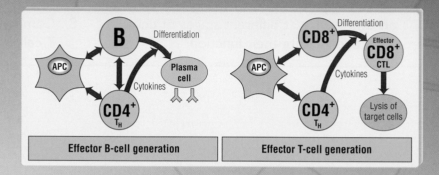

Some of the basic concepts of cell-cell interaction and cooperation in immune responses were introduced in Chapter 2. We also learned, in Chapters 7 and 8, how T-cell receptors (TCRs) recognize antigen only when presented by major histocompatibility complex (MHC) molecules on antigen-presenting cells (APCs) (an example of the requirement for cell-cell interaction in generating an immune response). In addition, the need for costimulatory signals provided by interaction with other cells for the full activation of B and T lymphocytes was introduced as a concept in Chapter 11 and further discussed in Chapter 15. At this point, it is appropriate to bring these concepts together and, as illustrated in the overview figure above, to explain the critical role of cell-cell interaction in generating the signals required to produce effector B cells (plasma cells) and effector T cells (T-helper cells and cytotoxic T lymphocytes [CTLs]).

■ GENERATION OF STIMULATED (OR PRIMED) B AND T CELLS

Foreign antigen, collected at sites of infection, is typically brought to secondary lymphoid organs, such as the spleen and lymph nodes (see Chapter 13), by dendritic cells (DCs). Naive B and T cells circulate through the lymphoid organs and monitor for the presence of antigen (see Chapter 13). Cytokines released by activated DCs and other APCs (such as macrophages) can function as signals of infection and stimulate circulating leukocytes to adhere to high endothelial venules (HEVs), extravasate, and transmigrate into the secondary lymphoid tissue (see Chapter 12). This proc-

ess brings B and T cells into proximity with APCs bearing foreign antigen and stops their migration. B cells with a B-cell receptor (BCR) that is specific for available antigen then take up the antigen via receptor-mediated endocytosis (see Chapter 10). Antigen processing takes place with the eventual display of antigenic peptides on the B-cell surface in association with MHC class II molecules (see Chapter 10; Fig. 16.1). In this regard, B cells can function as APCs for T cells.

T cells constantly scan for APCs displaying appropriate MHC-antigenic peptide complexes; when they are detected, a T cell–APC cell-cell interaction takes place. Contact with an MHC-foreign peptide antigen complex results in signaling through the TCR (see Chapter 11), which, in addition to activating biochemical pathways in the cell, strengthens the adhesive bond between the cells by inducing expression of cell adhesion proteins. Some of the most important receptor-ligand pairs involved in the T cell–APC interaction are illustrated in Figure 16.2. The stable interaction between a T cell and an APC, such as in Figure 16.2, is sometimes referred to as conjugate formation. After antigen recognition, there is a redistribution of molecules in the membranes of the respective cells. The cell's cytoskeleton proteins are actively involved in redistribution of transmembrane proteins in the lipid bilayer of the cell surface membrane so that receptor-ligand pairs migrate into the area of close contact between the cells, and form a supramolecular cluster known as the **immunological synapse**. Among the molecules that form the synapse are those shown in Figures 16.2 and 16.3—for example, TCR, CD4 or CD8, lymphocyte function-associated antigen 1 (LFA-1), CD28, CD154 on the T cell and MHC,

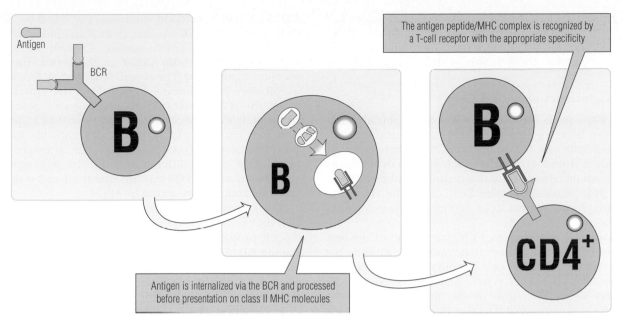

The antigen peptide/MHC complex is recognized by a T-cell receptor with the appropriate specificity

Antigen is internalized via the BCR and processed before presentation on class II MHC molecules

Figure 16.1 B-cell presentation of antigen to T-helper (T$_H$) cells.

intercellular adhesion molecule 1 (ICAM-1), CD80, and CD40 on the APC.

Lymphocyte-DC interactions take place in the T-cell zone of a secondary lymphoid organ, for example, of a draining lymph node (see Chapter 13) At this point, we have reached the stage where there are activated B and T cells, specific for the same antigen, in the same zone of a lymph node.

■ GENERATION OF EFFECTOR CELLS

A major activity of CD4$^+$ T helper (T$_H$) cells is the release of cytokines. Cytokines released from T$_H$ cells can help drive the immune response in the direction of immunoglobulin (Ig)E antibody synthesis—a T$_H$2 response—or in the direction of enhanced bactericidal activity of macrophages and IgG synthesis—a T$_H$1 response. Box 16.1 provides

Figure 16.2 The major cell-surface molecules involved in the interaction of T cells with antigen-presenting cells (APCs). ICAM-1, intercellular adhesion molecule 1; LFA-1, leukocyte function-associated antigen 1.

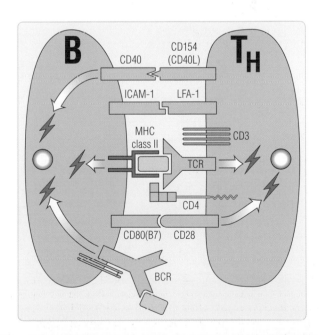

Figure 16.3 Formation of a B cell–T-cell conjugate. ICAM-1, intercellular adhesion molecule 1; LFA-1, leukocyte function-associated antigen 1.

 MHC II

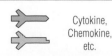 Cytokine, Chemokine, etc.

 Complement (C′)

 Signaling molecule

a description of cytokine expression by these T-helper sub-sets. Box 16.2 provides an example of the difference that a preponderance of a T_H1 response rather than a T_H2 response can make to the outcome of an infection (leprosy).

CD4⁺ T_H Interaction with B Cells

B cells expressing MHC class II-antigenic peptide complexes can be recognized by CD4⁺ T_H cells and a B-cell–T-cell conjugate (see Fig. 16.3) forms. Next, there is release of cytokines from the T cell, and delivery of costimulatory signals from membrane-bound receptor-ligand pairs. These signals, plus signals from the BCR, cause the B cells to differentiate into plasma cells secreting IgM (a primary response).

As discussed in Chapters 13 and 14, some of the activated B cells do not differentiate into plasma cells but instead initiate formation of a germinal center in the lymphoid follicles. These B cells have received a costimulatory activation signal by virtue of the interaction between CD40 on the B cell and CD154 (formerly known as CD40L or CD40 ligand) on the T cell. CD154-CD40 interaction, and the resulting costimulatory signal delivered to the B cell, are required for the transition from a B cell producing a low-affinity IgM response to a B cell producing a high-affinity antibody of a different class (e.g., IgG). Prevention of CD154–CD40 interaction leads to greatly diminished antibody responses to typical protein antigens.

Figure 16.4 illustrates the steps in B-cell–T-cell interaction leading to a secondary immune response. Stimulation of the T cell through the TCR induces CD154 on the T cell.

CD154–CD40 interaction stimulates the B cell (or APC) to induce expression of another critical costimulatory molecule on the B cell (APC) surface: CD80(B7). The CD80 molecule interacts with CD28 on the T cell (they are a receptor-ligand pair). The signal delivered by CD28 to the T cell after it encounters CD80(B7) is the critical signal along with TCR signal transduction that causes activation of the gene for interleukin (IL)-2 and eventual T_H proliferation (see Fig. 16.4). CD80 molecules are only found on professional APCs (see Chapter 2) such as macrophages, activated B cells, and dendritic cells. The requirement for costimulation via CD28 ensures that the T cell is only activated by antigens presented by APCs.

The costimulatory receptor-ligand pairs CD40-CD154 (CD40L) and CD80(B7)-CD28 act synergistically to enable T_H-cell proliferation. A mutation in the human gene encoding CD154 exists, and this causes a syndrome known as X-linked hyper-IgM. This disease (Box 16.3) demonstrates the critical role of the CD40–CD154 interaction in the response to T-dependent antigens (see Chapter 14).

Proliferation of T_H2 cells helps the germinal center B cells to differentiate into plasma cells secreting a higher affinity and different class of immunoglobulin than the low-affinity IgM typical of the primary response. For example, IL-4 released from T_H2 cells causes class switching (see Chapters 6 and 14) to IgE production.

The germinal center B cells are subject to rapid somatic mutation in their variable region gene segments and they undergo selection to retain those that have a higher affinity immunoglobulin (affinity maturation; see Chapter 14). Class switching may then occur, and a high-affinity immuno-

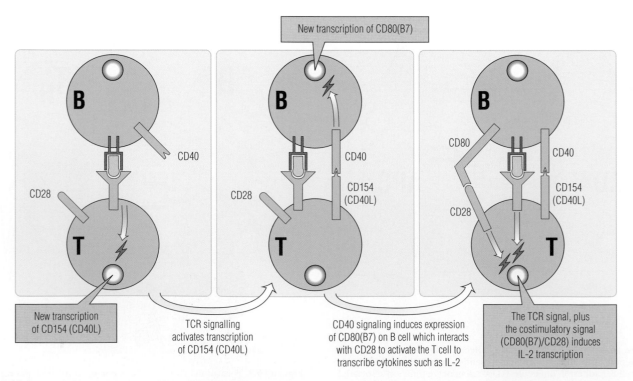

Figure 16.4 Costimulatory signals in B–T interactions.

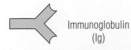

globulin of the IgG, IgA, or IgE type can be produced. These plasma cells then secrete antibody until the antigen is eliminated or until they die. Plasma cells typically survive from a few days up to a few weeks.

A few of the activated germinal center B cells become long-lived quiescent memory B cells, as described in Chapter 17. Similarly, some of the activated T cells become memory T cells (see Chapter 17). Subsequent encounter with antigen by these memory cells leads to a more rapid, and more effective, secondary, tertiary, or subsequent, immune response.

CD4$^+$ T$_H$ Interaction with CD8$^+$ T Cells

CD8$^+$ CTLs kill virally infected cells and tumor cells, among others. CD8$^+$ T cells require activation signals before they can differentiate into effector CTLs with the full range of cytotoxic granule proteins, perforin and other molecules required to kill a target cell (see also Chapter 21). The required activation signals are recognition of antigen (i.e., MHC-viral antigenic peptide complexes) and costimulatory signals from virus-specific CD4$^+$ T$_H$ cells. This is another example of the requirement for cell-cell interaction to generate an immune response, in this case a cell-mediated immune response. As shown in Figure 16.5, CD4$^+$ T$_H$ cells recognize viral antigen displayed on APCs; activation of the CD4$^+$ T$_H$ cell causes release of IL-2, which stimulates viral antigen-specific CD8$^+$ T cells. TCR recognition of viral antigen, plus a second signal via the IL-2 receptor (IL-2R) (see Fig. 16.5), stimulates differentiation of the CD8$^+$ T cell into an effector CTL, capable of cell

killing on encountering a virally infected target cell. CTLs kill target cells by exchanging granule contents and eventually inducing apoptosis (see Chapter 21).

■ PROVIDING THE MOST APPROPRIATE IMMUNE RESPONSE FOR A GIVEN PATHOGEN

The cell-cell interaction and cooperation described earlier allows the immune system to make the appropriate response for a particular pathogen. For example, a pathogen (e.g., a virus), multiplying in the cytoplasm of any given cell, will generate peptide antigens that are carried to the cell surface by MHC class I molecules (see Chapter 10). CD8$^+$ T cells with appropriate TCRs will encounter the MHC class I–viral antigen complex and be activated, eventually becoming mature effector CTLs capable of killing the virally infected cell (see Fig. 16.5).

By comparison, peptide antigens derived from pathogens growing in intracellular vesicles of macrophages, or peptide antigens derived from ingested toxins or extracellular microbes, will be picked up and carried to the cell surface by MHC class II molecules (see Chapter 10). Because MHC class II molecules are scanned by CD4$^+$ T cells, T cells of the T$_H$1 or T$_H$2 subsets may be activated. If T$_H$1 cells are generated, these cells will either activate the bactericidal action of macrophages through release of interferon-γ (IFN-γ) or cause B cells to switch to IgG synthesis, thereby facilitating opsonization and clearance

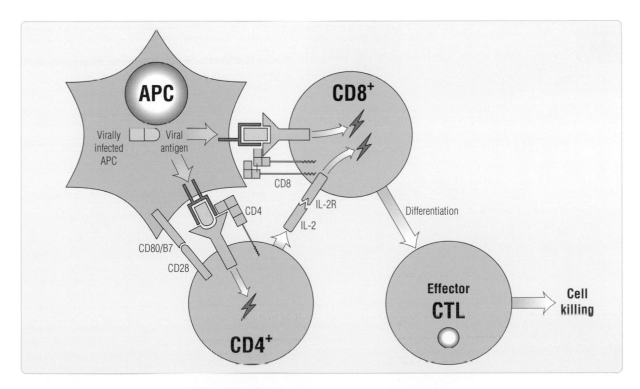

Figure 16.5 Interaction of CD4$^+$ T cells and CD8$^+$ T cells in the maturation of effector cytotoxic T cells.

 MHC II

 Cytokine, Chemokine, etc.

 Complement (C')

 Signaling molecule

of extracellular bacteria. If T_H2 cells are activated, they can activate B cells to make IgE antibody, and activate mast cells and eosinophils to aid in parasite elimination. Consequently, infection by viruses or intracellular bacteria tends to result in production of cytokines that favor the generation of T_H1 cells (Fig. 16.6). The T_H1 cells are then able to activate the appropriate protective response—that

is, macrophages or CTLs. Parasitic infections (e.g., worms) generate cytokines that favor T_H2 cell production. The T_H2 cells are then able to activate mast cells or eosinophils, or cause B cells to switch to IgE synthesis and thereby generate an appropriate protective response resulting in elimination of the worm (parasite).

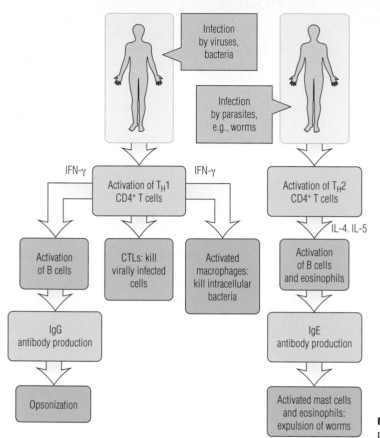

Figure 16.6 T-cell subsets and their role in responses to different pathogens.

 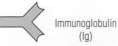 T cell receptor (TCR)   Immunoglobulin (Ig)   Antigen   MHC I

BOX 16.1 Cytokine Expression by Human CD4⁺ T-cell Subsets

As we have seen in Section III of this book, the activities of CD4$^+$ T cells can be critical in mediating effector cell function in the immune response. For example, CD4$^+$ T cells help B cells to differentiate into antibody-secreting plasma cells, and CD4$^+$ T cells provide stimuli for the differentiation of CD8$^+$ T cells into CTLs capable of killing virally infected cells. The CD4$^+$ T cells mediate their activities via cytokine release and by cell-cell contact, with the involvement of receptor-ligand pairs that activate signal transduction pathways. Given that cytokine production is such an important aspect of CD4$^+$ T-cell function, extensive studies to characterize the cytokines released by CD4$^+$ T cells have been carried out. CD4$^+$ T cells can be separated into two distinct subsets—the T helper 1 (T_H1) and T helper 2 (T_H2) subsets—on the basis of the cytokines they express. It should be noted that these designations are based on in vitro analyses. It is also important to note that although human T cells can be separated into T_H1 and T_H2 subsets, the distinction between T_H1 and T_H2 cells in terms of cytokine profiles is less clear in humans than in mice. Figure 16.7 lists the cytokines that predominate in each subset in humans.

Cytokines such as interferon-γ (IFN-γ) and tumor necrosis factor-β (TNF-β) enhance CD8$^+$ cytotoxic T cells and activate macrophages and natural killer cells. IFN-γ also facilitates B cell switching to IgG production and because IgG is an efficient opsonizing antibody, this also facilitates bacterial clearance. IL-4 and IL-5, however, activate B cells and eosinophils and induce IgE-type responses. T_H2 cells are dominant in parasitic infections (e.g., worms) and allergy. T_H1 cells are dominant in responses to microbial infection. Subset-specific cytokines can also have regulatory effects on the other subset; for example, IFN-γ inhibits the generation of T_H2 cells and IL-4 inhibits the generation of T_H1 cells.

FIG. 16.7 Cytokine Expression by Activated Human CD4⁺ T-Cell Subsets

Cytokine	T_H1	T_H2
Interferon-γ	+	-
Tumor necrosis factor β (lymphotoxin)	+	-
Interleukin 4	-	+
Interleukin 5	-	+

 MHC II   Cytokine, Chemokine, etc.   Complement (C')   Signaling molecule

BOX 16.2 Leprosy

A few years after arriving in the Midwestern United States from Asia, a 35-year-old man (A.M.) presented at the local teaching hospital emergency department with multiple nodules and lesions on the arms, hands, and buttocks. These lesions had been present for more than 1 year but now he was also experiencing considerable loss of sensation in his hands, and had been having difficulty functioning in his job as a waiter in a busy restaurant in Chicago. A skin biopsy demonstrated acid-fast bacilli that were identified as *Mycobacterium leprae*. Further examination by hematoxylin and eosin staining of tissue taken from an arm lesion showed numerous bacteria in macrophage-like cells (Fig. 16.8), as well as disseminated infection into local nerves. Leprosy was diagnosed, and treatment begun with the drugs dapsone, rifampicin, and clofazimine. After about 12 months of this drug treatment regimen, A.M.'s lesions and neurologic symptoms were substantially reduced. The final diagnosis was borderline lepromatous leprosy.

There are several forms of leprosy (see Fig. 16.8). Often, as in the case described, the disease is somewhere in between the two polar extremes, tuberculoid leprosy, and lepromatous leprosy. The immune status of the individual seems to determine the outcome of infection by *M. leprae*. In an individual where the immune system is triggered in the direction of a T_H2-type response (i.e., IgE antibody production, IL-4 cytokine release and little cell-mediated immunity) then lepromatous leprosy (see Fig 16.8A) results. In this form of the disease, infection is widely disseminated, the antibody response is ineffective, and the bacilli continue to grow in macrophages. In the absence of drug treatment, there is a poor clinical picture with extensive damage to connective tissues and peripheral nerve tissue.

On the other hand, in an individual who triggers a T_H1 response to infection by *M. leprae* the organism is substantially localized to macrophages, and bacterial growth is controlled by the T_H1 T cells that activate macrophage killing of the bacilli. In this so-called tuberculoid form (see Fig. 16.8B) of the disease, there is usually a less severe clinical picture, especially if there is drug treatment. In tuberculoid leprosy, there is some inflammation and granuloma formation with localized peripheral nervous tissue damage but nothing as severe as in the lepromatous form of the disease.

More often than not, leprosy presents as intermediate between the two extremes of tuberculoid and lepromatous, as in the case of A.M. What produces the different forms of leprosy in different individuals is not clear. However, this organism can cause two very different disease outcomes, depending on the type of immune response that is triggered in the infected host.

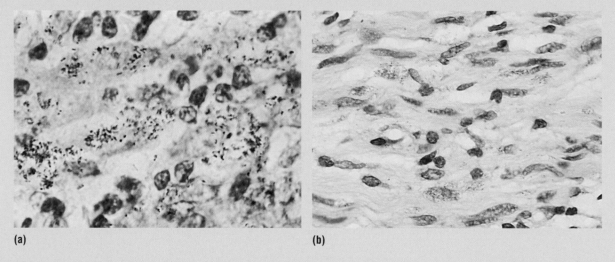

(a)   (b)

Figure 16.8 Leprosy. (A) A biopsy from a patient with lepromatous leprosy. There are many mycobacteria but very little immune reaction. (With permission from Cotran RS, Kumar V, Collins T: Pathologic Basis of Disease, 6th ed. St. Louis: WB Saunders, 1998.) (B) In tuberculoid leprosy, there are far fewer mycobacteria but much more reaction in the form of macrophages and T cells. (Courtesy of Professor Umberto De Girolami, Brigham & Women's Hospital, Boston.) Compare this with Figure 22.5 showing *M. tuberculosis* infection.

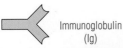 T cell receptor (TCR)   Immunoglobulin (Ig)   Antigen   ⊥ MHC I

BOX 16.3 B-Cell–T-Cell Interaction: CD40-CD154 and X-Linked Hyper-IgM Syndrome

A 10-month-old child had a series of bacterial chest and sinus infections since he was about 6 months of age. He was found to have low IgG and IgA but high IgM. These abnormalities are consistent with the hyper-IgM syndrome, and the diagnosis was confirmed when his T cells were shown not to express CD154 (CD40 ligand). He can only produce IgM because his T cells are unable to offer appropriate help to induce B cells to switch Ig class. He was started on Ig replacement and responded well, with a decreased frequency of chest and sinus infectious. Hyper-IgM syndrome also affects T-cell function: because CD154 is absent, T cells cannot communicate normally with APCs.

Boys with hyper-IgM syndrome are especially vulnerable to protozoal infections of the liver and gastrointestinal tract. At the age of 8 years, this child showed evidence of infection with *Cryptosporidium*. Fortunately, he has a sister with an identical human leukocyte antigen (HLA) type and she was able to act as a bone marrow donor for the patient (see Chapter 33). This is a prolonged and unpleasant procedure, but it was his only hope of improving T-cell function. Over the next few months, his condition improved steadily (Fig. 16.9), and at the age of 11 years he was competing in national skiing championships!

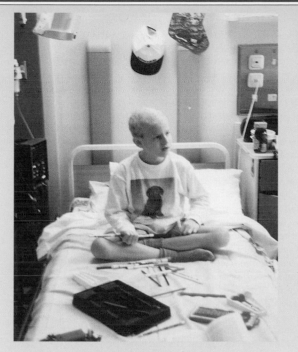

Figure 16.9 A boy with hyper-IgM syndrome recovering from bone marrow transplant. His hair loss is a consequence of the conditioning chemotherapy required for BMT (see Chapter 33).

 MHC II

 Cytokine, Chemokine, etc.

Complement (C')

 Signaling molecule

BOX 16.4 Exploiting Our Knowledge of B-T Cooperation to Prevent Bacterial Meningitis with a Conjugate Vaccine

Until the advent, in about 1990, of national vaccination programs that utilized a conjugate vaccine, meningitis caused by the bacterial pathogen *Haemophilus influenzae B* was a serious concern. The disease peaks in infants of 10 to 11 months of age, because until about ages 18 to 24 months, children are unable to mount the effective T-independent response required for protection against the bacterial pathogen, and in severe cases there may be neurologic damage, or even death. The original vaccine was a purified capsular polysaccharide, a T-independent antigen that did not function well in infants younger than the age of about 20 months. Consideration of the knowledge immunologists had gained about T-dependent immune responses, and about B cell–T cell cooperation in immune responses, led to the development of a vaccine in which the bacterial polysaccharide was coupled covalently to a protein. This conjugate vaccine (so-called Hib vaccine) induced far better responses than the unconjugated vaccine, even in very young children. Several proteins have been used for the conjugate, including the protein component of tetanus toxoid. In countries where this conjugate vaccine is being used, the incidence of meningitis has dramatically declined.

In the United States, the incidence of meningitis declined by approximately 80% 1 year after introduction of the national Hib vaccination program, and since 1993, the incidence of Hib-mediated meningitis has declined by 95% in US children younger than the age of 5 years.

The theory behind the vaccine is that B cells with immunoglobulin receptors for the bacterial capsular polysaccharide component of the vaccine take up the conjugate by receptor-mediated endocytosis. The protein component of the conjugate can then be processed and presented on the surface of the B cell associated with MHC class II molecules. The MHC class II–vaccine peptide complex can then be recognized by a T_H cell of the appropriate specificity. The T_H cell then activates the B cell to make antibody against the bacterial polysaccharide. The general principle is as illustrated in Figure 16.10, except that the "antigen" is a conjugate of a B-cell epitope (the polysaccharide component) and a T-cell epitope (the tetanus toxoid protein). The structure of the vaccine and its interaction with the B cell is illustrated in Figure 16.10.

The conjugate Hib vaccine has been so successful that other glycoconjugate vaccines (covalent conjugates of a bacterial capsular polysaccharide antigen and a protein) have been developed, and more are in development to help control encapsulated bacteria that cause infectious disease. For example, a pneumococcal conjugate vaccine has shown considerable success and a meningococcal polysaccharide—diptheria-toxoid conjugate vaccine was approved for use in the United States in 2005. These vaccines, based on polysaccharide-protein conjugates, offer promise of a more effective response to certain infectious diseases.

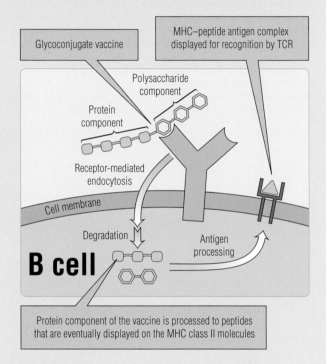

Figure 16.10 B-cell processing of a glycoconjugate vaccine.

LEARNING POINTS Can You Now ...

1. Describe how naive B and T cells are primed by cell-cell interactions with antigen-presenting cells?

2. Draw the cell-cell interactions involved in the generation of plasma cells and memory B cells?

3. Draw the cell-cell interactions involved in the generation of cytotoxic T lymphocytes (CTLs)?

4. Describe the difference between a T_H1 response and a T_H2 response in terms of disease outcome?

5. Describe how a glycoconjugate vaccine induces a protective response?

  T cell receptor (TCR)   Immunoglobulin (Ig)   Antigen   MHC I

CHAPTER 17

Immunological Memory

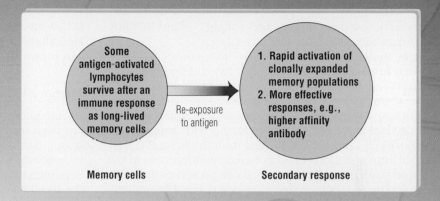

Some antigen-activated lymphocytes survive after an immune response as long-lived memory cells

Re-exposure to antigen

1. Rapid activation of clonally expanded memory populations
2. More effective responses, e.g., higher affinity antibody

Memory cells **Secondary response**

One of the hallmarks of the adaptive immune system is that it "remembers" previous encounters with antigen (see Chapter 2). As shown in the overview figure above, in this chapter we describe how memory cells are established and how the memory response is generated, and explain the advantages of immunologic memory to the individual who re-encounters a pathogen. Immune memory is very important in protection from infectious agents. Immune memory allows the host to initiate the **secondary immune response** on subsequent encounters with a pathogen. This secondary immune response was initially discussed in Chapter 2 and allows the immune system to make a more vigorous (e.g., more antibody production) and a more effective response (e.g., higher affinity specific antibody) on re-exposure to previously encountered antigens (Figs. 17.1 and 2.4).

As described in Chapters 2 and 4 (see also Chapter 24), vaccination takes advantage of immunologic memory. Vaccines against infectious diseases, such as smallpox and poliomyelitis, have been some of the most important achievements of medical science. Vaccines, along with improved hygiene and sanitation, have saved countless lives, and they have been responsible for dramatically improving the quality of life for literally millions of people throughout the world. However, although great successes have come from taking advantage of the existence of immunologic memory, we still have much to understand about how immunologic memory is established and maintained. In this chapter, we present a summary of what is most important about long-term immunologic memory.

LONG-TERM IMMUNOLOGICAL MEMORY

Long-term immunological memory refers to the capacity to generate an enhanced and more effective immune response to an antigen that was last encountered some considerable time ago. Long-term memory is thought to result from the presence of clonally expanded, antigen-specific B and T lymphocytes that persist in a resting state for many years and, in some cases, life-long. For example, vaccinia virus-specific T cells have been demonstrated in individuals vaccinated up to 50 years ago. Studies of human populations living in isolated island communities have shown antibody-mediated protection against measles virus that persisted for more than 65 years.

It has been difficult to distinguish memory cells unequivocally from other lymphocytes, although there is now general agreement that there is a memory cell phenotype with both qualitative and quantitative differences from other lymphocytes (Fig. 17.2).

Memory B Cells

Naive B cells when activated by antigen differentiate into effector B cells (plasma cells) that secrete antibody (see Chapter 14). In a primary response, the plasma cells secrete an immunoglobulin (Ig)M antibody of relatively low affinity, whereas in a secondary response a higher affinity antibody, usually of a different class (i.e., IgG, IgA, or IgE), is secreted. Somatic hypermutation takes place during the

FIG. 17.1 Contrasting Aspects of Primary and Subsequent Antibody Immune Responses*

	Primary Response	Subsequent Response
Time period to response (days)	5–10	1–3
Major antibody class	IgM	IgH (IgA or IgE)[†]
Affinity for antigen	Low	High

*Activated B cells differentiate to become memory B cells, which, on re-encountering antigen, can generate a faster, and more effective, protective antibody immune response
[†]Usually the antibody is IgG. However, depending on the nature of the antigen and the route of antigen entry, the response may be IgA or IgE (see Chapter 14)

secondary response to generate a higher-affinity binding site for antigen (see Chapters 6 and 14).

It is thought to be likely that the memory B cell is derived from an activated B cell that has undergone genetic changes (somatic hypermutation) in variable region *V* gene segment DNA to create a more effective antibody (Fig. 17.3). Clearly, this cell is qualitatively different from the original naive cell that first reacted with antigen. This memory cell can be distinguished from the naive B cell by the somatic mutations that have created differences in the Ig gene sequences. The memory B cell preserves the more useful antigen receptor that has been derived by sequential somatic genetic changes. On subsequent exposure to antigen, it is this memory cell that responds, not another naive cell. Evidence that this is true comes from the following observation. Individuals exposed to a pathogen early in life—for example, measles virus—respond to the same epitopes on the pathogen when re-exposed later in life, and they do not respond to new epitopes present on the pathogen, even though they are antigenic. This observation is consistent with secondary and subsequent exposure to antigen activating preexisting memory cells rather than inducing the differentiation of new naive cells. The advantage to the host is that a secondary response

(i.e., a more rapid and higher affinity response) is generated, allowing the infection to be eliminated sooner than if a new primary response were generated.

Memory T Cells

Unambiguously defining the memory phenotype of T cells has been much more difficult than for B cells. Part of the reason for this has been that the genes for the T-cell receptor do not undergo the qualitative changes, somatic hypermutation, and class switching, that occur in genes for the B-cell receptors (immunoglobulins). However, a memory T-cell effect has been observed. There is a quicker, more efficient T-cell response on subsequent exposure to antigen, and the number of T cells that respond to antigen is increased.

With respect to T cells, it has been observed that there is a subset of T cells that is similar to effector CD4+ or CD8+ T cells, but has some differences (see Fig. 17.2), and overall has a phenotype consistent with a memory T cell. Defining marker proteins that distinguish unambiguously between naive, effector, and memory T cells has been very difficult. There are differences in cell-surface proteins, perhaps the most significant being changes in certain cell-adhesion

FIG. 17.2 Phenotype of Memory Cells

	Memory Cell	Naive Cell	Effector Cell
B lymphocytes			
Response time to antigenic stimulation	Fast	Slow	Responding
Antigen receptor: Immunoglobulin class expressed	IgG (IgA or IgE)	IgM	IgG (IgA or IgE)
Affinity of antibody secreted	High	Low	Increases during response
Effector function	None	None	Antibody secretion
T lymphocytes			
Response time to antigenic stimulation	Fast	Slow	Responding
Expression of L-selectin (CD62L), the receptor that facilitates homing to peripheral lymph nodes	Variable	High	Low
Recirculation pattern	Circulate through tissues for which they have homing receptors then migrate to site(s) of infection	Constantly circulates from blood to lymph nodes and other lymphoid organs to scan for antigen	Migrates to site(s) of infection, usually in the periphery
			Help (cytokine release) or target-cell killing
Effector function	None	None	

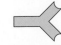
T cell receptor (TCR)

Immunoglobulin (Ig)

Antigen

MHC I

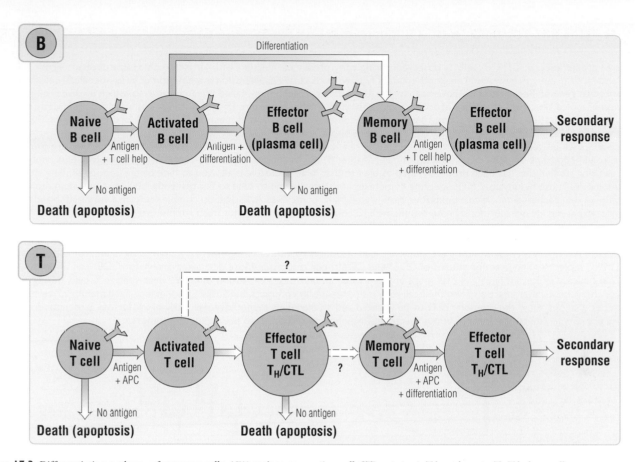

Figure 17.3 Differentiation pathway of memory cells. APC, antigen-presenting cell; CTL, cytotoxic T lymphocyte; T$_H$, T helper cell.

molecules. The adhesion molecule, L-selectin (see Chapter 13), is expressed at high levels on naive T cells but is generally found at a much lower level on most T cells of a memory phenotype. This may help to explain the observation (see Chapter 13) that T cells with a memory phenotype recirculate between blood and tissues, whereas naive T cells recirculate between blood and lymph nodes.

A technique known as the tetramer assay (Box 17.1) can visualize and enumerate T cells based on their binding to specific fluorescent MHC-peptide antigen complexes. This is being used to improve characterization of subsets of antigen-specific T cells. This technology will undoubtedly also help in the characterization of memory T cells and their distinction from naive or effector T cells.

■ LYMPHOCYTE HOMEOSTASIS

Given that it is possible for us to retain immunologic memory of every foreign antigen encounter we have ever had, even if the number of memory cells generated in each immune response were small (and it is usually substantial!), there would eventually be an issue of availability of appropriate body sites to maintain and nurture these cells. The blood and lymphoid tissues have space for only a

finite number of cells! Fortunately, like other lymphocytes, most memory cells appear to die eventually—probably by programmed cell death (**apoptosis**). The mechanisms involved in apoptosis are further described later and in detail in Chapter 21. Cell death maintains a balance (homeostasis) between the need for vast clonal expansion of lymphocytes in primary responses to new antigens, and the need for maintaining memory cells, with the limited number of suitable sites for lymphocytes.

The concept that is currently favored by immunologists with regard to lymphocyte homeostasis and the persistence of memory cells is as follows. Most activated effector cells die as antigen is eliminated. Clones of antigen-specific memory cells survive for longer periods. For these memory cells to survive, they need to compete for space in a nurturing environment with available growth factors (e.g., cytokines). Given that these are in finite supply, it is possible that memory cells from some antigenic encounters do not survive long-term. Conceivably, some memory cells are better adapted for survival under these conditions. For example, they have a reduced need for cytokines/growth factors and, therefore, they are more competitive in terms of ability to survive. This could mean that immunologic memory of some antigens may be more stable than memory of some other antigens.

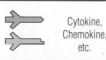 MHC II

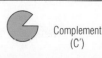 Cytokine, Chemokine, etc.

Complement (C')

 Signaling molecule

BOX 17.1 In Situ Detection of T-cell Immunity

Extensive proliferation of CD8+ T cells is observed during early phases of infection with viruses such as Epstein-Barr virus (EBV) and HIV. Recently, experimental attempts to identify how much of this proliferation is a function of virus-specific T cells, as opposed to general T-cell activation, have been made. Relatively new technology, called tetramer analysis, which involves using fluorescent-labeled tetramers of major histocompatibility complex (MHC) molecules (Fig. 17.4) to stain specific T cells directly, and allows direct visualization of tetramer-stained cells by flow cytometry, suggests that as much as 10% to 20% of the activated CD8+ T cells can be virus-specific in certain situations.

Once an exact antigenic peptide/MHC molecule binding relationship has been established, tetramer-MHC complexes are prepared as follows. Soluble domains of MHC class I molecules (see Chapter 8) are biotinylated on the C-terminus of the molecule. A peptide from the virus being studied that has been predetermined to bind to that MHC molecule is allowed to bind to the peptide-binding cleft of the MHC molecule. These biotinylated MHC-peptide complexes are then allowed to bind to fluorescently labeled streptavidin molecules in a 4:1 ratio, so that each avidin molecule binds four biotinylated MHC complexes. Avidin-biotin complexes form a very tight bond that survives most experimental manipulations. These tetramer-MHC complexes are mixed with fresh lymphocytes and bind tightly to T-cell receptors expressed on T cells that are specific for the MHC-peptide combination. For example, if the peptide was an EBV peptide, the cells responding specifically to EBV would bind the tetramer and could be visualized and enumerated by flow cytometry (see Chapter 5).

The use of tetramers is revolutionizing the study of T-cell responses to infection. Tetramers are now being made from both class I and class II MHC molecules and used for studies of CD8+ and CD4+ T-cell responses. More data are available for CD8+ cell responses at this time. One clinically important finding is that there appears to be an enormous expansion of CD8+ virus-specific T cells during the first 7 days, or thereabouts, after infection. Then the T-cell response dramatically contracts, and finally a pool of long-lived memory T cells remains.

Tetramer analyses allow the memory cells to be isolated and studied. This technology will likely allow further understanding of the memory phenotype as well as inform us about cytotoxic T-lymphocyte responses to pathogens and tumors.

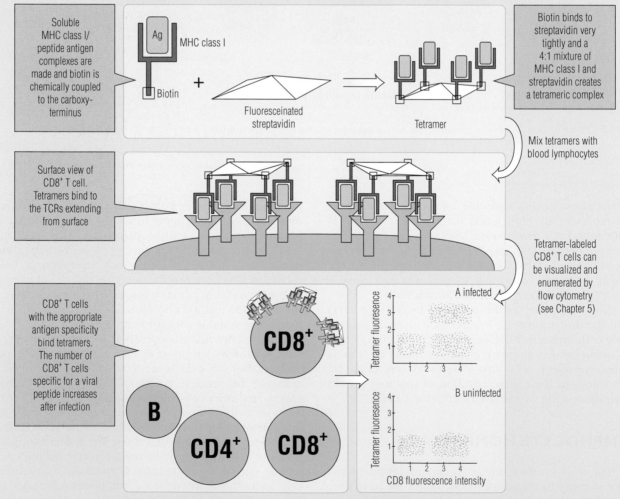

Figure 17.4 Tetramer assay to identify T cells. Tetramers (four base units) bind to T-cell receptors (TCRs), thus linking the presence of TCR on a cell with fluorescent intensity. Flow cytometry can then assess cell number. There is clearly a new population of T cells in viral infection (**A**) compared with the uninfected state (**B**). The flow cytometric analysis shows that there are more CD8+ cells binding the fluorescent tetramer in the infected sample. Ag, antigen; MHC, major histocompatibility complex.

 T cell receptor (TCR)

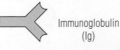 Immunoglobulin (Ig)

 Antigen

 MHC I

■ APOPTOSIS

Apoptosis is triggered through receptor-ligand interactions —mainly the Fas-Fas ligand interaction (Fig. 17.5). Binding of Fas ligand (e.g., expressed on a killer T cell) to Fas (e.g., expressed on a target cell) triggers a cascade of intracellular biochemical changes in the target cell. Fas interacts with several proteins in the "death pathway" eventually to activate a proteolytic enzyme known as **caspase**. Caspase is critical in activating several more proteolytic enzymes in the caspase cascade. This proteolytic cascade is somewhat analogous to the kinase cascade of cell activation (see Chapter 11). The critical step of the caspase cascade is activation of a cytoplasmic enzyme, caspase-activatable DNAse (CAD), which can then migrate to the nucleus and cleave DNA into the small fragments that are a characteristic end point of apoptosis (see Fig. 17.5 and Chapter 21).

Several genes have been found to promote cell death, and there are also several genes that inhibit cell death (Box 17.2). The family of death-inhibiting genes includes the *bcl* genes. A gene, *bcl-2*, initially detected in B cell lymphomas (see Chapter 34), is typical of the death-inhibiting or antiapoptotic genes. One explanation that has been proposed for the survival of long-term memory cells is that they have a higher than usual level of expression of the Bcl family of proteins. This characteristic protects them from antigen-induced cell death and facilitates their long-term survival.

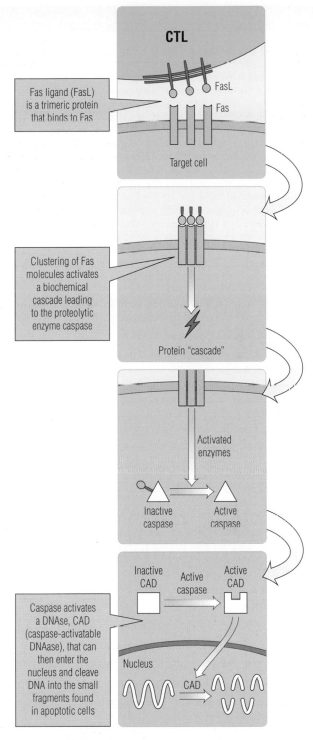

Figure 17.5 Cell death pathway: the role of receptor-ligand interactions (Fas-Fas L) to activate caspase and, finally, caspase-activatable DNAase (CAD), which degrades DNA.

 MHC II   Cytokine, Chemokine, etc.   Complement (C')   Signaling molecule

BOX 17.2 Apoptosis-Programmed Cell Death

Apoptosis is a mechanism for the elimination of excess or damaged cells. It is an evolutionarily conserved process that is initiated by the dying cell and represents a form of controlled cellular destruction. Several genes have been identified that either promote or inhibit apoptosis (Fig. 17.6). Antiapoptotic genes could confer characteristics such as longer than usual survival. The most important of the antiapoptotic genes appears to be *bcl-2*. Antiapoptotic genes of the *bcl-2* type appear to work by raising the so-called apoptotic threshold of a cell, that is, the dose of apoptosis initiator required for a cell expressing the Bcl-2 protein is greater than in the absence of Bcl-2.

The gene *bcl-2* was originally detected as a mammalian oncogene involved in a human chromosomal translocation between chromosomes 14 and 18 that is detected in more than 70% of lymphomas. The chromosomal translocation results in increased expression of Bcl-2, and this imparts a relative resistance to apoptosis on the resulting B tumor cells (see Chapter 34).

FIG. 17.6 Death-Inhibiting/Death-Promoting Genes

Antiapoptotic (Death-Inhibiting) Genes	Proapoptotic (Death-Promoting) Genes
bcl-2	*bax*
bcl-X$_L$	*bak*
bcl-w	*bcl-X$_S$*

LEARNING POINTS Can You Now ...

1. Recall examples of the major medical triumphs that resulted from artificial induction (by vaccination) of immunologic memory?

2. List the major differences between a primary and a secondary immune response?

3. Draw a model for the differentiation pathway of memory lymphocytes?

4. List the qualitative and quantitative changes that distinguish memory from naive lymphocytes?

5. Draw the principal features of the apoptotic pathway?

6. List the characteristics of memory cells that help to ensure their survival?

 T cell receptor (TCR)

 Immunoglobulin (Ig)

 Antigen

 MHC I

CHAPTER 18

A Brief Review of Immune Physiology

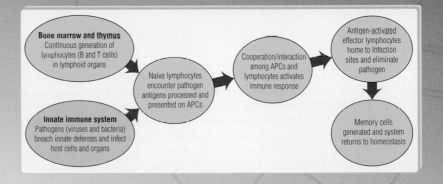

Section III of the book has principally focused on the physiology of the adaptive immune response. After a discussion of the genes and molecules involved in antigen recognition in Section II, we moved in Section III to a discussion of cells, tissues and organs, and a more integrated, physiological system view of the adaptive immune response.

By this point in the book, you should have gained a good understanding of the following important topics (which are also illustrated in the overview figure above):

- How a repertoire of antigen receptors is developed
- How antigen-presenting cells (APCs) process and display antigens for recognition by T cells
- How naive B and T lymphocytes recognize antigen and are then activated to differentiate into effector cells
- How APCs, and B and T lymphocytes, interact and cooperate in an adaptive immune response
- How lymphocytes home to lymphoid tissues and recirculate to the periphery to protect against invading pathogens
- How memory of a previous response is maintained, allowing a more rapid and effective response on reencountering a pathogen.

We established in Chapter 10 that antigen associates with the αβ T-cell receptor (TCR) only after handling by specialized APCs. Most importantly, you should recall that the route of antigen processing (cytosolic versus vesicle bound) determines whether an antigen is presented by MHC class II molecules to a TCR on a CD4$^+$ T-helper (T$_H$) cell, or by major histocompatibility complex (MHC) class I molecules to a TCR on a CD8$^+$ cytotoxic T cell.

By themselves, the αβ (or γδ) TCR protein chains, and the membrane-bound immunoglobulin (Ig) molecule, are poor receptors—that is, they are ineffective at delivering a message to the interior of the cell that a stimulus (antigen) has been received. Chapters 11 and 16 described:

- The structure and function of the B-cell receptor (BCR) and the TCR
- The role of co-receptor and costimulatory molecules in optimizing the function of the antigen receptors
- The connection between the antigen receptors and the signal transduction machinery of B and T lymphocytes.

This should have given you an understanding of how lymphocytes become effector cells and the processes involved in lymphocyte activation.

In Chapters 14 and 15, we discuss how the repertoire of B-cell and T-cell specificities is developed. We learned that there are orderly processes of gene rearrangement that take place in different cell types during B-cell and T-cell development in the adult bone marrow and thymus, respectively. How thymocytes and B-cell precursors mature into T and B effector cells, respectively, with an appropriate repertoire of antigen receptors was also described. There are many similarities in the development of B and T lymphocytes and their respective repertoires of antigen-specific receptors. The greatest difference between the two lineages is that the BCR is subject to continued improvements after exposure to antigen. Thus, the processes of affinity maturation and class switching are used to generate a higher-affinity, more effective antibody molecule during the immune response. Although the TCR does not change in structure during an immune response, clonally expanded memory T cells are better able to mount a faster and more effective response when they encounter antigen, for example, after memory T-lymphocyte circulation to the peripheral tissues (see Chapter 17). Amongst the other important topics that you should recall from these chapters are:

- How T-dependent and T-independent B-cell activation occurs
- The mechanism of tolerance induction in B-cell and T-cell populations
- The changes in cell surface protein expression during B-cell and T-cell development
- Positive and negative selection mechanisms

Studies of the adaptive immune response have shown that not only must the lymphoid cells cooperate to mount an effective immune response (see Chapter 16) but also that any immune response takes place in a physiological system of organs and tissues connected by the lymph and blood (see Chapters 12 and 13) and, consequently, is subject to influence by other organ systems. Lymphocytes recirculate throughout the body, homing to particular lymphoid organs and moving out of the blood into sites of infection as they respond to cytokines and other molecules released from or expressed on the cell surface of activated lymphoid and other cells (particularly APCs). Cell adhesion molecules (see Chapter 13) are particularly important in the trafficking of lymphocytes—the constant patrolling of lymphocytes, particularly naive T lymphocytes, in search of antigen.

It is important that you also recall the following topics from these chapters:

- The critical roles of growth factors and colony-stimulating factors, for example, in the developmental pathways to lymphoid and myeloid cells
- The characteristics of the major lymphoid and myeloid cell types
- The cellular organization and major functions of the lymphoid organs
- The cell-cell interactions involved in generating effector B and T cells

Chapter 17 describes immunologic memory and also pointed out the existence of mechanisms that maintain lymphocyte homeostasis. Unless there is a response to antigen (e.g., during an infection), the number of lymphocytes in a human is maintained within a relatively narrow range. There are ordered pathways to generate new lymphocytes when they are required (see Chapters 12, 14, and 15), and there are ordered and regulated pathways for lymphocyte death. Chapter 17 briefly describes the process of programmed cell death (apoptosis) and explains how this may be balanced by antiapoptotic molecules encoded by the so-called death-inhibiting family of *bcl* genes. This topic will be expanded on in Chapter 21. You should also recall:

- The major differences between a primary and a secondary immune response

- The changes that distinguish memory from naive lymphocytes

■ THE INTEGRATED IMMUNE SYSTEM: CONNECTIONS BETWEEN THE ADAPTIVE AND INNATE RESPONSES

This chapter is also a bridge chapter between consideration of the adaptive response and the innate response, and between a section of the book that has been chiefly concerned with molecules, and one in which a more system-wide treatment of immunology is presented. The remainder of this chapter is designed to help the reader cross that bridge.

The immune response takes place in an organism, and the immune system has to be integrated with the other physiological systems. The immune system does not work alone, and there is still much to understand about the immune response in the context of the whole organism. It seems likely that such an integrative view will be important for further medical advances based on exploiting our knowledge of immunology. This integrated view of the immune system is a topic for Chapter 36, but the topic of connections between different aspects of the immune system is also central to the next section of the book (Section IV), which otherwise predominantly describes **innate immunity**.

To aid in learning a complex subject such as immunology, we generally break up the topic into pieces. However, as students of human immunology, we have to remember to put the pieces back together again! As in other things, the whole of immunology is definitely more than the sum of the parts. One way in which to demonstrate that this is true is to consider the connections between the innate and adaptive immune response. For some time, immunologists who studied aspects of the adaptive immune response, such as B-cell ontogeny or TCR gene rearrangement, carried out their research largely oblivious to the results of studies of the innate immune response—for example, studies of the activation of neutrophils, or studies of the details of the inflammatory response in constitutive defense reactions to microbes. However, the two aspects of the immune response, adaptive and innate, are interconnected in important ways. The innate response complements the adaptive response. For example, the innate response includes physical barriers and first line of defense responses to external pathogens (see Chapter 2). If the defenses of the innate system are breached, the adaptive system is triggered. However, the innate response is not separate from the adaptive response. Rather, there are overlapping and connecting molecules (e.g., cytokines) and cells (e.g., macrophages) that integrate the two. It is perhaps more appropriate to view the adaptive and innate responses as stages, but somewhat seamless stages, of the same system, wherein a primary adaptive immune response generally depends on previous activation and participation of the innate immune system.

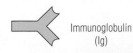 T cell receptor (TCR) — Immunoglobulin (Ig)

 Antigen — MHC I

As is developed more fully in the next section of the book, an excellent example of the connection between the innate and adaptive systems is the role played by pattern-recognition molecules (PRMs), such as the Toll-like receptors (Box 18.1), of the innate system. The concept of PRMs was introduced in Chapter 2 in connection with mannan-binding lectin and the lectin pathway of complement activation. PRMs can bind to molecules that are shared among infectious microbes but are not found in vertebrates—for example, the complex carbohydrates called mannans found in the cell walls of yeasts, and the lipopolysaccharide (LPS) cell wall components of gram-negative bacteria. LPS is an activator of the innate immune response through stimulation of macrophages (see Box 18.1). Mammals use several pattern-recognition molecules, such as complement components and lung surfactant protein, for innate host defense reactions (see Chapter 19). These molecules (PRMs) distinguish between mammalian self and microbial nonself in a nonmicrobe-specific way (see Box 18.1 and Chapter 2).

It is the coordinated action of the innate and adaptive immune responses that counters attacks by pathogens. The next section of the book describes the innate response in more detail.

BOX 18.1 The Role of Toll-like Receptors as a Link Between The Innate and Adaptive Immune Systems

Certain pattern-recognition molecules (PRMs) found on antigen-presenting cells (APCs) function as receptors for pathogen-specific molecules, such as lipopolysaccharide (LPS), and transduce activation signals on binding these molecules (Fig. 18.1). The activated APCs then send signals (e.g., cytokines) that alert and activate lymphocytes. The PRMs that do this were identified as cell surface receptors after a search for mammalian equivalents of molecules called Toll receptors, which have critical roles in the immune systems of insects (see Chapter 20). The fruit fly, *Drosophila melanogaster*, and other insects have well-characterized innate immune systems that confer resistance to microbial infections. A major aspect of host defense in *Drosophila* is release of antimicrobial peptides. Humans have been shown to possess molecules that are homologs of Toll, for example, the family of molecules referred to as TLR (for Toll-like receptor). Several human cell types including macrophages, dendritic cells, and neutrophils express members of the family of Toll-like receptors. They function as PRMs and bind entities such as LPS. LPS binding triggers the Toll-like receptor, then the cytoplasmic domain of the TLR initiates a signaling cascade that leads to the production of cytokines (e.g., tumor necrosis factor-α, interleukin [IL]-1, IL-6, and IL-12), chemokines (e.g., IL-8), and costimulatory molecules (Fig. 18.1). The cytokines attract antigen-specific lymphocytes and bring the adaptive immune response into play.

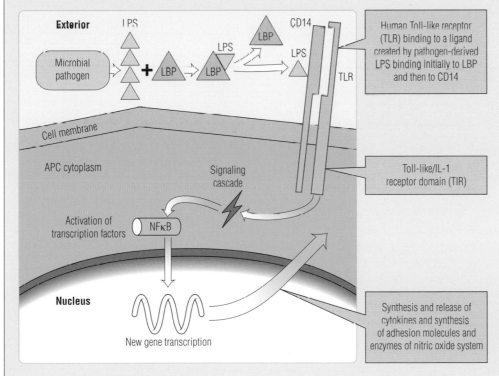

Figure 18.1 Toll-like receptors in activation of antigen-presenting cells (APCs) by microbes. LBP, LPS-binding protein; LPS, lipopolysaccharide; NF-κB, nuclear factor kappa B.

 MHC II

 Cytokine, Chemokine, etc.

 Complement (C′)

 Signaling molecule

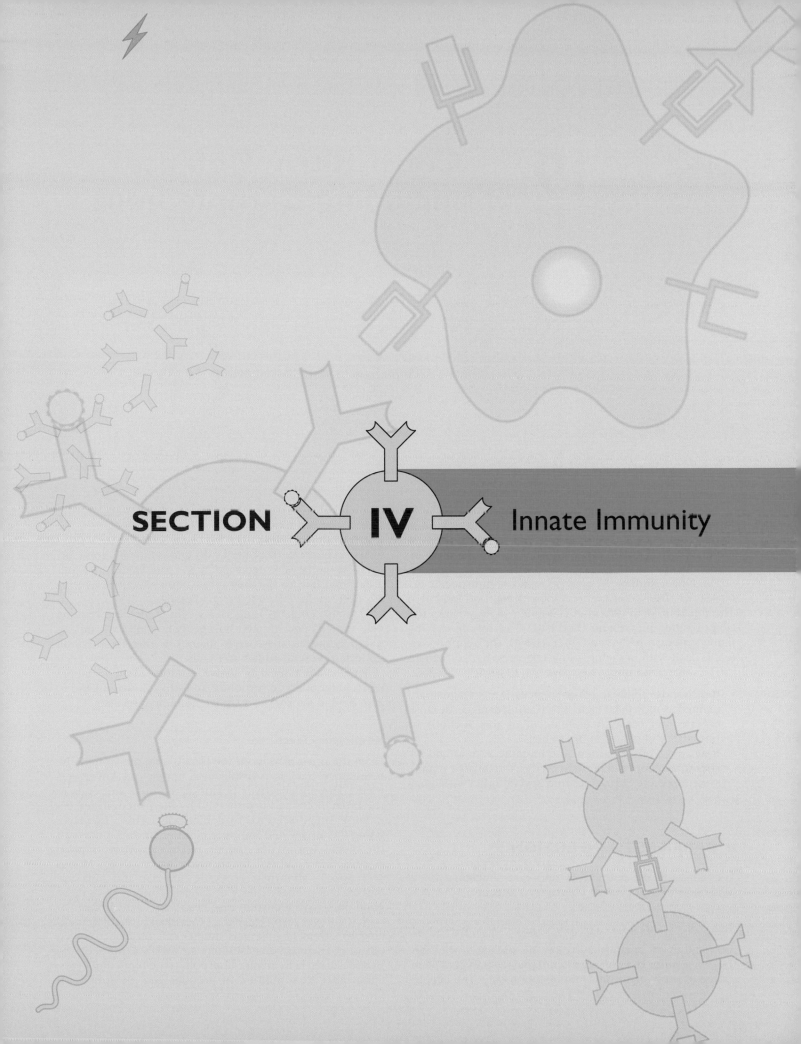

SECTION IV

Innate Immunity

19 Constitutive Defenses Including Complement

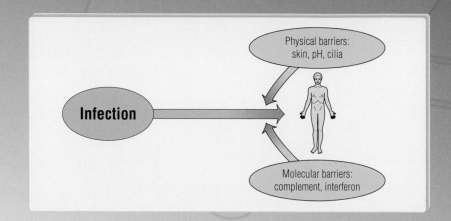

Infections that manage to break through the body's physical barriers activate the molecular barriers of innate immune system. Two of these are the interferons and the complement system.

The innate immune system is a series of nonspecific defenses that are in constant readiness to fight off infection. The innate system differs in a number of ways from the adaptive immune system (Fig. 19.1). The way innate immune systems operate and interact with the adaptive system is dealt with in the next four chapters.

The innate immune system has two key roles:

- It responds rapidly to danger signals. Danger signals are defined as molecular signals indicating damage, because of infection (described in detail in this section) or physical or chemical injury to cells
- It activates other parts of the immune system and tissues throughout the body. To do this, the innate immune system secretes cytokines and several other inflammatory mediators.

■ BARRIERS TO INFECTION

The skin, and the respiratory and gastrointestinal tracts have evolved as specialized barriers to infection.

Skin

Although many organisms live on the surface of the skin, the dense outer layer of dead keratinocytes prevents penetration of these organisms into deeper tissues. The deeper-layer living keratinocytes are active components in the innate immune system. These keratinocytes secrete cytokines such as interleukin-8 (IL-8) and tumor necrosis factor (TNF) if they are damaged in any way. These cytokines are responsible for the inflammation that occurs following exposure to, for example, ultraviolet light.

Skin also contains Langerhans cells, which are sentinel cells of the dendritic cell lineage. Following exposure to microorganisms, these cells migrate to the local lymph node and present antigen to T cells.

The skin is typical of innate immune system components in its ability to respond rapidly to stimulation and to activate and inform the adaptive immune response.

Respiratory Tract

From the point of view of the innate immune system, the respiratory tract is divisible into upper and lower segments. The upper airway begins at the nose and ends in the bronchioles and is protected by the **mucociliary escalator**. Mucus secreted by goblet cells forms a fine layer lining the airway and trapping microorganisms. Cilia waft the mucus toward the mouth and nose, where trapped organisms are cleared by sneezing or coughing. Mucus secretion is abnormal in cystic fibrosis, and cilia are defective in primary ciliary dyskinesia. Patients with these conditions have recurrent respiratory-tract infections.

In the lower respiratory tract (terminal bronchioles and alveoli), layers of cilia and mucus can obstruct oxygen diffusion. The main defenses here are **surfactants** secreted by specialized cells lining the alveoli—type II pneumocytes. Surfactants are a mixture of proteins and phospholipids

FIG. 19.1   Differences Between the Innate and Adaptive Immune Systems

Innate system	Adaptive system
Distinguishes danger from homeostasis	Distinguishes self from nonself
Preformed (constitutive) or rapidly formed components	Relies on genetic events and cellular growth
Responds within minutes to infection	Response develops over days
No specificity: the same molecules and cells respond to a range of pathogens	Very specific; each cell is genetically programmed to respond to a single antigen
Uses pattern-recognition molecules	Uses antigen-recognition molecules
Uses germline genes to produce collectins (mannan-binding lectin, surfactant), complement, C-reactive protein and Toll-like receptor	Uses hypervariable regions in immunoglobulin and T-cell receptors and genetic recombination to produce immunoglobulin and T-cell receptors
Probably fewer than 100 receptors exist	Possibility of up to 10^{18} different receptors
Pattern-recognition molecules detect molecules unique to pathogens, for example, lipopolysaccharide	Recognizes comformational structures (immunoglobulin) or short, peptides bound to MHC molecules (T-cell receptor)
No memory: the response does not change after repeated exposure	Immunological memory; on repeated exposure the response is faster, stronger and qualitatively different
The older system, seen in all members of the animal kingdom	Evolved in early vertebrate kingdom, many millions of years after the innate immune system
Can only recognize molecules signalling infection or injury	Cannot distinguish host from pathogens
Rarely malfunctions	Frequently malfunctions and may cause autoimmunity

that prevent alveoli from collapsing during expiration. Surfactant also contains pathogen-binding proteins, which are members of the **collectin** family (Fig. 19.2). The collectins have globular lectin-like heads that can bind to sugars on microorganisms and long collagen-like tails that bind to phagocytes or complement. These molecules have a **pattern-recognition** role.

Both segments of the respiratory tract are also reliant on immunoglobulins, as shown by the frequency of respiratory infections in patients with antibody deficiency.

The Gastrointestinal Tract

The low pH of the stomach is one of the main defenses against infection of the gut. For example, patients who are unable to secret gastric acid have a high risk for *Salmonella* infection. The lower gut is colonized by trillions of bacteria, which are normally harmless and inhibit the growth of pathogenic bacteria.

■ EXTRACELLULAR MOLECULES OF THE INNATE IMMUNE SYSTEM

The innate immune system relies on families of proteins that can provide a very rapid response to infection. The **type I interferons** (IFNs) are produced locally in response to infection and directly inhibit the growth of pathogens. **Collectins**, **complement**, and the **C-reactive protein** (CRP) are constitutively produced proteins, although they are found at higher levels during infections, and bind onto pathogens.

Type I Interferon

Interferons are so named because cells treated with interferon become resistant to viral infection; interferon inter-

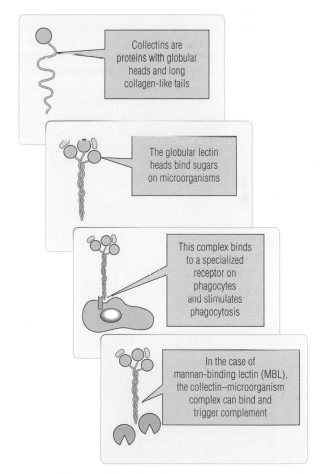

Collectins are proteins with globular heads and long collagen-like tails

The globular lectin heads bind sugars on microorganisms

This complex binds to a specialized receptor on phagocytes and stimulates phagocytosis

In the case of mannan-binding lectin (MBL), the collectin–microorganism complex can bind and trigger complement

Figure 19.2 The collectin family includes surfactant proteins and mannan-binding lectin (MBL); both are important pattern-recognition molecules. C1q is a related protein. These proteins have both lectin-like and collagen-like domains. Lectins are sugar-binding proteins that can bind to microorganisms. The collagen-like domains bind to cellular receptors or activate complement.

 MHC II

 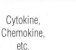 Cytokine, Chemokine, etc.

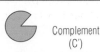 Complement (C')

 Signaling molecule

feres with viral replication. The antiviral effects are most potent with type I IFN (IFN-α and IFN-β) and less so with IFN-γ. Interferons also activate the T_H1 arm of the adaptive immune response.

- Type I IFNs are secreted by a wide range of cells at frontline tissues, for example, epithelial cells lining the gut. Many cells produce IFNs in response to nonspecific injuries, such as trauma or radiation injury. However, the most efficient producers of type I IFNs are a type of antigen-presenting cell (APC) called plasmacytoid dendritic cells, which secrete IFNs in response to infection. These specialized APCs, described in Chapter 12, secrete type I IFNs in response to double-stranded RNA, which they recognize using a pattern-recognition molecule called Toll-like receptor 3, which is discussed in Chapter 20. Double-stranded RNA is not present in mammalian cells, but is produced by viruses during intracellular infection of cells. Double-stranded RNA is a good example of the type of molecule detected by pattern-recognition molecules; its presence indicates that viral infection is taking place, but not the exact type of virus. Type I IFNs have a range of actions (Fig. 19.3).
- Inhibition of viral replication by activation of two intracellular enzyme pathways that degrade the viral genome and inhibit transcription of viral messenger RNA. This effect of type I IFNs is effective only on neighboring cells. Such a short-range effect is described as a paracrine action.
- Stimulation of activity of TAP (transporter-associated with antigen presentation) peptide transporters and proteasomes (see Chapter 10) and increased expression of MHC class I (see Chapter 8); these increase the availability of peptides for binding to MHC class I and promote the effects of CD8+ T cells.

- Promotion of the development of T_H1 cells (Chapter 15).
- Activation of natural-killer cells (see Chapter 21)

Within hours of viral infection, type I IFN secretion is induced, inhibiting viral replication and arming natural-killer cells to destroy infected cells. Although IFNs improve antigen presentation on MHC class I, primary T-cell and antibody responses may take as long as a week to develop. Consequently, IFNs provide a rapid response that bridges the period required to initiate the innate immune response.

IFN-α is used to treat viral hepatitis. In hepatitis B virus infection, IFN-α improves liver function and reduces viral replication in 40% of patients. Treatment is less successful in hepatitis C infection, when only 20% of patients respond. The benefits of IFN-α are mediated mainly by its antiviral effects and partly through stimulation of the adaptive immune system. IFN-α has also been used to treat malignancies, most often chronic myeloid leukemia. The exact mode of action is unclear, although IFN seems to induce either apoptosis or maturation of malignant cells. Recombinant IFNs can be synthesized in high quantities in mammalian cells. Some of the clinical side effects and manufacturing problems are discussed in Chapter 35.

During infections, macrophages and other innate immune system cells secrete other cytokines such as IL-1, IL-6, and TNF. These cytokines activate the specific immune system and cause the **acute phase response** (see Box 19.1).

Complement

Although there are a large number of complement components, the overall system is simple and easy to understand. There are nine basic complement components, C1 to C9. When they become activated, complement components are split into small and large fragments; the small

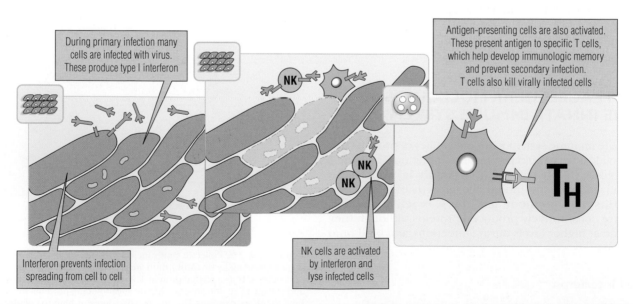

Figure 19.3 Type I interferons include α, γ, and β forms. Inferferon γ has more potent immunostimulatory effects and less potent direct effects on viral replication. NK, natural killer.

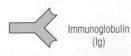 T cell receptor (TCR)   Immunoglobulin (Ig) Antigen MHC I

fragments are referred to as C3a, C4a, and so on. A simple way of remembering an overview of complement is that three different activators detect pathogens and activate a key component, C3, which is required to switch on three different types of effector molecule (Fig. 19.4).

Complement can be activated by interactions between antibody and antigen. Complement facilitates the effects of antibody and is so named because antibody alone will not kill most bacteria; these molecules are required to complement the bactericidal effects of antibody.

Activation of Complement

There are three ways in which C3 can be activated (Fig. 19.5).

Lectin Pathway

Mannan-binding lectin (MBL) is a collectin that is able to bind, through its lectin portions, onto carbohydrates pres-

ent on bacteria. Although MBL has no enzyme activity of its own, after the lectin portions bind to bacteria, the MBL collagen-like domain indirectly activates the next complement components C2 and C4, which together activate several hundred C3 molecules.

The Classical Pathway

This is so named because it was discovered first, although it was probably the last to evolve. The classical pathway is triggered by immune complexes of antibody and antigen. C1 is the initiating protein and is able to recognize the Fc portion of immunoglobulin molecules when sufficient Fc portions are in close enough proximity. This is most likely to occur when an antigen binds several immunoglobulin (Ig) molecules. Because it has five Fc portions, IgM is particularly good at C1 binding. C1 also has no enzyme activity, but after binding to an Fc, it is able to activate C2 and C4, which in turn activate multiple C3 molecules.

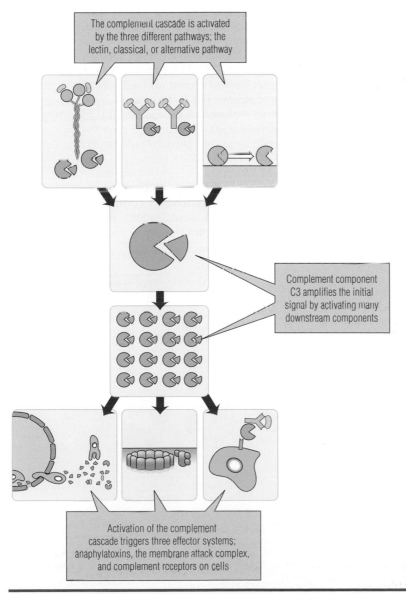

Figure caption (within figure):
The complement cascade is activated by the three different pathways; the lectin, classical, or alternative pathway

Complement component C3 amplifies the initial signal by activating many downstream components

Activation of the complement cascade triggers three effector systems; anaphylatoxins, the membrane attack complex, and complement receptors on cells

Figure 19.4 An overview of the complement cascade.

 MHC II
 Cytokine, Chemokine, etc.
 Complement (C')
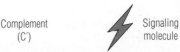 Signaling molecule

The Alternative Pathway

C3 is not a stable molecule and is constantly undergoing spontaneous low-level activation. Spontaneous activation of C3 is most likely to happen on surfaces (although normal cells express surface complement inhibitors) that prevent C3 activation. The surfaces of pathogens lack complement inhibitors. Any cell surface that is not protected by complement inhibitors will be attacked by complement.

Alternative pathway complement activation has proven to be a special challenge in the transplantation of organs from other species (xenotransplantation), which could otherwise relieve the shortage of human donor organs. Kidneys transplanted from pigs to primates die within minutes. This is in part mediated by alternative pathway complement activation. Pig cells act as a surface on which the spontaneous activation of C3 is promoted. Although pig cells express complement inhibitors, these will not inhibit human complement. Thus "molecular incompatibility" leads to widespread complement activation and destruction of the kidney. To overcome molecular incompatibility, nuclear transfer and cloning techniques are being used to insert human complement inhibitor genes into pigs (see Chapter 33).

The early part of complement system can also detect cells dying as a result of necrosis, usually secondary to physical or metabolic damage. Cell death from necrosis is an uncontrolled process, and dying cells appear to leak several types of molecules that are able to activate the complement cascade. In this way, some inflammation is a consequence of any type of damage done to tissues. You will read about another type of cell death, apoptosis, in Chapter 21. This process is strictly controlled and does not activate complement in the same way as necrosis. Inflammation is thus not a consequence of apoptosis.

Summary of Complement Activation

The alternative pathway activates complement on the surface of any cell that lacks complement inhibitors, whereas the lectin and classic pathways provide focused complement activation to molecules that have been bound by MBL or antibody.

Amplification Steps

Each complement component is constantly present in blood and, on activation, becomes capable of activating several downstream components. Complement activators are sensitive to small stimuli, such as very few bacteria, and the subsequent amplification steps ensure a dramatic, but usually local, response. This is obtained through the enzyme activity of complement components throughout the complement cascade: C2, C4, C3, C5, and C6. These molecules are activated by cleavage into small and large fragments (Fig. 19.6). The large fragments may become enzymes themselves and cleave and activate the next molecule in the cascade. These fragments may also interact with inhibitors that switch off the amplification steps.

The small fragments of C3 and C5 have biologic activity and are known as anaphylatoxins (see later).

Complement Effectors

Activation of complement produces a number of effector molecules: the anaphylatoxins, complement fragments binding and activating complement receptors, and the membrane attack complex.

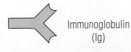

Figure 19.5 Activation of C3 can take place through any one of three pathways.

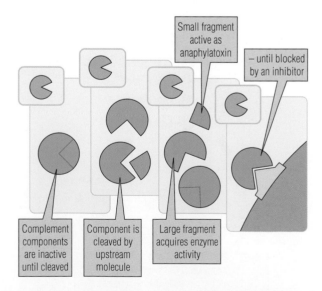

Figure 19.6 After cleavage, fragments of complement components C2, C4, C3, C5, and C6 acquire enzyme activity and activate downstream components.

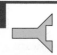 T cell receptor (TCR)

 Immunoglobulin (Ig)

 Antigen

MHC I

Anaphylatoxins

The activation of complement components C3 and C5 produces small fragments C3a and C5a. Because they have a low molecular weight, these peptides diffuse away from the site of complement activation and cause the effects shown in Figure 19.7. The C2a low-molecular-weight peptide is cleaved to produce a small kinin, which has marked effects on making endothelial cells contract, increasing vascular permeability.

Complement Receptors

There are several complement receptors (CR) present on a variety of cells; these bind early complement components (MBL, C1, and activated C4 and C3). Complement receptors serve the following functions (Fig. 19.8).

- Opsonization. This is the process by which bacteria and other cells are made available for phagocytosis. Molecules that help to bind pathogens to phagocytes and stimulate phagocytosis are known as opsonins. Because so much activated C3 is produced during complement activation, it is the most important opsonin and binds to three different receptors present on a range of phagocytes. IgG can also act as an opsonin, when it binds to Fc receptors on phagocytes. Because phagocytes do not have Fc receptors for IgM, complement-mediated opsonization is particularly important during a primary antibody response, when an IgM response dominates.
- B-cell stimulation. Binding of C3 to the CR2 receptor on B cells provides costimulation and decreases the threshold for B-cell activation a thousand-fold (Chapter 11). Hence, complement binding to antigen promotes the production of antibody. CR2 has been subverted by the Epstein-Barr virus (see Chapter 34), which uses it as its receptor.
- Immune complex clearance. Immune complexes are insoluble lattices of antigen bound to antibody that can form in tissues or in the blood. These trigger inflamma-

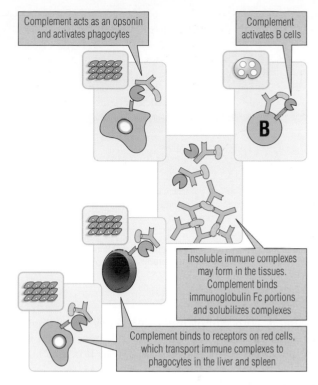

Figure 19.8 Complement receptors.

tion, and immune complex disease (see Chapter 29) will occur if they are not removed. Complement helps to remove immune complexes in two ways.

- Large insoluble complexes are particularly difficult to remove from tissues; high numbers of activated C3 interrupt the lattice of the immune complex, making them soluble
- C4 and C3 present in solubilized immune complexes can bind onto complement receptor CR1 on red cells, which transport the immune complexes to organs that are rich in fixed phagocytes, such as the liver and spleen. Using their own complement and Fc receptors, these phagocytes remove the immune complexes from red cells, phagocytose, and destroy them. The red cells are not harmed by this process.

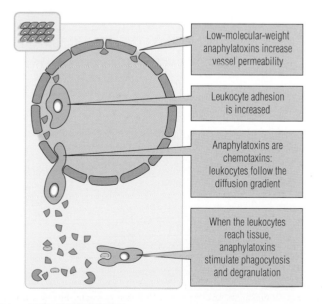

Figure 19.7 Anaphylatoxins.

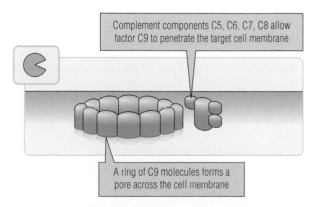

Figure 19.9 The ring of C9 molecules forming a pore in the attacked cell is very similar to perforin, a substance produced by natural-killer cells.

 MHC II

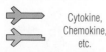 Cytokine, Chemokine, etc.

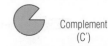 Complement (C')

 Signaling molecule

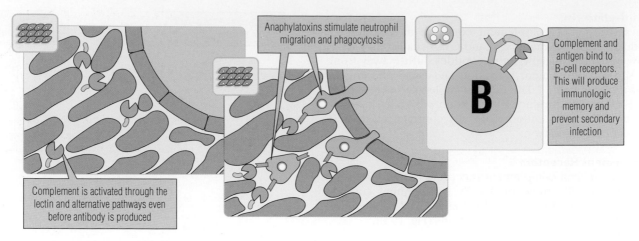

Anaphylatoxins stimulate neutrophil migration and phagocytosis

Complement and antigen bind to B-cell receptors. This will produce immunologic memory and prevent secondary infection

B

Complement is activated through the lectin and alternative pathways even before antibody is produced

Figure 19.10 Complement is particularly important in dealing with bacterial infections. There are some parallels with the ways by which interferons inhibit viral infections. Both complement and interferon can directly attack pathogens, and each recruits different cells of the innate and adaptive immune response.

- Patients with complement deficiency are at high risk for disease caused by immune complexes, such as systemic lupus erythematosus (SLE) (see Box 19.2).

Membrane Attack Complex

Activated C3 activates the final part of the cascade of complement components C5 through C9. These components form the membrane-attack complex. C5 and C6 have enzyme activity, which allows components C7, C8, and C9 to insert themselves into the plasma membrane of the target cell. A group of 10 to 16 molecules of C9 form a ring, which creates a pore in the plasma membrane (Fig. 19.9). This allows free passage of water and solutes across the membrane, killing the cell. The membrane attack complex attacks pathogens directly but in humans only appears to be crucial for defenses against *Neisseria* (see Box 19.2).

Figure 19.10 summarizes how complement is involved in the response to bacterial infection.

Complement Inhibitors

Complement tends to undergo spontaneous activation, especially by the alternative pathway. Excessive complement activation is undesirable because it causes inflammation and widespread cell death. To prevent inadvertent complement activation, eight complement inhibitors exist. Their site of action is shown in Figure 19.11.

The importance of these inhibitors is indicated by the fact that deficiency can lead to illness, for example, hereditary angioedema (Box 19.3).

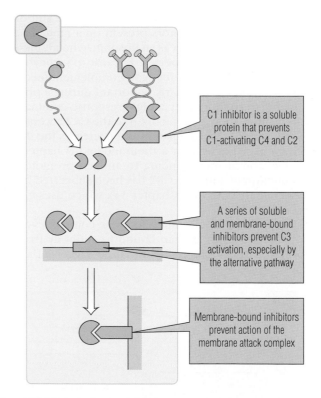

C1 inhibitor is a soluble protein that prevents C1-activating C4 and C2

A series of soluble and membrane-bound inhibitors prevent C3 activation, especially by the alternative pathway

Membrane-bound inhibitors prevent action of the membrane attack complex

Figure 19.11 Complement inhibitors.

 T cell receptor (TCR)

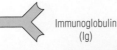 Immunoglobulin (Ig)

Antigen

 MHC I

BOX 19.1 Acute Phase Response

An 11-year-old girl presents at the emergency department late at night because of a 12-hour history of abdominal pain and vomiting. On examination, her temperature and pulse are normal (Fig 19.12), and the only sign in the abdomen is some tenderness in the right iliac fossa. The attending surgeon orders some blood tests: the results are shown in the table (Fig 19.13). He thinks that appendicitis is possible, but is not certain. In any case, the girl has eaten in the last few hours, and a general anesthetic would not be safe. The patient is kept on the observation ward overnight.

The following morning, her temperature and pulse are up slightly, and the nurses on the ward ask the surgeon to review the patient. Tenderness is still the only sign in the abdomen, but repeat blood tests show an elevated neutrophil count, raised C-reactive protein (CRP), and raised erythrocyte sedimentation rate (ESR). These are all characteristics of an acute-phase response. The acute-phase response is often used clinically to distinguish inflammation from other types of clinical problem. In this case, the presence of an acute-phase response convinces the surgeon that he needs to do a laparotomy, during which he finds and removes an inflamed appendix. The girl recovers over the next few days.

The acute-phase response is triggered by the release of interleukin-1 (IL-1), IL-6, and tumor necrosis factor (TNF) from macrophages. These have a direct effect on the hypothalamus (Fig 19.14), increasing the body temperature, which impairs pathogen reproduction. This effect is mediated by these cytokines, inducing the synthesis of prostaglandin in the hypothalamus. Aspirin can block prostaglandin synthesis and prevent fever. IL-1, IL-6, and TNF also stimulate the production of a series of proteins by the liver:

- Innate immune system molecules: C3, C4, and CRP
- Damage-limiting proteins: α_1-antitrypsin, haptoglobin
- Clotting factors: fibrinogen

Granulocyte-colony stimulating factor (G-CSF) produced during the acute-phase response leads to a rapid increase in the production of neutrophils in the marrow. The acute-phase cytokines also contribute to a general activation of the adaptive immune response leading to an increase in the production of polyclonal immunoglobulins.

CRP is a protein produced in the liver, which binds to phospholipids on the surface of bacteria (such as *Pneumococcus*). CRP then acts as an opsonin-stimulating phagocytosis. CRP also activates the complement system through the lectin pathway. CRP production is increased dramatically during inflammation through the actions of TNF and is a particularly good indicator of inflammation. For example, CRP levels are increased up to 1000-fold in acute inflammation, such as appendicitis, and fall rapidly after the appendix has been removed. CRP is also increased by noninfectious diseases. For example, CRP is increased in the autoimmune disease rheumatoid arthritis and provides a good way of monitoring disease activity and response to treatment.

The increased synthesis of the proteins mentioned above increases plasma viscosity, which is reflected by an increased ESR. Measuring the ESR is one of the simplest ways of showing an acute-phase response. The ESR takes longer than CRP to become abnormal during an inflammatory response.

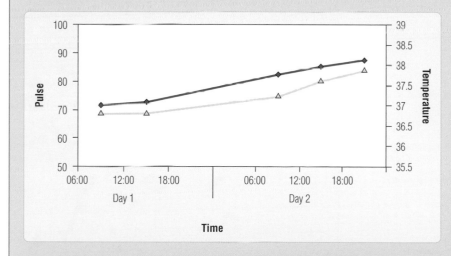

Figure 19.12 This chart shows the vital signs for the patients described in this box. *Blue squares* are the pulse and the *yellow triangles* are temperature (in Centigrade).

FIG. 19.13   This Table Shows the Results of Blood Tests Done on the Patient in This Box

	Day 1, 12:00 AM	Day 2, 8:00 AM	Normal range
ESR	12	38	Less than 7
CRP	4	122	Less than 12
Neutrophil count	5.1×10^3/ml	13.4×10^3/ml	$3–6 \times 10^3$/ml

Continued

 MHC II   Cytokine, Chemokine, etc.   Complement (C')   Signaling molecule

BOX 19.1 Acute Phase Response—cont'd

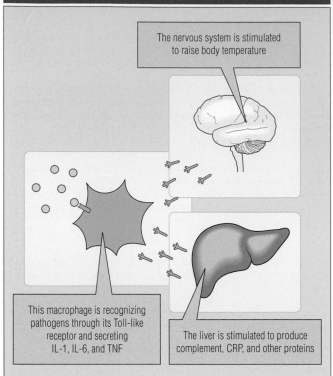

The nervous system is stimulated to raise body temperature

This macrophage is recognizing pathogens through its Toll-like receptor and secreting IL-1, IL-6, and TNF

The liver is stimulated to produce complement, CRP, and other proteins

Figure 19.14 The acute-phase response has widespread effects throughout the body.

BOX 19.2 Complement Deficiency

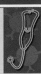

A 16-year-old boy presents at the emergency department with severe headache. He is found to be pyrexial (having a fever of 39.2° C—normal below 37.0° C) and has marked neck stiffness. The attending doctor thinks he might have meningitis and does blood cultures and a lumbar puncture. The cerebrospinal fluid (CSF) should be clear, but in this case, it is slightly cloudy. Examination of the CSF shows dramatically increased numbers of neutrophils, some of which contain diplococci (Fig 19.15). The doctor starts the patient on intravenous broad-spectrum antibiotics, and the boy improves over the next few hours. The following day, culture of the CSF sample confirms infection with *Neisseria meningitidis*.

When the doctor talks to the patient's parents the next day, he finds that two of the boy's siblings have also had *N. meningitidis* infection. This type of family history is typical of hereditary complement deficiency. Further tests confirm deficiency of C8 in the patient and his two affected brothers.

Deficiencies of complement components cause recurrent bacterial infection, partly because the innate immune system clears opsonized bacteria and partly because complement is involved in initiating antibody production (Fig. 19.16). Deficiencies of the membrane attack complex lead to a specific higher risk for infection with *Neisseria* species, as in this case.

Deficiencies in the early lectin and classic pathways cause type III hypersensitivity (immune-complex disease), because immune complexes cannot be solubilized or transported to phagocytes (see Chapter 29). Deficiency of early complement components can cause the autoimmune disease systemic lupus erythematosus (SLE).

Low levels of complement are more usually the result of consumption rather than reduced production of complement components in the liver. Complement is consumed when immune complexes are produced, for example, during infections or autoimmune diseases.

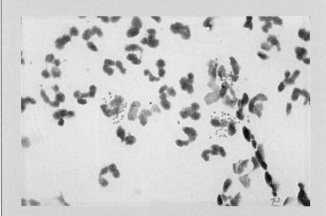

Figure 19.15 This is a Gram stain of the cerebrospinal fluid (CSF) taken from the patient described in this box. Normal CSF contains fewer neutrophils. In addition, three neutrophils in this image can be seen to contain intracellular diplococci, which is characteristic of *Neisseria meningitidis*.

Continued

 T cell receptor (TCR)

 Immunoglobulin (Ig)

 Antigen

 MHC I

BOX 19.2   Complement Deficiency—cont'd

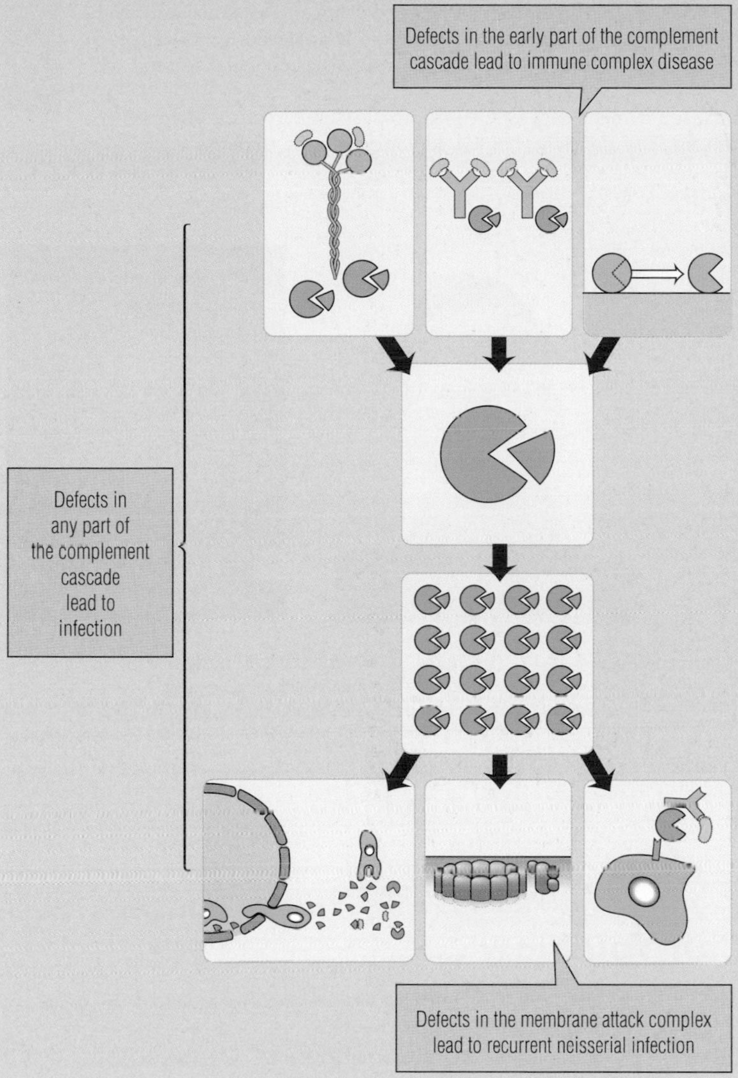

Defects in the early part of the complement cascade lead to immune complex disease

Defects in any part of the complement cascade lead to infection

Defects in the membrane attack complex lead to recurrent neisserial infection

Figure 19.16 The clinical features of complement deficiency depend on exactly which components are defective.

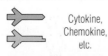 Cytokine, Chemokine, etc.

 Complement (C')

 Signaling molecule

MHC II

BOX 19.3 Hereditary Angioedema

A 20-year-old man has had several bouts of facial swelling (Fig. 19.17). He has had bouts of facial swelling and unexplained severe abdominal pain throughout life. His complement C4 level is low, although C3 is normal. A sample is analyzed for levels of C1 inhibitor, which is found to be very low. A diagnosis of hereditary angioedema is made, and, on this occasion, he is treated with purified C1 inhibitor. His swelling subsides over a few hours.

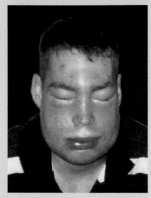

Hereditary angioedema is an autosomal-dominant disease caused by deficiency of C1 inhibitor. C1 inhibitor is a member of a plasma protein family called serpins—serine proteases inhibitors. The deficiency of C1 inhibitor means that the early complement cascade is very easily activated. The activation of the complement cascade is halted at the level of C3, because an appropriate surface for complement activation is missing. C4 and C2 are cleaved in the activation and excessive amounts of the C2a kinin are produced. C1 inhibitor also normally inhibits the production of another kinin, bradykinin, from kininogen. In patients with hereditary angioedema, activation of the complement and kinin cascades by minor triggers, such as trauma, infection, or even psychological stress, cannot be inhibited by C1 inhibitor. The result is excessive amounts of C2a kinin and bradykinin production, leading to increased capillary permeability at any site, causing painful, and sometimes life-threatening, swelling.

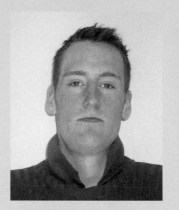

Purified C1 inhibitor can prevent and treat attacks of hereditary angioedema (this is not currently licensed in the United States). An alternative is to give anabolic steroids, which increase C1 inhibitor levels.

Another important serpin is α_1-antitrypsin, which normally releases proteases released by phagocytes. Patients who inherit genes for abnormal α_1-antitrypsin develop emphysema (lung destruction caused by the unopposed action of proteolytic enzymes) and liver disease (caused by the accumulation of abnormal α_1-antitrypsin molecules).

Figure 19.17 This figure shows the patient in the box as he normally appears and how he appears during an attack of angioedema. (From Helbert M: Flesh and Bones Immunology. Edinburgh, Mosby, 2006.)

LEARNING POINTS Can You Now ...

1. List the differences between the innate and adaptive immune response?
2. Explain how interferons work, and give two examples of how they are used as treatments?
3. Draw a diagram of the complement system?
4. List two consequences of complement deficiencies?
5. Describe how the acute-phase response can best be measured?

 T cell receptor (TCR)

 Immunoglobulin (Ig)

 Antigen

MHC I

20 Phagocytes

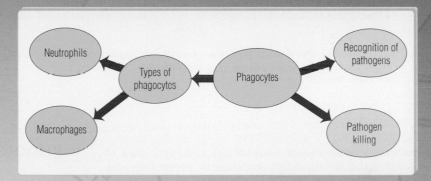

In this chapter, you will learn about the next component of the innate immune system, phagocytes. You will understand the differences between the two types of phagocytes, neutrophils and macrophages, and how they recognize and kill pathogens

Phagocytosis is the internalization of particulate matter by cells into cytoplasmic vesicles. Phagocytosis is triggered when phagocytes recognize pathogens. Phagocytes contain lysosomes: granules containing enzymes that fuse with the vesicles and degrade the particulate matter. In addition, activation of a cascade of phagocyte enzymes leads to the production of toxic molecules (the respiratory burst), which is necessary to kill phagocytosed organisms. Phagocytes are, therefore, mainly concerned with clearing small extracellular pathogens, such as bacteria, protozoans and fungi, and cellular debris. A second important role is that phagocytes can also produce cytokines and cell-surface molecules, which alert the adaptive immune system to the presence of infection. Phagocytes also recognize dying cells and participate in the clearance of cellular debris. In the case of cells undergoing apoptosis, phagocytes do not secrete cytokines that trigger inflammation. However, in the case of cells undergoing necrosis, phagocytes secrete pro-inflammatory cytokines and participate (with complement) in activating inflammation.

■ PHAGOCYTIC CELL TYPES

Phagocytes are bone marrow-derived (myeloid) cells. A range of phagocytic cells have evolved in humans, each with specific functions.

Neutrophils

Neutrophils are the most numerous white cells in blood (Fig. 20.1A). Neutrophils migrate rapidly into sites of infection, where they kill pathogens. Pus formed at the site of infection is largely composed of dead neutrophils. Neutrophils play a crucial part in early defenses against bacterial infections; consequently, patients with defective neutrophils or low levels of neutrophils (neutropenic) are at particular risk for serious bacterial infection (see Clinical Box 20.1 at the end of this chapter).

Monocytes/Macrophages

Monocytes (Fig. 20.1B) are also myeloid cells but are very different from neutrophils (Fig. 20.2). Monocytes in the blood are immature cells migrating to their site of activity. Monocytes migrate into tissues where they mature into macrophages (Fig. 20.1C) and take on a number of specialized forms (Fig. 20.3). All macrophage forms have long life spans, surviving in the tissue for months or years.

Tissue Macrophages

These are found in a wide range of sites. They are large cells with specialized granules and cytoplasmic compartments. In some tissues (bone marrow, lymph nodes), these active macrophages are referred to as histiocytes.

Giant and Epithelioid Cells

In sites of chronic inflammation, macrophages undergo further maturation and become multinucleated giant cells or epithelioid cells, under the influence of T-cell cytokines. Epithelioid and giant cells are characteristic of

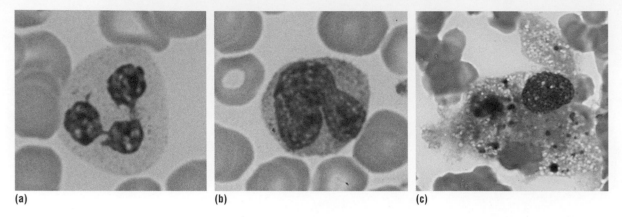

(a)   (b)   (c)

Figure 20.1 Phagocytic cells. **A,** Neutrophils have a very distinct appearance because of their granules, which contain proteolytic enzymes. They can easily be counted by automated instruments when the acute phase response is being measured. **B,** Monocytes are immature macrophages, which (C) have a much more distinctive appearance.

granuloma formation (see Chapter 22) and participate in prolonging the inflammatory response by presenting antigen to T cells and by secreting cytokines. Unlike neutrophils, macrophages live for many years and pus is not formed during this type of inflammation.

Fixed Macrophages
These specialized phagocytes line sinusoids in the spleen and liver. In the liver, these macrophages are referred to as Kupffer cells. Their role is to phagocytose circulating particulate matter (see Fig. 19.8) and, in some situations, phagocytose entire cells (see hemolytic anemia in Chapter 28).

Alveolar Macrophages
These contribute to the lung's innate defenses. They are involved in disease processes such as chronic obstructive pulmonary disease.

Glial Cells
These are long-lived macrophages resident in the nervous system. They are involved in clearing dead neuronal cells.

Osteoclasts
The most specialized macrophages are the osteoclasts in bone, which participate in regulating calcium metabolism by resorbing bone and releasing calcium into the blood.

■ PHAGOCYTE PRODUCTION

Neutrophils and monocytes are produced from the same stem cells in the bone marrow (see Fig. 20.3 and Chapter 12). Many more neutrophils are produced each day than monocytes. This rapid production is especially vulnerable to the effects of cytotoxic drugs, which can give rise to neutropenia and vulnerability to infection (Box 20.1). Production of these cells is stimulated by colony stimulating factors (CSFs), which are produced by tissue macrophages as part of an acute-phase response. CSFs ensure that neutrophils are produced in increasing numbers during infection. Recombinant granulocyte CSF (filgrastim, lenograstim) can be used to boost neutrophil numbers—for example, following stem cell transplant.

■ PHAGOCYTE RECRUITMENT

Monocytes constantly migrate into healthy tissue and differentiate into the specialized macrophages mentioned earlier. Macrophages remain in a resting state unless they are stimulated by signals binding to their receptors, described later. Although neutrophils make up the majority of phagocytes circulating in the blood, they are absent from normal tissues and will only migrate into inflamed

FIG. 20.2 Differences Between Neutrophils and Monocytes/Macrophages

Neutrophils	Macrophages
Rapid increase in production during the acute	Slight increase in blood levels during inflammation phase response
Only found in inflamed tissues	Found in healthy tissues
Single mature form	Variety of mature forms
Rapidly form pus	Slowly form granuloma-with T-cell help
Short lived–die after phagocytosis	Long lived–survive after phagocytosis

 T cell receptor (TCR)   Immunoglobulin (Ig)   Antigen MHC I

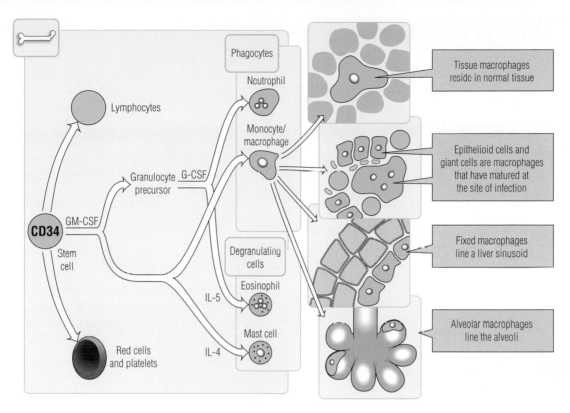

Figure 20.3 Neutrophil production is increased during the acute-phase response by granulocyte colony-stimulating factor (G-CSF). Macrophages are produced constantly at low levels and develop into specialized types in different tissues. GM-CSF, granulocyte-macrophage colony-stimulating factor (see Chapter 12).

tissue (Fig. 20.4). Resident macrophages recruit neutrophils to sites of inflammation using signals similar to those already discussed in Chapter 13 in relation to lymphocyte trafficking. For example, cytokines produced by local macrophages stimulate endothelial cells in local capillaries to increase expression of P selectin and integrins such as intercellular adhesion molecules (ICAMs).

Chemokines are low-molecular-weight chemotactic cytokines that direct cells to specific sites. There are a dozen or so chemokines and a similar number of chemokine receptors. Macrophages at the site of infection secrete chemokines, such as interleukin-8 (IL-8). These modify neutrophil integrins to make the neutrophils more adherent. This allows them to bind to endothelium and undergo diapedesis (passage through intact vessel walls into tissues) (see Chapter 13). The final chemokine-mediated step is chemotaxis: the directional migration of cells along a gradient of chemokines. The net result of chemokine secretion is the attraction of neutrophils into tissues. Interestingly, the same chemokines that attract neutrophils into inflamed tissue stimulate the departure of local dendritic cells for lymph nodes to stimulate the adaptive immune system.

Anaphylatoxins (see Chapter 19) produced by activation of the complement cascade are also chemotactic for phagocytes.

To summarize, resident macrophages at the site of infection secrete cytokines and chemokines, which stimulate

neutrophil production, neutrophil and endothelium expression of selectins and integrins, neutrophil adherence to endothelium in local vessels, and, finally, chemotaxis to the site of infection.

■ RECEPTORS ON PHAGOCYTES

Phagocytes recognize danger signals by using receptors on their cell membranes during their journey through the tissues and their encounters with pathogens or damaged cells (Fig. 20.5).

- Receptors for chemokines and cytokines; these direct phagocytes to the site of inflammation and, once there, prepare them for action.
- The Toll-like receptors (see Chapter 18) are a family of at least 10 different membrane molecules, each of which recognizes different classes of pathogen molecules, as shown in the table (Fig. 20.6). The different Toll-like receptors (TLRs) have overlapping roles and it is likely that several different receptors would be triggered by any given infection. TLRs are found on macrophages and other antigen-presenting cells, such as dendritic cells and B cells, as well as other cells, such as epithelial cells, which have a role in recognizing infection. On binding to the pathogen molecule, TLRs initiate an intracellular signal, leading to cytokine production. The

 MHC II

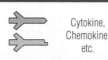 Cytokine, Chemokine, etc.

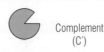 Complement (C')

 Signaling molecule

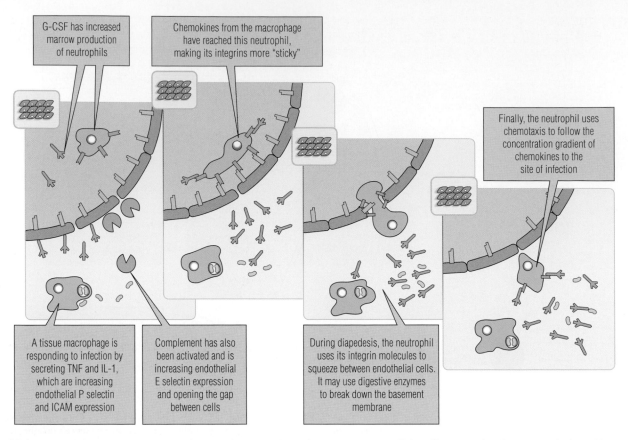

Figure 20.4 Neutrophil migration. G-CSF, granulocyte colony-stimulating factor; ICAM, intercellular adhesion molecule; IL-1, interleukin 1; TNF, tumor necrosis factor.

TLRs have such potent effects that they may have considerable roles as targets for drugs, as described in Box 20.2 at the end of this chapter.

• Another type of pattern recognition molecule found on the surface of cells of the innate immune system is the C-lectin receptor. These are defined as lectin (sugar-binding proteins) molecules that require calcium ions for binding. The sugars that C-lectin receptors recognize are carbohydrate-particular sequences on glycolipids or glycoproteins on pathogen cell surfaces or dying mammalian cells. Binding of C-lectin receptors activates the macrophages leading to cytokines production. They also firmly bind pathogens. In this way, the C-lectin receptors capture pathogens and then deliver them to

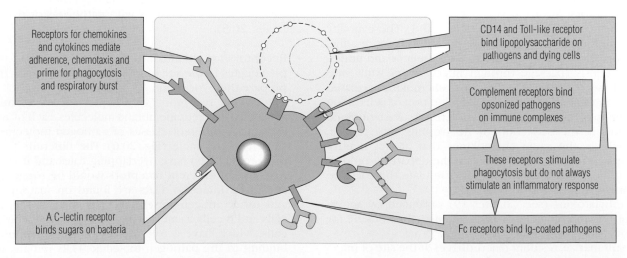

Figure 20.5 Phagocyte receptors. LPS, lipopolysaccharide.

 T cell receptor (TCR)

 Immunoglobulin (Ig)

Antigen

MHC I

FIG. 20.6 Knowledge of Several Toll-Like Receptors is Being Used to Develop New Drugs

TLR	Expressed on	Ligand	Associated pathogen
TLR2	Widespread	Sugars and lipoproteins	A wide range of bacteria
TLR3	Dendritic cells, epithelial cells	Double-stranded RNA	Viruses
TLR4	Macrophages	LPS (TLR4 forms a complex with CD14)	Gram-negative bacteria
TLR5	Macrophages	Flagellae	Wide range of motile bacteria
TLR7	Dendritic cells, macrophages	Single-stranded RNA	Viruses
TLR9	Dendritic cells, B cells	Unmethylated cytosine and guanine sequences—CpG	Bacteria

endocytic pathways. In professional antigen-presenting cells such as macrophages and dendritic cells, C-lectin receptors are required for the degradation of pathogens and subsequent presentation to T cells.

- Receptors for complement components. Complement may bind onto pathogens and cellular debris released from cells undergoing necrosis (see Chapter 19). Opsonized bacteria generally stimulate an inflammatory response, for example, when they are being phagocytosed by neutrophils inside an abscess. By comparison, immune complex clearance by fixed macrophages in the liver and spleen takes place with no inflammation.
- Receptors for immunoglobulin (Ig). Phagocytes can recognize IgG through their Fc receptors. IgG stimulates phagocytosis and thus acts as an opsonin.
- Receptors for apoptotic cells (see Box 21.6). Cells that have undergone apoptosis have done so as part of a physiologic process and are phagocytosed without eliciting an inflammatory response. Phagocytes use CD14 and complement receptors to recognize apoptotic cells.

■ ACTIONS OF PHAGOCYTES

Once they have arrived in the tissues and are stimulated through their receptors, phagocytes kill and clear pathogens through phagocytosis, respiratory burst, and the release of proteolytic enzymes.

Phagocytosis

Phagocytosis is a metabolically active process that is triggered by binding through one of the receptors mentioned above. Phagocytosis is most effectively triggered by pathogens that have been opsonized by complement or IgG (Fig. 20.7). A phagosome is formed by the ingestion of particulate matter. A number of pathogens have developed defense mechanisms to avoid destruction by phagocytes.

Respiratory Burst

Following phagocytosis, three interrelated enzyme pathways are activated that produce toxic molecules, which further damage pathogens (Fig. 20.8). The enzymes produce hydrogen peroxide (phagocyte NADPH oxidase), hypochlorous acid (bleach; myeloperoxidase), and nitric oxide (inducible nitric oxide synthetase).

The phagocyte NADPH oxidase enzymes are defective in a type of primary immunodeficiency, chronic granulomatous disease (Box 20.3). Myeloperoxidase is one target of the autoantibodies antineutrophil cytoplasmic antibodies (ANCA) (see Fig. 28.9).

Nitric oxide is a special molecule because, as well as being toxic to pathogens, it also acts as an important messenger. Nitric oxide is constitutively produced at low levels by neuronal and endothelial cells and has a role as a neurotransmitter and in maintaining vascular tone. Phagocytes can produce high levels of nitric oxide when inducible nitric oxide synthetase is activated. High levels of nitric oxide reduce vascular tone and cardiac output and contribute to the low blood pressure of septic shock (see Box 20.1). There is also evidence that nitric oxide acts as a messenger molecule and can promote the effects of T cells, contributing to chronic inflammation.

Proteolytic Enzymes

Macrophages contain enzymes in lysosomes, which can be regenerated during the long life of these cells. In neutrophils, the proteolytic enzymes are contained in granules, which give the cell its characteristic appearance. Neutrophils cannot regenerate granules, and when these have

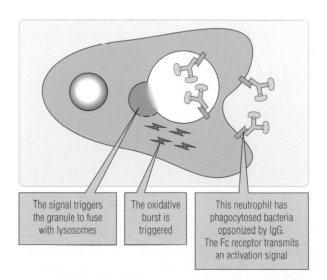

The signal triggers the granule to fuse with lysosomes

The oxidative burst is triggered

This neutrophil has phagocytosed bacteria opsonized by IgG. The Fc receptor transmits an activation signal

Figure 20.7 Phagocyte killing.

 MHC II
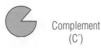 Cytokine, Chemokine, etc.
 Complement (C')
 Signaling molecule

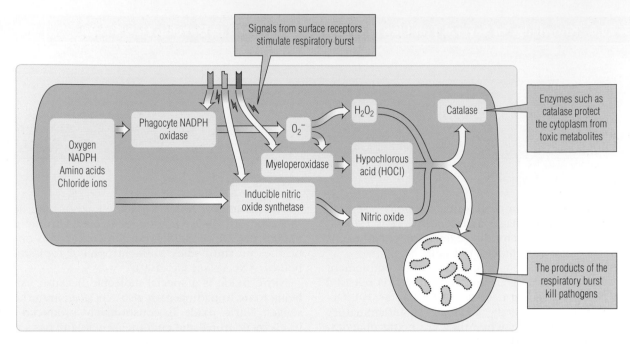

Figure 20.8 Respiratory burst.

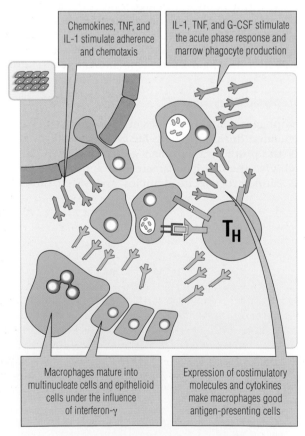

Figure 20.9 The result of mediator release by macrophages can be granuloma formation. A granuloma is a site of chronic inflammation in which macrophages may mature into giant cells or epithelioid cells. Lymphocytes are also present and support macrophages by secreting interferon-γ. G-CSF, granulocyte colony-stimulating factor; IL-1, interleukin 1; TNF, tumor necrosis factor.

been used up, the cell dies. The main enzymes present are proteolytic and are able to digest bacteria in the acid pH of the lysosomes.

In the case of macrophages, the digested peptides can be presented to T cells.

The proteolytic enzymes are usually held retained in lysosomes. Enzymes that leak out of phagocytes are usually prevented from damaging tissues by serpins, such as α₁-antitrypsin (see Box 19.3).

Other substances are released into the phagosome, including defensins and lactoferrin. Defensins are low-molecular-weight peptides that punch holes in bacteria. Lactoferrin binds onto iron, depriving bacteria of this important nutrient.

Inflammatory Signaling

Neutrophils and macrophages produce inflammatory mediators called prostaglandins and leukotrienes. These are discussed in Chapter 21. Although neutrophils secrete chemokines and nitric oxide, their short life span prevents them from contributing to a stable, long-lasting inflammatory response. Instead, a short-lived response is produced, usually with pus formation. This type of response may be called a pyogenic (pus-forming) reaction. By comparison, macrophages have a key role in stimulating chronic inflammation, largely through secretion of soluble messengers with local and systemic effects. Macrophages are also important antigen-presenting cells because they process antigen, secrete cytokines, and express high levels of costimulatory molecules and major histocompatibility complex (MHC) class II molecules (see Chapters 16 and 8, respectively). If antigen is not cleared, the inflammation becomes chronic, and a granuloma is the result.

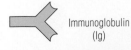
T cell receptor (TCR)

Immunoglobulin (Ig)

Antigen

MHC I

Granulomata are discussed more fully in Chapter 22, but Figure 20.9 shows how mediators produced by macrophages and T cells contribute to chronic inflammation.

Acute-Phase Response

Macrophages secrete IL-1, IL-6, and tumor necrosis factor (TNF) after they have recognized pathogens using pattern-recognition molecules. These cytokines increase production of complement and arm the adaptive immune system (see Chapter 19). TNF has direct effects on metabolism and increases the breakdown of fat in the body's stores. IL-1, IL-6, and TNF also affect the central nervous system through receptors in the hypothalamus. The main response is an increase in body temperature, which is seen very rapidly after the beginning of the response to infection. The role of increased body temperature is to inhibit the replication of viruses and bacteria. There is also an increased metabolic rate and anorexia, all contributing to the weight loss that is a characteristic of serious infection.

Macrophages also secrete cytokines that activate other parts of the immune system. IL-8 is a chemoattractant and attracts neutrophils to the site of infection. These cytokines all predominantly activate the innate immune system, but dendritic cells stimulated through their TLRs can secrete IL-12, which has a role in activating nearby T cells of the adaptive immune system. IL-12 alerts the adaptive immune system to the presence of infection.

■ PHAGOCYTE DEFECTS

Primary disorders of phagocytes are rare but include important problems, such as chronic granulomatous disease (see Box 20.3). Secondary phagocyte defects are much more common. The most important is neutropenia, where numbers of neutrophils are reduced, usually as a result of drug treatment (see Box 20.1). Phagocyte function is impaired secondary to a number of other disorders, such as diabetes and renal failure, and during corticosteroid treatment (Fig. 20.10).

■ MOLECULAR RECOGNITION BY THE INNATE AND ADAPTIVE IMMUNE SYSTEMS

It is useful at this point to review the ways in which the two arms of the immune system recognize different molecules. The adaptive immune system can recognize many millions of possible antigens, using MHC molecules, T-cell receptors, and Ig molecules, and can distinguish self from

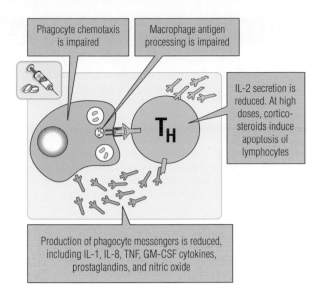

Figure 20.10 Effects of corticosteroids on phagocyte function. GM-CSF, granulocyte-macrophage colony-stimulating factor; IL, interleukin; TNF, tumor necrosis factor.

nonself. However, cells of the adaptive immune system are incapable of distinguishing the normal homeostatic environment from danger. This means that if the adaptive immune system was able to initiate a response autonomously, it could react to self-peptides and initiate autoimmunity (see Chapter 27). By comparison, the innate immune system recognizes "danger," whether it is due to tissue damage or infection. The pattern-recognition molecules used by the innate system can only recognize pathogen molecules. Recognition systems, such as the Toll-like receptors, activate the cells expressing them, such as macrophages, to express increased amounts of MHC molecules and costimulatory molecules such as B7, and to secrete cytokines. Only then can T cells respond to antigen. Thus, the innate immune system alerts the adaptive system. However, macrophages can be dependent on the adaptive immune system, particularly T_H1 T cells. For example, T_H1 help is required to produce IgG, the most effective Ig at opsonizing bacteria for recognition by the Fc receptor. Additionally, interferon-γ produced by T_H1 is required to support and maintain macrophages during chronic infections, as you will discover in Chapter 22.

Many students make the mistake of believing that the more recently evolved adaptive immune system acts autonomously of the older innate system. We have seen now that this is not correct. Antigen-presenting cells must first detect invading pathogens before they can costimulate T cells.

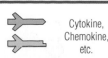 MHC II

 Cytokine, Chemokine, etc.

Complement (C')

 Signaling molecule

BOX 20.1   Neutropenic Sepsis Leading to Septic Shock

A 12-year-old girl has been receiving cytotoxic chemotherapy for acute lymphoblastic leukemia. Although there is evidence that the leukemia is responding to the drugs, she has become neutropenic (neutrophils were less than 0.5×10^6 mL). Early in the evening, she complained of shivering (rigors) and chills and was found to be pyrexial. Within half an hour, she collapsed and was found to have the features of shock (tachycardia and hypotension) along with warm peripheries. When she is examined by the physician, there are no signs of focal organ involvement (such as pneumonia) and a diagnosis of neutropenic sepsis complicated by septic (endotoxic) shock is made.

Blood is taken for culture (these later grow *Escherichia coli*), and she is started on broad-spectrum antibiotics and fluid replacement. She gradually improves during the next 12 hours (Fig. 20.11).

Neutrophils play a crucial role in the early part of bacterial infection. When neutrophils are present and can function normally, they limit infection to the site of entry and produce pus. This creates physical signs, such as pneumonia or abscess formation. In neutropenic patients, neutrophils cannot localize infection, which rapidly spreads to the blood and then to other tissues. Other cells of the immune system (particularly macrophages) are able to function normally; for example, this patient was able to mount an acute-phase response with fever and rigors. Septic shock is an exaggerated part of the normal innate response to infection. Septic shock is an acute state of hypotension caused by the effects of bacterial endotoxins. The shock is a result of decreased vascular tone and impaired cardiac output. Septic shock is common in neutropenic patients but may be seen in patients with normal immune responses who are overwhelmed by infection, for example after a ruptured bowel. Most cases are caused by gram-negative organisms, and lipopolysaccharide is typically the endotoxin implicated.

Endotoxin release triggers the innate immune response by activating macrophages through Toll-like receptors. Consequences of macrophage activation include the secretion of TNF, prostaglandins, and nitric oxide. The TNF triggers more nitric oxide production by smooth muscle and endothelial cells. The very high levels of nitric oxide are responsible for the decreased vascular tone and cardiac output (it should be remembered that normal levels of nitric oxide help maintain vascular tone). Endothelial cell activation may also trigger the clotting cascade.

Septic shock is often complicated by widespread organ failure, especially when the clotting cascade is also activated. The multi-organ failure is not a direct consequence of the initial infection, but is caused by the innate immune system's response to the infection. The syndrome of multiorgan failure consequent to exaggerated innate immune system activation is sometimes referred to the systemic inflammatory response syndrome (SIRS), and has a mortality of over 70%. Attempts at blocking the effects of gross activation of the innate immune system have largely been unsuccessful (Fig. 20.12).

Toxic shock syndrome is a different entity, mediated by cytokines secreted from T cells.

This example illustrates how important it is to respond promptly to very early symptoms of infection in neutropenic patients.

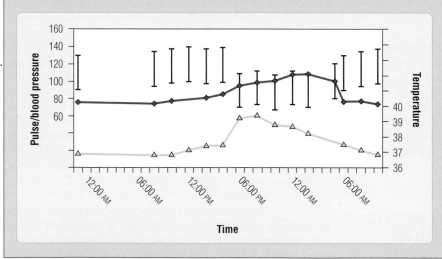

Figure 20.11   This chart shows the vital signs for the patients described in this box. *Blue squares* are the pulse, *black bars* are the blood pressure, and the *yellow triangles* are temperature.

Continued

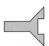 T cell receptor (TCR)

 Immunoglobulin (Ig)

 Antigen

 MHC I

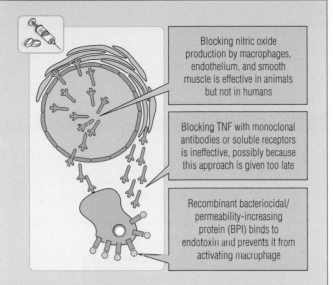

Blocking nitric oxide production by macrophages, endothelium, and smooth muscle is effective in animals but not in humans

Blocking TNF with monoclonal antibodies or soluble receptors is ineffective, possibly because this approach is given too late

Recombinant bacteriocidal/permeability-increasing protein (BPI) binds to endotoxin and prevents it from activating macrophage

Figure 20.12 Various attempts have been made to reverse the effects of septic shock. None has been very successful, possibly because by the time shock is diagnosed, the mechanisms have often become reversible.

Stimulation of Toll-like receptors has potent activating effects on many components of the immune system. In clinical medicine, there are two areas where it is desirable to increase the immune response. These are cancer and vaccines, discussed further in subsequent chapters. Suffice it to say at this point that because cancer and vaccines are not infections, they are not good at producing danger signals, and very often the immune system does not respond as well as we would like it to. Two Toll-like receptor ligands, unmethylated cytosine and guanosine sequences (CpG motifs) and imiquimod, can safely mimic infections and have been tested in these settings.

CpG motifs are found in bacteria and are absent in human cells. They potently stimulate dendritic cells expressing TLR9 to secrete IL-12, which promotes T_H1 responses and boosts the subsequent production of both IgG and cytotoxic T cells (Fig 20.13). When combined with existing vaccines, CpG can improve antibody and T-cell responses. CpG have also been found to be effective in clinical trials for some cancers, when combined with conventional treatments. CpG appears to have very few side effects.

Imiquimod is a synthetic drug that mimics single-stranded RNA and stimulates TLR7, also on macrophages and dendritic cells. These then secrete a wide range of cytokines, with stimulatory effects on the innate and adaptive immune system. Imiquimod is widely used to treat wart infections. Like many chronic viral infections, the wart virus is able to replicate slowly inside cells and does not produce a strong danger signal. Imiquimod painted onto warts can be a very effective treatment. Imiquimod can potentiate the effects of vaccines and has been used to treat tumors. It has the advantage that it can be painted directly on to some skin tumors with considerable effects.

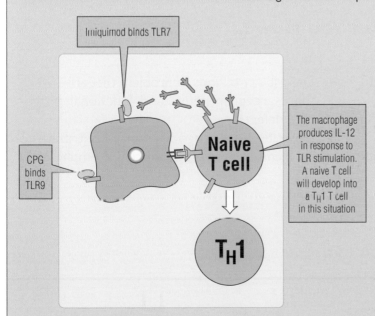

Imiquimod binds TLR7

CPG binds TLR9

Naive T cell

The macrophage produces IL-12 in response to TLR stimulation. A naive T cell will develop into a T_H1 T cell in this situation

T_H1

Figure 20.13 CpG and imiquimod mimic danger signals and boost T_H1 responses to antigens. CpG, cytosine and guanine sequences; T_H, T helper.

BOX 20.3   Chronic Granulomatous Disease

A 4-year-old boy presents with a high fever and signs of fluid in the left pleural cavity. A sample from the pleural cavity shows pus, from which *Staphylococcus aureus* is grown.

The child has a history of growth retardation and perianal abscesses. He has no siblings and the only family history is of the death of a maternal uncle from infection in his teens.

Blood examination shows a marked neutrophilia of 23×10^6 mL when the normal range is 3 to 6×10^6 mL. A nitro blue tetrazolium (NBT) test is carried out to determine whether his neutrophils are capable of mounting a respiratory burst (Fig. 20.14). The patient's neutrophils are unable to produce a respiratory burst, consistent with a diagnosis of chronic granulomatous disease (CGD).

CGD is a primary immunodeficiency affecting neutrophil function. This disease is characterized by recurrent bacterial and fungal infections in the presence of a neutrophilia. It is caused by mutations in the genes for NADPH oxidase or its regulatory proteins. CGD is usually X-linked. Although neutrophils are produced in abundance and are able to migrate to sites of infection, they cannot produce superoxide radicals and kill pathogens. Pathogens (such as the fungus *Aspergillus* and the bacterium *Staphylococcus*), which would normally lead to short lived pus forming infections, are not cleared and lead to the formation of granulomata, typical of chronic infection (see Chapter 22).

Infection in children with CGD can be prevented by the use of prophylactic antibiotics and antifungal agents, although other approaches, such as stem cell transplant, have been tried.

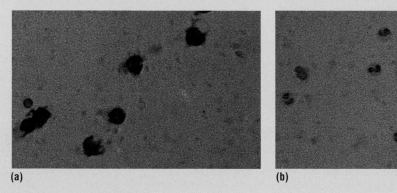

(a)　　　　　　　　　　　　　　　　(b)

Figure 20.14   The nitro blue tetrazolium (NBT) test. NBT is a pale-yellow color, but changes to purple in cells that have undergone an oxidative burst. **A**, Neutrophils from a normal donor have been stimulated the NBT has produced a black color. **B**, Neutrophils from a patient with chronic granulomatous disease are unable to change the color of the dye. There is no cytoplasmic staining, and it is possible to see the multilobed nucleus.

LEARNING POINTS　Can You Now ...

1. List the differences between the roles of neutrophils and macrophages?

2. List the different types of macrophage and their specialist functions?

3. Describe how the innate immune system activates the adaptive immune system?

4. Describe two kinds of problem that arise when there are quantitative and functional phagocyte defects?

5. Describe how phagocytes may contribute to problems such as septic shock and emphysema?

 T cell receptor (TCR)　　 Immunoglobulin (Ig)　　 Antigen　　 MHC I

21 Killing in the Immune System

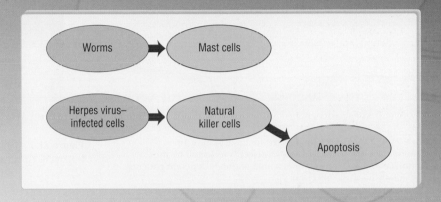

The immune system has to destroy a wide range of pathogens and uses the mechanisms shown in the figure above, and Figure 21.1, to achieve this. In this chapter, you will learn how two special types of pathogen, worms and some viral infections, have driven the adaptive immune system to develop specialist killing cells—mast cells and natural killer (NK) cells. You will also learn more about apoptosis, a generic killing mechanism used by many parts of the immune system.

RESPONSE TO PARASITE WORMS

During human evolution, parasitic worms were a major threat to the species. Probably because of improved sanitation, worms are no longer considered a problem to people in the developed world, although a third of the world's population is still infested with these parasites. Worms come in a variety of shapes and sizes (from 1 mm to 1 m) and tend to have complicated life cycles involving eggs, larvae, and adult forms. Worm eggs are resistant to low pH and proteolytic digestion in the stomach and do not hatch until they reach the lower gut. Adult worms living inside the lower gut are protected from many of the components of the immune response. To overcome this, mast cells and eosinophils evolved to respond to worms living in the gut. Essentially, on activation these cells discharge toxic substances into the gut lumen, increase mucus secretion, and cause smooth muscle contraction, resulting in expulsion of

the worm; these responses are summarized in Figure 21.2. The same mechanisms evolved in the airways.

MAST CELLS

Mast cells are derived from an unknown precursor cell in the bone marrow, under the influence of the T helper 2 (T_H2) cytokines interleukin (IL)-3 and IL-4. Rather like macrophages, mast cells home into a range of normal tissues, including the submucosa, skin, or connective tissue (Fig. 21.3). Recruitment to these frontline sites is increased during worm infestations.

Like macrophages, mast cells reside in the tissues for several weeks. During this time, mast cells produce granules containing a range of mediators. They also acquire immunoglobulin (Ig)E on their specialized Fc receptors (FcεRI). FcεRI have a very high affinity for IgE, and, therefore, even IgE produced at a very low level elsewhere in the body will bind with mast cells. Consequently, the mast cells can bind a range of IgE molecules against a number of different antigens. Mast cells become activated when these surface IgE molecules are cross-linked by antigen (Fig. 21.4). Mast cell FcεRI are different from other types of Fc receptor; they bind Ig that is not bound to antigen and do not induce activation until they have been cross-linked by antigen. Mast cells are also activated by anaphylatoxins C3a and C5a (see Chapter 19) and by a number of drugs, including opiates.

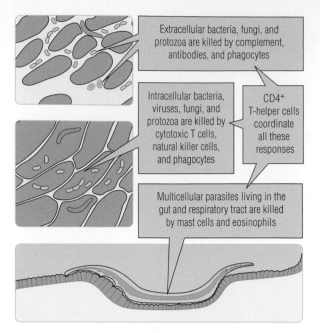

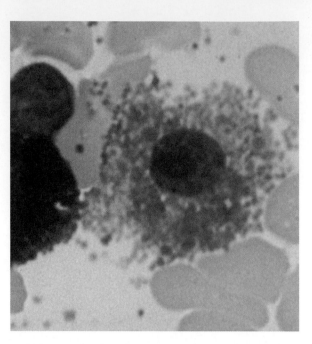

Figure 21.1 Targets for killing by the immune system. In immunodeficiency states, the type of defect is reflected by the infections patients develop. For example, antibody-deficient patients suffer mainly bacterial infection.

Figure 21.3 Mast cell. The granules in this mast cell contain cytokines, histamine, and proteolytic enzymes.

Mast cell activation results in degranulation and release of preformed substances from the granules and activation of arachidonic acid metabolism to produce a range of freshly made mediators (Fig 21.5).

Granule Contents

Mast Cell Enzymes
Mast cell granules contain a number of proteolytic enzymes, including tryptase and chymotrypsin. These enzymes in-

crease mucus secretion and smooth muscle contraction in, for example, bronchi. In addition, they cleave and activate components of the complement and kinin pathways, which promotes inflammation.

Histamine
Histamine causes smooth muscle contraction in the gut and lungs in an attempt to expel worms. Histamine increases vascular permeability by causing endothelial cell contraction, leading to a widening of intercellular gaps

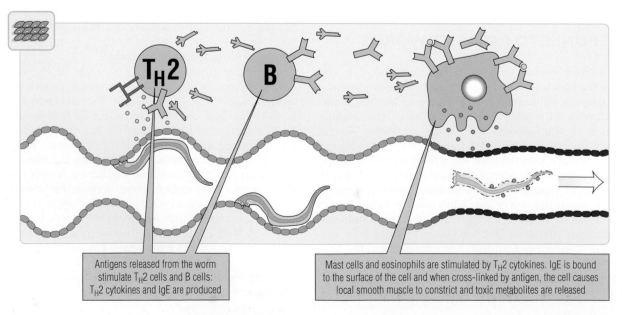

Antigens released from the worm stimulate T_H2 cells and B cells: T_H2 cytokines and IgE are produced

Mast cells and eosinophils are stimulated by T_H2 cytokines. IgE is bound to the surface of the cell and when cross-linked by antigen, the cell causes local smooth muscle to constrict and toxic metabolites are released

Figure 21.2 Summary of the response to a gut-dwelling worm.

 T cell receptor (TCR)

 Immunoglobulin (Ig)

 Antigen

 MHC I

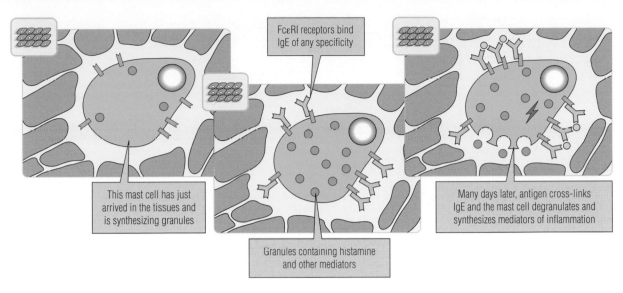

Figure 21.4 Mast cell activation.

and subsequent tissue edema. Histamine provides a chemotactic signal to attract more white cells to the site of worm infestation. Histamine causes marked itching in the skin, possibly to draw the attention of an infested host to the presence of skin parasites.

Cytokines

Like activated macrophages, mast cells produce a range of cytokines to promote and extend the inflammatory response. Tumor necrosis factor (TNF) is preformed and present in granules and will activate local endothelium to enhance diapedesis of more inflammatory cells. Mast cells also produce other cytokines after stimulation, and, unlike those produced by macrophages, these stimulate T_H2 responses. IL-4 activates T_H2 cells, and IL-3 and IL-5 stimulate eosinophil production and activation. IL-4 and IL-5 also

skew the adaptive immune response away from a T_H1 response.

Arachidonic Acid Metabolites

Metabolites of arachidonic acid metabolism are produced by mast cells and also by phagocytes. Arachidonic acid metabolism is activated by mast cell exposure to antigen and can follow two different pathways (Fig. 21.6).

- The cyclo-oxygenase pathway produces **prostaglandins**, which act within seconds to stimulate vasodilatation, increased vascular permeability, and constriction of smooth muscle in the gut and bronchi. Prostaglandins may have other slower effects, such as inhibiting T_H1 cells.

FIG. 21.5 Mast Cell Mediators*

Mediator			Actions
Preformed mediators present in granules	Proteolytic enzymes: tryptase and chymotrypsin		Activates components of the complement and kinin pathways (for examples cleaving kininogen to bradykinin), which promote inflammation.
	Histamine		Smooth muscle contraction in the gut, lungs, and blood vessels. Increases vascular permeability.
	Cytokines	Tumor necrosis factor (TNF) IL-4 IL-3 and IL-5	Activates endothelium to enhance diapedesis. Activates T_H2. Stimulate eosinophil production and activation
Arachidonic acid metabolites	Cyclooxygenase pathway	Prostaglandins, thromboxane	Vasodilatation, increased vascular permeability and constriction of smooth muscle in the gut and bronchi.
	Lipoxygenase pathway	Leukotrienes, platelet activating factor	Bronchial and gut smooth muscle contraction. Chemotactic stimuli for neutrophils and eosinophils.

*The main effects of the release of mast cell mediators are vasodilation and increased vascular permeability (causing tissue swelling) and smooth muscle contraction and mucous secretion

 MHC II

 Cytokine, Chemokine, etc.

Complement (C')

 Signaling molecule

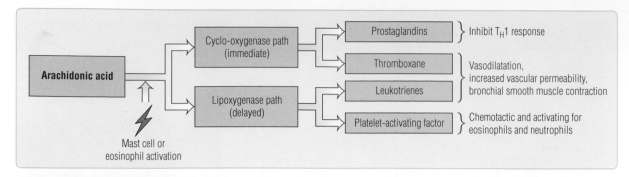

Figure 21.6 Arachidonic acid metabolism. Several of these pathways are affected by drugs. For example, aspirin and other "nonsteroidal anti-inflammatory" drugs inhibit the cyclo-oxygenase pathways, blocking the immediate effects of mast cell degranulation. However, these drugs do not block the lipoxygenase pathway and can lead to increased production of leukotrienes, which can exacerbate the delayed features of mast cell degranulation.

- The lipoxygenase pathway produces leukotrienes. These have rather slower effects than prostaglandins but contribute to bronchial and gut smooth muscle contraction. In addition, leukotrienes act as chemotactic stimuli for neutrophils and eosinophils and thus contribute to increasing the cellularity of the immediate reaction and converting it to a delayed or chronic reaction.

Mast cells reside in a number of tissues that are at the front line for parasitic infection. Although activation of mast cells is dependent on preformed IgE antibodies, they respond very rapidly to antigen stimulation. The immediate response is caused by histamine, proteolytic enzymes, and prostaglandins, and consists of smooth muscle contraction, increased vascular permeability, and mucus secretion. The cytokines and leukotrienes promote a late-phase response to antigen. This is characterized by an influx of eosinophils and T_H2 cells. This late-phase inflammation may become chronic but is distinct from the granulomata, which are characterized by the presence of macrophages and T_H1 cells.

Eosinophils

Eosinophils are broadly similar to mast cells; however, two factors make them unique: they are specifically recruited to tissues during some types of inflammation, and their granules contain particularly toxic substances.

Eosinophils are derived from precursors that are similar to neutrophils, and their production is stimulated by IL-3 and IL-5. Eosinophils are normally present in blood in small numbers, but their numbers increase dramatically in response to IL-3 and IL-5 secreted by T_H2 cells and mast cells. The causes of increased numbers of eosinophils in the blood—eosinophilia—are discussed in Box 21.1. Eosinophils are recruited to parasite-infested sites by the chemokine **eotaxin**, which is produced by epithelium cells and leukotrienes produced by mast cells.

Eosinophils are activated by cytokines, chemokines, and, perhaps, cross-linked IgE on FcεRI. Activated eosinophils release the same mediators as mast cells (except histamine) and, in addition, three special mediators:

- A peroxidase that is released onto the surface of parasites and then generates hypochlorous acid
- Major basic protein, which damages the outer surface of parasites (and host tissues!)
- Cationic protein, which damages the parasite's outer surface and acts as a neurotoxin, damaging the simple nervous system of the parasite.

Immediate (Type I) Hypersensitivity

Because the effects of eosinophil or mast cell degranulation are so rapid, this type of response is sometimes referred to as immediate (type I) hypersensitivity, although the cytokines and other mediators released can also set up delayed and chronic inflammatory responses.

People living in the developed world are no longer challenged by worms. In these populations, mast cells and eosinophils cause immediate hypersensitivity in response to innocuous antigens such as pollens—the hallmarks of allergy (see Chapter 26). Eosinophils and mast cells secrete a wide range of mediators, many of which are targets in the treatment of allergy.

■ NATURAL KILLER CELLS

NK cells have two important roles. As their name suggests, they are excellent killers of cells infected by some viruses, but, like macrophages, they have an additional role of stimulating the adaptive immune response.

NK cells are part of the innate immune system and fill a potential gap in the specific immune response. Most cells infected with viruses, for example, influenza, are killed when cytotoxic T lymphocytes (CTLs) recognize viral peptides bound to major histocompatibility complex (MHC). Some infectious agents, notably members of the herpes virus family, downregulate MHC expression on infected cells to evade detection by T cells. Herpes viruses can also block intracellular antigen presentation pathways (see Chapter 10). These evasion mechanisms prevent cytotoxic T-cell recognition, but NK cells are still able to recognize and kill cells infected with herpes viruses, because they

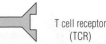 T cell receptor (TCR)

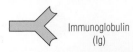 Immunoglobulin (Ig)

 Antigen

 MHC I

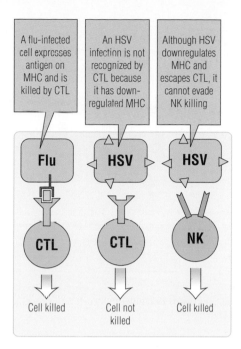

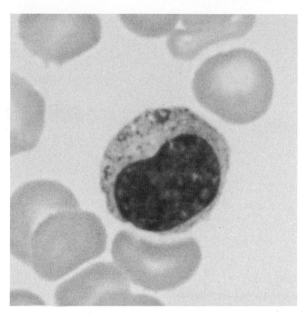

Figure 21.8 The granules in natural killer cells contain perforin and granzyme.

Figure 21.7 Comparison of the killing of influenza and herpes simplex (HSV) infected cells. Because herpes simplex downregulates MHC expression, cytotoxic T cells (CTLs) cannot kill infected cells. NK cells are stimulated by the absence of MHC and kill the infected cell as a result.

have evolved to recognize and kill cells with low MHC expression (Fig. 21.7). Similarly, some tumor cells have acquired mutations that result in decreased MHC expression and are able to evade tumor-specific T cells.

NK cells develop and acquire their receptors in the bone marrow. Although they are not generated in the thymus, they share some characteristics with T cells. For example, they share some T-cell surface molecules (such as CD2) and have a similar appearance to lymphocytes. (An alternative name for NK cells is large granular lymphocyte; Fig. 21.8). NK cells also use the same generic killing mechanisms as cytotoxic T cells. However, NK cells do not have rearranged T-cell receptor molecules and are thus classified as belonging to the innate immune system. NK cells also share some characteristics of macrophages— they are capable of recognizing antibody coated target cells, but they do not kill these by phagocytosis.

NK cells arise from the same lymphoid progenitor cells as T and B cells, although it is not clear how their production is regulated. NK cells constitute approximately 5% to 15% of lymphocytes in peripheral blood. They are activated by cytokines (Fig. 21.9), but killing itself is regulated by signaling through special receptors.

Antibody-Dependent Cellular Cytotoxicity

In NK cells, a special Fc receptor, FcγRIII, recognizes IgG-bound viral antigen on the surface of infected cells and triggers killing. IgG-mediated NK killing is referred to as antibody-dependent cellular cytotoxicity and is illustrated in Figure 21.10. FcγRIII is also expressed by some macro-

phages, in which case IgG acts as an opsonin and triggers phagocytosis.

Natural Killer Receptors

NK cells can recognize and kill cells that express lower than normal levels of MHC. To do this, NK cells have two types of specialized receptor for MHC. **Killer immunoglobulin-like receptors** (KIRs) are members of the immunoglobulin superfamily and recognize specific MHC α-chains. **NKG2/CD94** are C-lectin molecules that recognize the nonclassic human leukocyte antigen (HLA)-E molecule.

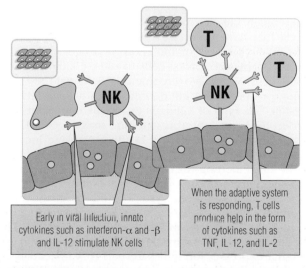

Early in viral infection, innate cytokines such as interferon-α and -β and IL-12 stimulate NK cells

When the adaptive system is responding, T cells produce help in the form of cytokines such as TNF, IL-12, and IL-2

Figure 21.9 Cytokine regulation of natural killer (NK) cells. Like T cells, NK cells proliferate in response to interleukin (IL)-2. TNF, tumor necrosis factor.

 MHC II

 Cytokine, Chemokine, etc.

 Complement (C')

 Signaling molecule

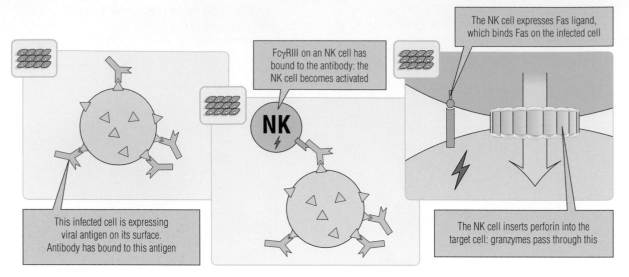

The NK cell expresses Fas ligand, which binds Fas on the infected cell

FcγRIII on an NK cell has bound to the antibody: the NK cell becomes activated

NK

This infected cell is expressing viral antigen on its surface. Antibody has bound to this antigen

The NK cell inserts perforin into the target cell: granzymes pass through this

Figure 21.10 Antibody-dependent cellular cytotoxicity. Binding of antibody to FcεRIII stimulates the natural killer (NK) cell. This process is similar to opsonization by IgG.

Both types of receptor are special because they can inhibit killing. When an NK cell encounters a virally infected cell, two outcomes are possible (Fig. 21.11).

- The NK cell recognizes that the cell is infected, using an innate immune system pattern-recognition molecule. The NK cell uses its receptors to check that MHC is present on the surface of the cell. If MHC is present at an adequate level, the receptor delivers a negative signal, which prevents the NK killing. Because the virally infected cell expresses MHC, it will in any case be killed by a CTL.
- If the NK recognizes that a cell is infected by a virus and confirms that levels of MHC are reduced, it will go ahead and kill the target cell.

The balance between the stimulatory and inhibitory signals determines the outcomes of NK cell activation; NK preferentially kill cells with absent MHC expression.

Cells may have absent MHC expression because of viral infection or because of mutation in cancer cells. Either process enables abnormal cells to escape killing by cytotoxic T cells. NK cells overcome this potential flaw in the immune response by killing cells with absent MHC expression. This type of killing is especially important when interferon-γ is present; this cytokine maximizes MHC expression by normal cells and at the same time increases NK cell activity. Reduced expression of MHC acts as a danger signal, alerting NK cells to the presence of infection.

NK cells have one more important role. They are the major cell of the immune system in the pregnant uterus. Uterine NK cells clearly have a role in preventing viral infection of the uterus and fetus during pregnancy. They have the added advantage of not attacking fetal tissue even though it expresses foreign (paternal) HLA molecules. NK cells are inhibited by cells that express normal levels of MHC, regardless of whether it is host or from another individual.

Cytotoxic T-Cell and Natural-Killer Cell Effector Mechanisms

The cytotoxic mechanisms used by NK cells are identical to those used by cytotoxic T cells. Both populations use perforin, granzyme, and Fas ligand expression and secre-

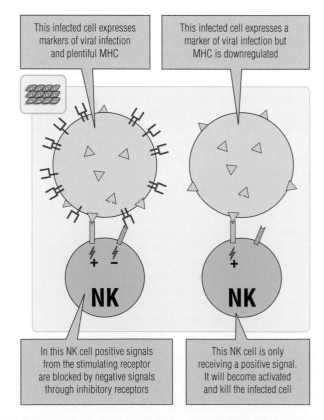

This infected cell expresses markers of viral infection and plentiful MHC

This infected cell expresses a marker of viral infection but MHC is downregulated

NK   **NK**

In this NK cell positive signals from the stimulating receptor are blocked by negative signals through inhibitory receptors

This NK cell is only receiving a positive signal. It will become activated and kill the infected cell

Figure 21.11 Natural killer (NK) receptors that inhibit killing may have a role in the treatment of a variety of diseases in the near future.

 T cell receptor (TCR)   Immunoglobulin (Ig)   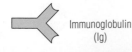 Antigen   MHC I tion of TNF, all of which can induce programmed cell death—**apoptosis**. NK cells and cytotoxic T cells also secrete immunoregulatory cytokines, such as interferon-γ, which promote the T_H1 inflammatory response.

Perforin

Perforin is contained within the cytotoxic granules of NK cells and cytotoxic T cells. When cytotoxic T cells or NK cells are activated, the actin cytoskeleton is reorganized so that perforin molecules are moved to the cell surface. Perforin polymerizes and forms a pore that is inserted into the target cell membrane, rather like the complement membrane attack complex (see Fig. 19.9). These pores allow salts and water to flow into the target cell and, more importantly, give granzyme access to the cytoplasm.

Granzyme

Granzyme is three separate proteolytic enzymes that are transported by the activated cytoskeleton and transferred into the target cell. As well as degrading host cell proteins, they specifically activate the **caspase** enzyme system, which results in apoptosis.

Fas Ligand

Fas ligand is a potent inducer of apoptosis and is used by NK cells and cytotoxic T cells to kill infected or tumor cells. Fas is a member of the same family of receptors as the TNF receptor (Fig. 21.12). Fas and Fas ligand are expressed on cells of the immune system during activation. Fas ligand expression is increased on cytotoxic T cells and NK cells when they become activated. Fas ligand binds Fas

on a target cell, which then undergoes apoptosis through the mechanisms described later. T cells may also express Fas and become targets of Fas-mediated killing. For example, cells in immunoprivileged sites, such as the testis, express Fas ligand. Any T cell that accidentally ends up in the testis will be exposed to Fas and will undergo apoptosis. T cells sometimes use Fas/Fas ligand during complex interactions that result in them killing one another—so-called fratricide. This kind of mechanism may seem obscure, but is used to destroy autoreactive T cells.

Fas ligand appears to be mainly involved in killing. It does not have the other more general effects of TNF receptor, for example, promoting inflammation or causing weight loss. The different members of the TNF family are described in detail in Chapter 23.

Although NK cells are very effective at killing in their own right, they also activate the adaptive immune response, by secreting cytokines that stimulate T_H1 responses. Macrophages behave in a similar way, and this is exactly what we expect from cells of the innate immune system. Both types of cell recognize families of pathogens rather than specific antigens. They attempt to eradicate the pathogen but also activate the adaptive immune system.

NK cells secrete interferon-γ when they encounter target cells. This cytokine stimulates T_H1 cells and inhibits T_H2 cells. A T_H1 response is especially effective at dealing with intracellular infection and can provide immunologic memory to guarantee a strong response should the host be exposed to the same pathogen again.

■ INTRACELLULAR MECHANISMS OF APOPTOSIS

In this chapter, we are most interested in apoptosis that has been induced through the ligation of receptors such as Fas or the TNF receptor (see Fig. 21.12). However, similar intracellular mechanisms lead to apoptosis, regardless of the many different triggers.

Fas and TNF receptor both have cytoplasmic tails (called death domains), which can activate the series of caspase enzymes (Fig 21.13). Caspases are proteolytic enzymes that cleave proteins after aspartic acid residues. The final result of activation of the caspase is activation of a specific DNase, which cleaves the DNA of the target cells into 200 base-pair fragments. Caspases are also activated when NK or cytotoxic T cells inject granzyme into the cell.

Another early effect of apoptosis is the disruption of mitochondria. Mitochondria become leaky, and the release of mitochondrial products further activates caspases. Bcl-2 is an antiapoptotic protein that binds to and stabilizes mitochondria and prevents upregulation of apoptosis (see Ch 17). Falling IL-2 levels reduce the intracellular concentration of Bcl-2 and can make apoptosis more likely to occur. This happens at the end of a successful immune response when antigen levels are falling and IL-2 secretion is diminished. However, other members of the Bcl-2 family of proteins can promote apoptosis, so, clearly, the regulation of apoptosis is complex and involves many interacting factors.

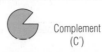

Figure 21.12 Fas and tumor necrosis factor (TNF) receptor can both induce cell death.

 MHC II   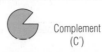 Cytokine, Chemokine, etc.   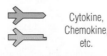 Complement (C')   Signaling molecule

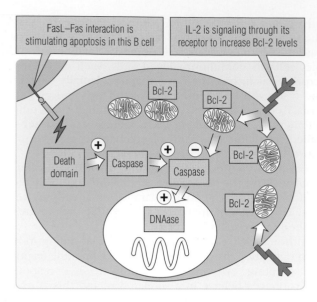

Figure 21.13 Whether or not this B cell undergoes apoptosis is determined by the balance of signals through Fas, caspases, interleukin-2 (IL-2), and Bcl-2.

Apoptosis in the Immune System

Apoptosis is the process of programmed cell death, whereby cells are deliberately killed as a part of physiologic processes. Apoptotic cells are recognized by phagocytes, which usually clear the cell remains without stimulating inflammation. By comparison, **necrosis** is the inadvertent death of cells, usually caused by exposure to metabolic insults, such as hypoxia or toxins. Necrosis does not result in DNA fragmentation and, because it activates the complement cascade, often results in an inflammatory response.

Apoptosis is an important physiologic process affecting many body systems. During embryonic life, for example, apoptosis is involved in remodeling tissues, such as the developing vascular system. In this way, apoptosis determines the shape of the developing fetus.

Apoptosis has a number of very important roles in shaping the adaptive immune repertoire. Autoreactive T and B cells undergo apoptosis very soon after they are generated in the thymus and bone marrow. Autoreactive lymphocytes that escape these central processes are forced to undergo apoptosis in the periphery. In these cells, recognition of self antigen by T- or B-cell receptor in the thymus or bone marrow triggers apoptosis. Additionally, after an immune response to a pathogen, redundant lymphocytes are also cleared by apoptosis. Each of these uses different mechanisms (Fig. 21.14), but the result is that the specificities of the immune response are shaped by apoptosis.

Apoptosis is also involved in some pathologic processes; for example, there is evidence that one of the ways that CD4+ T cells are destroyed by HIV infection is through induction of apoptosis. When apoptotic debris is not cleared adequately by phagocytes, it can become immunogenic. This can lead to the production of autoantibodies—for example, against DNA—and this may generate autoimmune disease—for example, systemic lupus erythematosus.

On the other hand, in some cases there is insufficient apoptosis for normal regulation. In the autoimmune lymphoproliferative syndrome, inherited defects in the apoptosis pathways cause defective B-cell apoptosis, leading directly to autoimmunity (Box 21.2). Defective apoptosis can also occur in clones of B cells that have increased levels of Bcl-2 through mutations or chromosome translocations may be protected from apoptosis and can develop into a B-cell malignancy (see Chapter 34). Defective apoptosis can also be acquired by infection with some herpes viruses. For example, Epstein-Barr virus evades apoptosis by producing a Bcl-2 like protein. This "immortalizes" the B cells that the virus infects and can also contribute to the development of B-cell malignancy.

FIG. 21.14 Apoptosis in the Immune System

Area involving apoptosis	Target	Mechanism
Negative selection in the thymus	T cells	
Peripheral T cell tolerance	Autoreactive T cells	Lack of costimulation?
At the end of an immune response when only a few cells are required to maintain memory	Responding T cells	Cytokine starvation leading to reduction in Bcl-2
Negative selection of B cells in bone marrow	B cells	
Low-affinity antibody production	B cells	Changes in Bcl-2
Peripheral B cell tolerance	Autoreactive T cells	Fas
Protection of immune privileged sites	T cells	Cells (e.g., testicular cells) express FasL, which kills incoming T cells
Intracellular infection	Any cells	Fas, tumor necrosis factor, granzyme
Malignancy	Malignant cell	Fas, tumor necrosis factor, granzyme

T cell receptor (TCR)

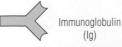

Immunoglobulin (Ig)

Antigen

MHC I

BOX 21.1 Eosinophilia

A 43-year-old man has returned from working as an overseas aid worker in Southeast Asia, where he has been involved in developing sewerage schemes (Fig. 21.15). On his return home, he is required to undergo a medical examination during which he is found to have a raised eosinophil count of 2.5×10^6 mL (the eosinophil count is normally below 0.35×10^6 mL) (Fig. 21.16) and to have abnormal liver function tests.

Although allergy is the most common cause of eosinophilia in the developed world, this patient has no signs or symptoms of allergies, such as asthma, rhinitis, or eczema. Neither does he have any features of the cancers, for example, lymphoma, sometimes associated with eosinophilia. A liver biopsy is performed, which shows parasite eggs surrounded by granulomata. A diagnosis of the parasitic worm infection, **schistosomiasis**, is made, and the patient responds well to treatment.

Schistosoma mansoni is a common parasite in some parts of the world. Humans are infected when larvae penetrate the skin from contaminated water supplies. Adult worms live in the portal veins and discharge eggs, which may lodge in the liver. Mast cells and eosinophils are able to kill schistosomiasis worms and their eggs, using the mechanisms described above. The marked eosinophilia is a reflection of the activation of these cells. As the eggs disintegrate, they release peptides that are processed and recognized as conventional antigens by T_H1 cells. Untreated schistosomiasis leads to chronic inflammation in the liver and is one cause of liver cirrhosis. It is not yet clear if this damage is caused by the eosinophil response to adult worms, the T_H1 cell response to worm eggs, or a combination of both.

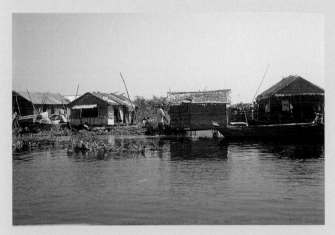

Figure 21.15 In this village in Cambodia, human feces are dropped straight into the water supply. The plant growing in the lake is water hyacinth, which provides the home for the snail that is the host to schistosomes. In this kind of environment, mast cells and eosinophils provide important defenses for the human population.

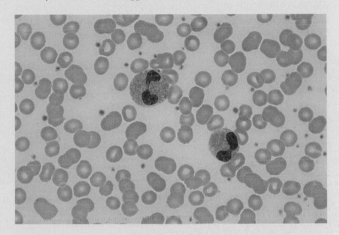

Figure 21.16 Eosinophils. The multilobed nuclei of these cells indicate how closely related they are to neutrophils (see Fig 20.1A). Note the red, coarse granules.

 MHC II

 Cytokine, Chemokine, etc.

 Complement (C')

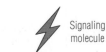 Signaling molecule

BOX 21.2 Auto Immune Lymphoproliferative Syndrome

A 2-year-old boy (A) is referred to the pediatric services after his family doctor has found him to have swollen lymph nodes. He is also found to have severe anemia and a reduction in his platelet count (thrombocytopenia). At first, the diagnosis appears to be acute leukemia, and a bone marrow sample is obtained. Fortunately, his marrow does not show any leukemic cells. There are increased numbers of red cell and platelet precursors in the marrow, consistent with autoimmune destruction of these cells in the blood (see Chapter 28). Another finding is that he has increased numbers of B cells in his blood. Through the use of B immuno-globulin gene rearrangement studies (see Chapter 14), the B cells are shown to be polyclonal.

The boy's diagnosis remains something of a mystery until his mother (B) mentions that various other family members have had blood problems. On further questioning, two family members died of lymphoma (C and D). The family history is shown in Figure 21.17. The family history reveals a typical autosomal dominant pattern of inheritance of the blood problems. The penetrance is poor, in other words, obligate carriers of the abnormal gene, such as our patient's mother, do not always develop the disease phenotype. This type of inheritance is typical of the autoimmune lymphoproliferative syndrome (ALPS). The Fas, Fas ligand, and caspase genes of our patient are sequenced. He is found to be heterozygous for a mutation in Fas. This is diagnostic of ALPS. Further testing shows that the patient's affected mother, uncle (E), and cousin (F) have the same mutation.

In ALPS, mutations in the Fas, Fas ligand, or caspase genes prevent apotosis from taking place normally. B cells are unable to undergo programmed death and accumulate in the lymph nodes and spleen, accounting for the swelling of these organs. In addition, the normal B-cell tolerance mechanisms that prevent auto antibody production are defective. ALPS patients produce autoantibodies against their own blood cells, causing all the blood problems this family experienced. The risk of lymphoma, a malignancy of lymphocytes, is also increased in ALPS patients.

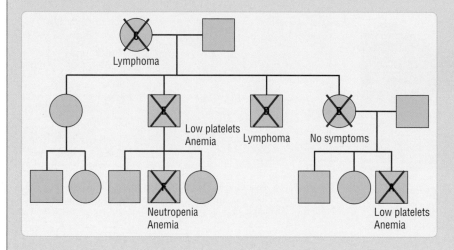

Fig 21.17 Family tree of family described in the box. *Circles* are female and *squares* are male. A *red cross* indicates carrier status.

LEARNING POINTS ... Can You Now ...

1. Identify the type of infection that mast cells and eosinophils respond to?
2. List the contents of mast cell and eosinophil granules?
3. Describe the consequences of arachidonic acid metabolism?
4. Describe two ways by which herpes virus family members avoid killing?
5. Describe NK cell receptors?
6. List NK cell killing mechanisms?
7. Draw the mechanism of apoptosis?
8. Give some examples of how defects in apoptosis can cause disease?

 T cell receptor (TCR)

 Immunoglobulin (Ig)

 Antigen

 MHC I

22 Inflammation

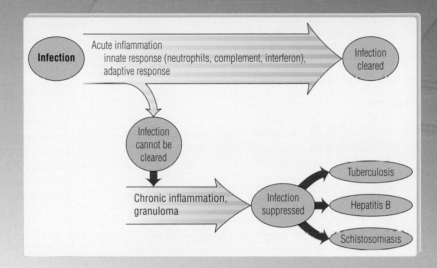

During infection, the innate and adaptive components of the immune systems generate inflammation. This clears most infections. Some infections cannot be cleared, and chronic inflammation results.

■ TYPES OF INFLAMMATION

Inflammation is clinically defined as the presence of redness, swelling, and pain. Histologically, it is defined as the presence of edema fluid and the infiltration of tissues by white cells. There are many causes of inflammation; for example, a burn will cause an acute inflammatory response, and although this is triggered by a physical stimulus, it is at least partially mediated by immunological mechanisms, such as the release of tumor necrosis factor (TNF) from damaged tissues.

If the offending stimulus cannot be rapidly removed, the inflammation tends to become chronic. Figure 22.1 shows some infections that result in either chronic or acute inflammation.

Acute reactions to bacteria result in pus formation; they are **pyogenic**. For example, you will be familiar with the pustules or larger abscesses in the skin usually caused by *Staphylococcus*. Yellow sputum also reflects pyogenic infection, this time in the chest, usually caused by *Pneumococcus* or *Haemophilus*. Meningitis due to *Neisseria meningitidis* is another type of pyogenic infection; recall all the neutrophils in the cerebrospinal fluid (CSF) sample in Figure 19.15. In pus and infected sputum, the yellow color is contributed by neutrophil granules. Although there may be severe damage in the short term, these infections often resolve with minimal scarring.

Chronic bacterial infections may lead to the formation of **granuloma**—collections of specialized macrophages surrounded by T cells. This occurs in tuberculosis (TB; the infection caused by *Mycobacterium tuberculosis*—Box 22.1). Chronic viral infection leads to more diffuse inflammation, although macrophages and T cells are still present. This typically occurs in infections with *Hepatitis B virus*, where acute inflammation occurs initially as a result of antiviral activity, and chronic inflammation can follow as the inflammatory response continues in a failed attempt to eliminate the pathogen. This chronic stage results in damage to the host organs (Box 22.2). Acute inflammation mediated by mast cells is characterized by edema; when it becomes more long lasting, eosinophils enter the inflamed tissue. A good example of chronic inflammation mediated by mast cells and eosinophils is **schistosomiasis**, discussed in Chapter 21. There is considerable overlap between the different types of inflammation as shown in Figure 22.2.

Pus formation can develop over a few hours. Granulomata take 2 to 3 days to develop because of the time it takes for the T-cell response to develop. Granulomatous reactions are sometimes referred to as delayed hypersensitivity. *Mycobacterium tuberculosis* elicits a typical **delayed hypersensitivity** reaction, as illustrated by skin testing for TB (see Box 22.1). Granuloma development requires T-cell involvement and, therefore, has characteristics

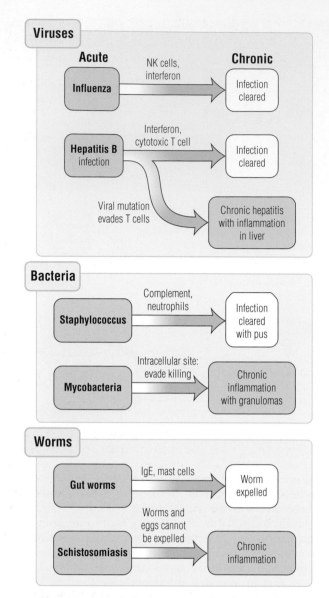

Figure 22.1 Acute or chronic inflammation depends on pathogen and host factors. In hepatitis B virus infection, both viral mutations and host human leukocyte antigen (HLA) type may determine whether chronic inflammation occurs. IgE, immunoglobulin E; NK, natural killer.

of adaptive immunity, such as antigen specificity and recall responsiveness.

■ CYTOKINE NETWORK IN INFLAMMATION

Cytokines are required to initiate acute inflammation and maintain chronic inflammatory responses. These responses require help from CD4+ T cells. The interaction between these and either macrophages or eosinophils is sometimes referred to as the **cytokine network**.

In Chapter 20 we described how macrophage cytokines and mediators initiate immune responses that even-

tually lead to granuloma formation. Macrophages secrete interleukin-1 (IL-1), TNF, and granulocyte-macrophage colony-stimulating factor (GM-CSF), which activate the acute-phase response and promote marrow production of neutrophils and monocytes. Macrophage-produced TNF and IL-1 increase adherence of leukocytes to local endothelium, and these leukocytes then follow the chemotactic signal of chemokines also produced by macrophages. Macrophages also produce cytokines that act on T cells, including IL-1 and IL-12. IL-1 is a general activator of T cells and, along with costimulatory molecules such as CD40, activates all classes of T cell. IL-12 preferentially activates T helper (T_H1) and natural killer (NK) cells, respectively.

In response to these macrophage-derived cytokines, T_H1 and NK cells secrete interferon-γ (IFN-γ) and more TNF. The major effects of IFN-γ are to:

- Increase expression of major histocompatibility complex (MHC) on macrophages and other local cells
- Increase antigen processing through proteasomes in macrophage
- Induce macrophage maturation
- Increase NK cell activity
- Inhibit T_H2 cells
- Cause mild antiviral effects (see Chapter 19).

The effects of IFN-γ on macrophages are to stimulate T_H1 cell activity further through antigen presentation and cytokine production. The exchange of cytokines between macrophages and T cells generates a strong positive feedback loop between these two populations and skews the immune response toward a T_H1 pattern (Fig. 22.3).

TNF, produced by macrophages and T cells, has a number of important roles in the developing inflammatory response. However, high local levels of TNF can cause negative effects, such as tissue destruction. TNF also has potent systemic effects—for example, fat catabolism, fever, and loss of appetite, leading to weight loss.

The feedback loop ultimately comes to a halt when phagocytes have cleared all residual antigen. Thus, stimulation of T cells ceases, and the level of IFN-γ falls. Costimulation by macrophages is reduced; the result is that T cells die through apoptosis.

The cytokine network is used to control several intracellular infections, most importantly bacteria of the *Mycobacterium* family. These range from organisms that have adapted to host immunity, for example, *Mycobacterium tuberculosis*, to usually harmless organisms, referred to as opportunist (or atypical) mycobacteria. The opportunist mycobacteria cause disease when the cytokine network has failed in a variety of separate situations:

- Rarely, some individuals inherit mutations in the genes for IL-12, IL-12 receptor, or IFN-γ receptor. These individuals are very prone to infection with all types of mycobacteria.
- More frequently, the cytokine network is disrupted by drugs. For example, monoclonal antibodies against TNF are used to treat rheumatoid arthritis (see Chapter 30). Mycobacterial infection is a recognized complication of anti-TNF treatment.

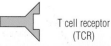
T cell receptor (TCR)

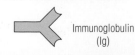
Immunoglobulin (Ig)

Antigen

MHC I

FIG. 22.2 Types of Inflammation

	Acute Inflammation (pyogenic)	Chronic Inflammation (granulomatus)	Acute Inflammation (immediate hypersensitivity)	Chronic Inflammation (eosinophil-mediated)
Typical triggers	Staphylococci	Mycobacterial infection, hepatitis B	Worms	Worms
Initiating cell	Macrophage	Macrophage	?	?
Effector cell in innate system	Neutrophil	Macrophage, natural-killer cell	Mast cell	Mast cell eosinophil
Effector cell in adaptive system	None involved	T_H1 cell	T_H2 cell, B cell	T_H2 cell, B cell
Mediators	Complement, GM-CSF, TNF, chemokines	TNF. IL-12, interferon-γ chemokines	Histamine, mast cell granule contents, leukotrienes	IL-3, IL-4, IL-5 chemokines
Systematic effects	Acute-phase respone; neutrophilia	Acute-phase response; chronic effects of TNF, neutrophilia may be present	May lead to anaphylaxis (Chapter 26)	Eosinophilia raised IgE
Type of lesion	Pus formation, abscesses	Granuloma may be present	Edema, mucus, smooth muscle contraction	Diffuse inflammation in mucosa or skin

GM-CSF, granulocyte-macrophage colony-stimulating factor; IL, Interleukin; TNF tumor necrosis factor

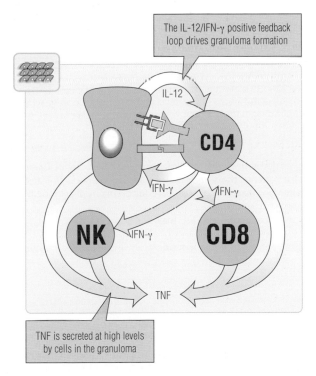

Figure 22.3 The cytokines interleukin-12 (IL-12), interferon-γ (IFN-γ), and tumor necrosis factor (TNF) drive granuloma formation.

• Most importantly, HIV infection is a very frequent cause of mycobacterial infection, particularly in Africa. This is because HIV infects and damages both T cells and macrophages, as discussed in Chapter 32. Early in HIV infection, when the immune deficiency is not severe, infection with mycobacterium tuberculosis is characteristic. In later HIV infection, with more severe immune deficiency, infection with opportunist mycobacteria is common.

■ "OVERZEALOUS" INFLAMMATION

During inflammation, granuloma formation and cytokines may have negative effects. The negative effects of TNF have already been mentioned. An example of an overzealous response is excessive granuloma formation in the lung in response to *M. tuberculosis*, which may produce necrotic lesions that subsequently cavitate. These cavities are produced when necrotic material is coughed up, which allows the mycobacteria contained to be spread from person to person. These infectious patients are described as having "open TB."

Another mycobacterium, *M. leprae*, can also stimulate the granulomatous reaction that controls the mycobacterial infection; hypersensitivity to *M. leprae* is discussed in Box 16.2. This form of leprosy is known as tuberculoid leprosy.

 MHC II

 Cytokine, Chemokine, etc.

Complement (C')

 Signaling molecule

BOX 22.1 Tuberculosis

Tuberculosis (TB) is relatively common in prison inmates. An infection control team is called into a prison after a prisoner has developed symptoms of TB. Her chest radiograph shows destruction of normal tissue and is suggestive of TB (Fig. 22.4). Culture of her sputum is positive for *Mycobacterium tuberculosis,* confirming the diagnosis and the very significant risk to other inmates. The index patient is transferred to the prison hospital for treatment and to prevent her from infecting other patients.

During her stay in prison, she has shared cells with 36 other prisoners. These prisoners require screening for exposure to TB and the development of infection. Because chest radiographs and sputum cultures are very insensitive to early TB infection, tests of immunity to *Mycobacterium tuberculosis* are used to screen individuals exposed to patients with "open TB." A blood test and a skin test are available and are described later in this box. In this case, four of the 36 prisoners show evidence of latent TB and are treated with combinations of antibiotics.

In the late 20th century, TB was thought to be under control. However, it has re-emerged as a major threat to global health and now kills 2 to 3 million individuals per year.

Mycobacterium tuberculosis stimulates macrophages by binding Toll-like receptors 2 and 4, which recognize mycobacterial lipoproteins and polysaccharides. This stimulates phagocytosis and secretion of inflammatory mediators, such as interleukin-12 and nitric oxide. Mycobacterial peptides presented by macrophages elicit strong T helper 1 (T_H1)-type responses. The most important of these are secretion of tumor necrosis factor (TNF) and interferon-γ (IFN-γ), which stimulate the formation of granuloma during primary infection.

Mycobacteria, such as *M. tuberculosis*, have waxy coats that block the effects of phagocyte enzymes. They also secrete catalase, which prevents the effects of the respiratory burst. Because it is hard to kill them, macrophages seal off mycobacteria inside phagosomes. This sealing off process requires help from T cells, in the form of T_H1 cytokines such as IFN-γ.

Initial exposure to TB results in primary infection. In most patients with primary TB, mycobacterial growth is contained within the granuloma (Fig. 22.5). Here, macrophages mature under the influence of IFN-γ into giant cells and epithelioid cells. Granulomata seal off infected macrophages so well that, occasionally, the center of a granuloma becomes hypoxic, and the cells may become necrotic. The necrotic area resembles cheese, and this caseous necrosis is a hallmark of TB infection.

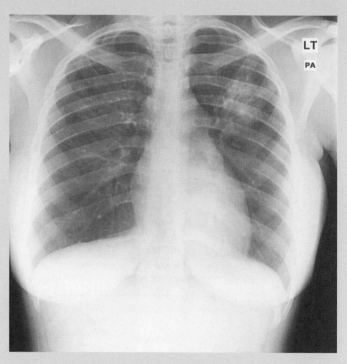

Figure 22.4 This chest radiograph shows typical changes of TB that tend to affect the apices of the lungs. You can easily see an opacity in the upper zone of the left lung. X ray courtesy of Dr Mark Woodhead, Manchester Royal Infirmary, UK.

Less than 10% of patients with primary TB have any symptoms, and even fewer develop widespread infection. In very young or immunodeficient patients, primary TB is not contained within the granuloma. In these patients, there may be widespread infection (miliary TB) (Fig. 22.6). Even when infection is contained and controlled in the lungs, many mycobacteria may survive inside macrophages or other cells for several years. This is referred to as latent infection.

Paradoxically, patients who respond to primary TB infection with excessive production of TNF may develop extensive local tissue damage and become infectious to other people.

Postprimary (reactivation) TB occurs in about 10% of patients, especially if macrophage function is moderately impaired. This commonly happens when patients are treated with high doses of corticosteroids or if there is malnutrition (for example in alcoholics). Reactivation of TB is also a common problem in HIV infection.

IMMUNOLOGIC TESTS FOR EXPOSURE TO TUBERCULOSIS

Two types of test are used to test for immunity to tuberculosis. They are most often used to screen individuals who have been exposed to patients with open TB. The older test is a skin test that relies on the delayed hypersensitivity reaction. Skin testing is gradually being replaced by a blood test that measures IFN-γ secreted in response to mycobacterial antigens (Fig. 22.7). This test is reliant on the presence of effector T cells circulating in the blood, which are able to secrete IFN-γ within 24 hours of the addition of antigen in patients with latent TB. Although it is being used less frequently, it is still important to be familiar with skin testing for immunity to TB because it illustrates some important immunologic principles.

Delayed hypersensitivity skin testing is carried out with intradermal injection of tuberculin: a sterile mixture of proteins and lipoproteins derived from *M. tuberculosis*. This type of skin test is also known as the **Mantoux** or **Heaf test**, depending on the type of injection technique used. The reaction starts when Toll-like receptors on dermal macrophages recognize the mycobacteria and in response secrete TNF and chemokines, which increase the expression of local endothelial adhesion molecules (Fig. 22.8). At the same time, dendritic cells migrate from the site of injection to draining lymph nodes.

Continued

 T cell receptor (TCR)

 Immunoglobulin (Ig)

 Antigen

 MHC I

BOX 22.1 Tuberculosis—cont'd

The migrating dendritic cells are loaded with mycobacterial antigens. This antigen can be presented to T cells in the draining lymph node, but only if adequate numbers exist from a primary response. Remember that the number of T cells for a specific antigen increases during the acquisition of immunologic memory. The activated T cells will subsequently migrate to the site of injection and interact with local activated macrophages. Macrophages will also accumulate and mature as a result of cytokines secreted by the T cells. When a strong response (Fig. 22.9) is produced at 48 hours, more than 80% of the cells present in the skin lesion are activated macrophages.

Delayed hypersensitivity tests assess immunologic memory for specific antigens; the intensity of the response depends on the extent of T-cell priming and the ability to make a T-cell recall response. T-cell priming can be brought about by latent TB infection or TB vaccine. TB vaccine is a live attenuated mycobacterium, bacille Calmette-Guérin (BCG), and is used routinely in many parts of the world, but not in the United States because of some concerns about its efficacy.

Interpretation of the skin test depends on whether the individual has been primed. Healthy individuals who have been vaccinated with BCG produce a moderate response to tuberculin testing at 48 hours. A response in an unvaccinated individual may suggest recent exposure to TB. Additionally, absence of a response in a patient who is known to have had BCG vaccine may suggest immunodeficiency, for example, secondary to HIV infection.

The blood test relies on the production of IFN-γ by T cells responding to *M. tuberculosis* peptides. It is hoped that this will make it more specific for TB exposure, because it is possible to incorporate peptides that are present in *M. tuberculosis* but not the BCG organism.

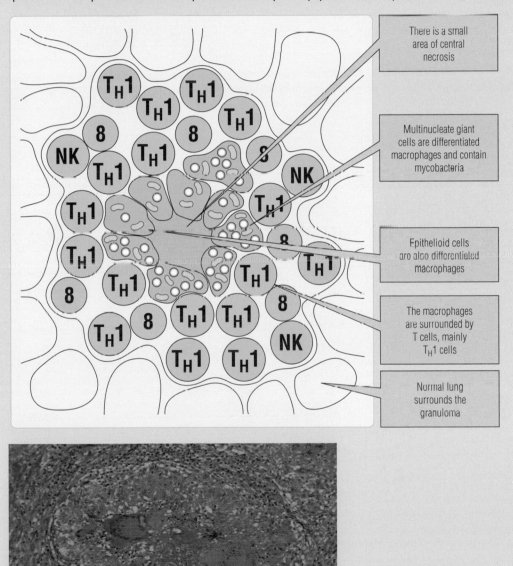

There is a small area of central necrosis

Multinucleate giant cells are differentiated macrophages and contain mycobacteria

Epithelioid cells are also differentiated macrophages

The macrophages are surrounded by T cells, mainly T$_H$1 cells

Normal lung surrounds the granuloma

Figure 22.5 A, This figure shows the major features of a tuberculous granuloma. In this particular case, there is not much necrosis. If necrosis becomes more severe, the granuloma will break down and *Mycobacterium tuberculosis* could be coughed up. NK, natural killer; T$_H$1, T helper 1. **B,** This is a micrograph of a tuberculous granuloma. Note the central necrosis, two giant cells on either side of this, and the cuff of lymphocytes in the periphery.

Continued

BOX 22.1   Tuberculosis—cont'd

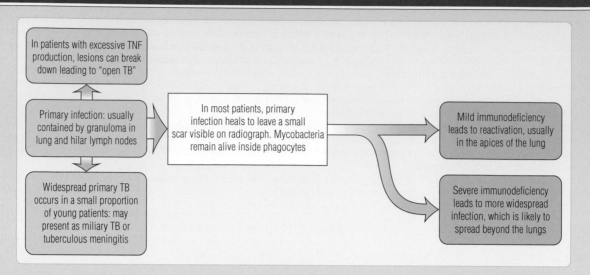

Figure 22.6 Infection with *Mycobacterium tuberculosis* can have a number of short- and long-term outcomes. TB, tuberculosis; TNF, tumor necrosis factor.

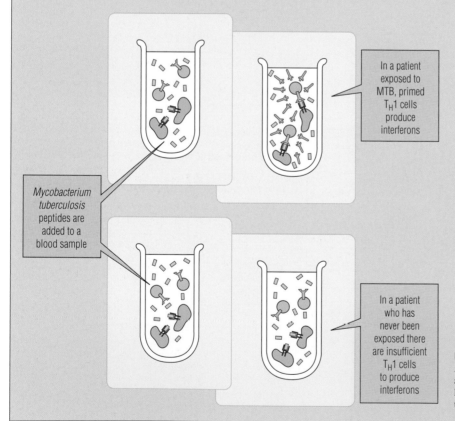

Figure 22.7 In the blood test for TB exposure, *Mycobacterium tuberculosis* (MTB) peptides are added to blood, which is then cultured for 12 hours. The amount of interferon-γ produced is then measured by ELISA.

Continued

 T cell receptor (TCR)   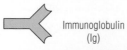 Immunoglobulin (Ig)   Antigen   MHC I

BOX 22.1 Tuberculosis—cont'd

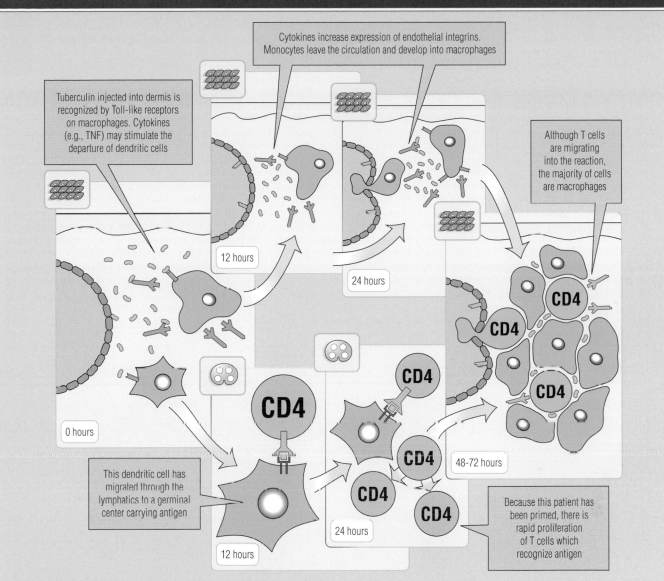

Tuberculin injected into dermis is recognized by Toll-like receptors on macrophages. Cytokines (e.g., TNF) may stimulate the departure of dendritic cells

Cytokines increase expression of endothelial integrins. Monocytes leave the circulation and develop into macrophages

Although T cells are migrating into the reaction, the majority of cells are macrophages

This dendritic cell has migrated through the lymphatics to a germinal center carrying antigen

Because this patient has been primed, there is rapid proliferation of T cells which recognize antigen

0 hours · 12 hours · 24 hours · 12 hours · 24 hours · 48-72 hours

Figure 22.8 Reactions occurring after an injection of tuberculin. After 48 hours, macrophages and T cells are accumulating in the dermis. TNF, tumor necrosis factor.

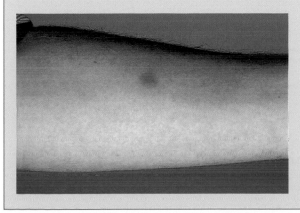

Figure 22.9 This is a positive tuberculin skin test in one of the prisoners described in the box, 48 hours after injection. This prisoner had never had TB vaccine, and, therefore, the positive test confirms exposure to TB and possible latent infection. TB, tuberculosis.

 MHC II Cytokine, Chemokine, etc. Complement (C′) Signaling molecule

BOX 22.2 Hepatitis B and Chronic Hepatitis

Hepatitis B infection is a major global infection with 350 million infected individuals across the world. The virus causes hepatitis, often leading to cirrhosis and liver cancer. *Hepatitis B virus* only replicates in hepatocytes but does not damage these cells directly; the virus is not cytopathic.

The immune response to *Hepatitis B virus* is important at two different stages. Antibodies to the *Hepatitis B virus* surface protein (HBsAg) can protect from infection; these antibodies are often the result of vaccination, as discussed in Chapter 24. Cellular immunity is important in people who do not have protective antibodies and in whom virus is already replicating in hepatocytes. *Hepatitis B virus* is susceptible to the antiviral effects of interferons, as described in Chapter 19. During hepatitis B infection, the specific immune system responds to infection with a T_H1-type response (as you would expect for a viral infection) and hepatitis B-specific $CD4^+$ and $CD8^+$ T cells migrate to the liver. These cells secrete interferon-γ (IFN-γ), and there is evidence that the antiviral effects of this cytokine inhibit viral replication. Although nearly all infected patients develop transient hepatitis, which is life threatening in less than 1%, most infected patients (80%–90%) manage to suppress viral replication through the antiviral effects of IFN-γ. Unlike the type I interferons, IFN-γ has potent stimulating effects on inflammation, and an inflammatory response develops, during which hepatocytes are damaged by the immune response, rather than by the virus itself. The result is acute hepatitis. In the majority of patients, viral replication is controlled. Although virus is not eradicated, ongoing T-cell responses are enough to minimize virus replication so that, for example, the patient stops being infectious to other individuals (Fig. 22.10).

In approximately 10% to 20% of infected people, the virus is not cleared through these means. This can happen when, for example, the initial inoculum of virus was particularly large. Alternatively, the virus may mutate so that antigenic epitopes change, and the virus evades the immune response. Host factors, for example the human leukocyte antigen (HLA) type, may affect the risk of not clearing virus. In these individuals, the inflammatory response persists, although it is unable to inhibit viral replication completely. Unlike TB, chronic hepatitis B infection does not produce granulomata. In hepatitis B patients, production of IFN-γ is a double-edged sword; it is the best hope for inhibiting viral replication but will promote a chronic inflammatory response. This results in chronic active hepatitis. The recruitment of natural killer cells, macrophages, and T cells that are not even specific for *Hepatitis B virus* eventually leads to chronic inflammation inside the portal areas. The resulting tissue destruction causes scars that can lead to liver cirrhosis and, through unknown mechanisms, can set the scene for liver cancer.

An understanding of hepatitis B infection has helped to develop strategies for preventing and treating this serious infection (Fig. 22.11).

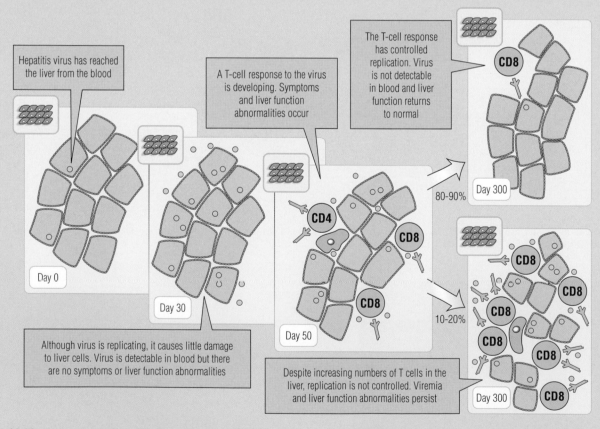

Hepatitis virus has reached the liver from the blood

A T-cell response to the virus is developing. Symptoms and liver function abnormalities occur

The T-cell response has controlled replication. Virus is not detectable in blood and liver function returns to normal

Day 0

Day 30

Day 50

Day 300

80–90%

10–20%

Day 300

Although virus is replicating, it causes little damage to liver cells. Virus is detectable in blood but there are no symptoms or liver function abnormalities

Despite increasing numbers of T cells in the liver, replication is not controlled. Viremia and liver function abnormalities persist

Figure 22.10 The outcome of hepatitis B virus infection depends on immunologic factors.

Continued

 T cell receptor (TCR)

 Immunoglobulin (Ig)

 Antigen

MHC I

BOX 22.2 Hepatitis B and Chronic Hepatitis—cont'd

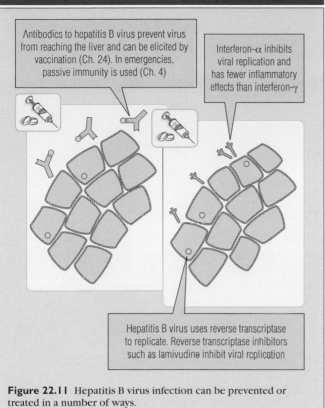

Antibodies to hepatitis B virus prevent virus from reaching the liver and can be elicited by vaccination (Ch. 24). In emergencies, passive immunity is used (Ch. 4)

Interferon-α inhibits viral replication and has fewer inflammatory effects than interferon-γ

Hepatitis B virus uses reverse transcriptase to replicate. Reverse transcriptase inhibitors such as lamivudine inhibit viral replication

Figure 22.11 Hepatitis B virus infection can be prevented or treated in a number of ways.

LEARNING POINTS Can You Now ...

1. Define inflammation?
2. Describe the outcomes of tuberculosis infection?
3. Describe the consequences of hepatitis B infection and how they are affected by the immune response?
4. Draw the cytokine network?
5. Write the sequence of cellular events in delayed hypersensitivity skin testing?

 MHC II

 Cytokine, Chemokine, etc.

 Complement (C')

 Signaling molecule

23 Cytokines in the Immune System

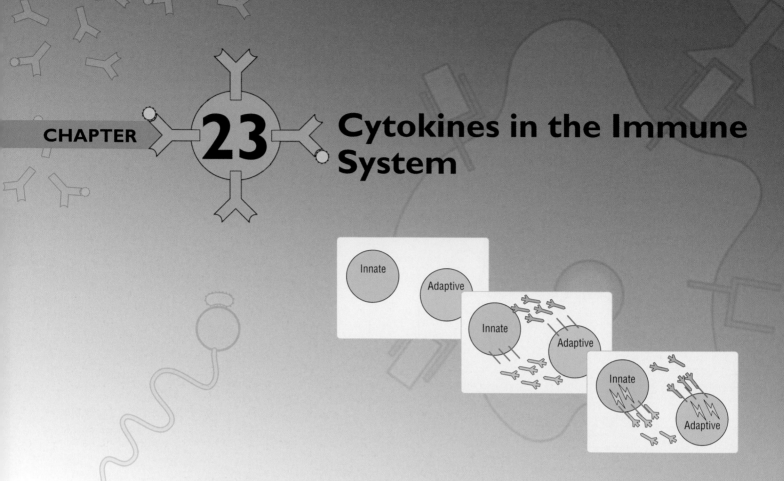

The cells of the adaptive and innate immune systems cannot function in isolation. Immune cells use cytokines to communicate. In this chapter, you will learn more about cytokines, how they are recognized by specific receptors, and how they activate special signaling molecules in their target cells.

■ INTRODUCTION

In this section, we review what you have learned so far about the adaptive and innate immune system and focus on the types, structure, and role of cytokines and their receptors. You will already be familiar with the some of the material in this chapter, but will need to develop a good working knowledge of cytokines because of their increasing significance in clinical medicine. Cytokines are sometimes measured in clinical tests (Fig. 23.1). Cytokines and cytokine antagonists are also already in widespread clinical use, and their role is likely to continue to develop.

■ DEFINITIONS AND SOME GENERAL NOTES ABOUT CYTOKINES

Cytokines are soluble messenger molecules usually secreted by cells of the immune system. Some cytokines (e.g., type I interferons [IFNs] and tumor necrosis factor [TNF]) are secreted by nonimmune cells (e.g., epithelial cells). Although some cytokines are constantly secreted at a low level (constitutively secreted), most are only secreted when cells become activated as part of the response to infection.

Cytokines are secreted at extremely variable levels. Adaptive immune system cytokines are secreted at very low levels and only affect neighboring cells (paracrine affects) or even the secreting cell itself (autocrine affects). This low-level secretion is to maintain the specificity of the adaptive immune system. For example, interleukin-2 (IL-2), secreted by activated T cells has potent effects that induce T-cell proliferation. Most of these effects are mediated on the cell that is secreting IL-2; if it were secreted at high levels, it might activate cells that were not recognizing specific antigen. Adaptive immune system cytokines are almost impossible to detect in fresh blood samples.

Cytokines of the innate immune system are often secreted at low levels over a short range (e.g., chemokines directed at attracting neutrophils to the site of infection), but can also be secreted at high enough levels to be measurable in blood samples. When they are secreted at high levels, they act like hormones of the endocrine system. For example, you have already read how IL-1, IL-6, and TNF secreted during an acute-phase response can have distant effects, such as the induction of fever (see Chapter 19).

Because most cytokines are secreted in response to infection, they are only secreted transiently. For example, IL-2 is only secreted by activated T cells for about 8 hours. Any longer secretion would cause inappropriate and potentially dangerous prolonged immune-system activation.

FIG 23.1   Clinical Uses of Cytokines

Cytokine measurement
TNF and IL-6 can be measured in blood samples in septic shock (see Chapter 20)
Interferon-γ is measured in blood samples incubated with mycobacterial peptides to diagnose latent TB (see Chapter 22)
Cytokine treatment
Innate immune system cytokines, such as interferon-α are used to treat chronic hepatitis virus infection (see Chapter 19)
Cytokines are **pleiotropic,** affecting many different types of cells, and mild side effects are common
Adaptive immune system cytokines are generally only secreted at very low levels, effective over short ranges. Their systematic use (at high dose) usually causes severe side effects
Cytokine blockade
Various strategies are used to block TNF and IL-I in the treatment of rheumatoid arthritis (see Chapter 30)
Because there is often **redundancy** in cytokine networks, blocking just one cytokine is often not 100% effective.
Basiliximab is used to block IL-2 binding to its receptor in the prevention of transplant rejection

Once infection is resolved, cytokine secretion tends to fall. In addition, toward the end of an immune response, inhibitory cytokines such as IL-10 and transforming growth factor β (TGF-β) may be produced to ensure the immune response does not continue.

Cytokine receptors are also often only expressed transiently. The complete IL-2 receptor is only transiently expressed by activated T cells. Again, this mechanism has evolved to prevent inappropriate activation of the immune system.

Cytokines have two more important features: redundancy and pleiotropism. Redundancy refers to the fact that generally several cytokines secreted during an immune response have very similar properties. For example, TNF and IL-1 have similar affects. These cytokines synergize with one another (have additive effects). This is important clinically, because attempts to block the effects of cytokines may not always guarantee clinical outcomes. Anti-TNF monoclonal antibodies are successful at preventing joint damage in rheumatoid arthritis, for example, but do not completely prevent disease because IL-1 is also mediating damage.

Pleiotropism refers to the fact that many cytokines affect several different types of cell. This is also clinically important: the antiviral effects of IFN-α are used to treat hepatitis B virus infection, but IFN-α makes patients feel unwell because it induces an acute-phase response. You can read more about how pleiotropism causes side effects of cytokine treatment in Chapter 35.

Cytokines act as part of a complex network. Apart from synergizing with one another, cytokines can also inhibit each other. For example, IFN-γ promotes T-helper 1 (T$_H$1) responses and also inhibits the development of T$_H$2 responses, mediated by IL-4. This can contribute to the unexpected effects seen when cytokines are administered or blocked during treatment.

Finally, the nomenclature of cytokines can be hard to follow. The largest group, interleukins, were so named because they were initially thought to act between leukocytes. In fact, they often have much wider affects on many different types of cell. The interleukins (IL-1, IL-2, etc.) were named in the order they were discovered, and their numbering has no relation to function!

Some of the originally discovered cytokines were named after their presumed function. IFNs, for example, were so named because they do interfere with viral replication, but they also have potent effects activating the immune system. TNF was so named because it can induce necrosis in cancers when injected into animals at high concentrations. Its effects *in vivo* are usually far more subtle.

In the table (Fig. 23.2), we have listed the important cytokines in order of their general effects. Note how many cytokines link the adaptive and innate immune systems.

■ CYTOKINE RECEPTORS AND SIGNALING MOLECULES

Most cytokines use one of three types of receptors that are linked to signal transduction molecules that convey signals from the receptor to inside the cell. These share some properties with the signal transduction machinery connected to T- and B-cell receptors (see Chapter 11). The three main types of receptor are the general cytokine receptor family, the chemokine receptor, and the TNF receptor.

Most cytokines use broadly similar receptor molecules (sometimes called the hemopoietin receptors). This includes cytokines that act as growth factors and the IFNs. These receptors consist of one or more transmembrane molecules with extracellular domains conferring specificity for particular cytokines (Fig. 23.3). The receptors for IL-2, IL-4, and IL-7 consist of three separate polypeptide chains, but share a common γ chain. The gene for the γ chain is defective in X-linked severe combined immunodeficiency disease (SCID). The clinical consequences of this are described in Box 12.2.

Most of these cytokine receptors are not expressed in high numbers in completely resting cells; they tend to be upregulated after a cell has been activated (e.g., after a T cell has been activated through its T-cell receptor). After upregulation, the cytokine receptors are normally spread across the surface of the cell. When cytokine binds to its receptor, it causes aggregation of the receptors at the cell surface. One of several tyrosine kinases, called JAKs, are

 MHC II
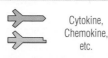 Cytokine, Chemokine, etc.
  Complement (C')
 Signaling molecule

FIG. 23.2 Important Cytokines*

General effects	Cytokine	Cells produced by	Cells affected	Receptor type	Mentioned in Chapter
Proinflammatory	Tumor necrosis factor	Macrophages T cells, and other cells	Many cell types	TNF receptor	12, 16, 19, 20, 21, 22
	IL-1	Macrophages	Endothelial cells, liver cells, hypothalamus	Immunoglobulin superfamily member	20, 22
	Chemokines (including IL-8)	Macrophages, endothelial cells, T cells	All leukocytes	Chemokine receptor	13, 20, 21, 22
	IL-12	Macrophages	T cells and NK cells	Cytokine receptor	15, 20, 22
	Type I interferons	Macrophages, many other cells	Many cell types		19, 22
	IL-6	Macrophages, T cells	Liver, B cells		15, 18, 19, 20
Growth factors	IL-7	Bone marrow stromal cells	Lymphoid progenitors		12
	IL-3	T cells	All hematopoietic cells		21
	G-CSF	Macrophages	Neutrophils		12, 20
	IL-2	T cells	T cells and NK cells		11, 12, 15 16, 21
T_H2 deviation	IL-4	T_H2 cells and mast cells	T cells, B cells and mast cells		12, 15, 16, 21, 22
	IL-5	T_H2	Eosinophils, B cells		15, 16, 21, 22
T_H1 deviation	Interferon-γ	T_H1	Macrophages, B cells, T cells, NK cells		16, 20, 21, 22
Inhibitory	IL-10	Macrophages, regulatory T cells	Macrophages		23
	TGF-β	T cells and macrophages	T cells and macrophages	Special receptor	23

*The type of secreting cell and target cell in this table are indicated by colors. Green indicates cells of the innate immune system, blue indicates cells of the adaptive immune system, and turquoise indicates cells of both systems.

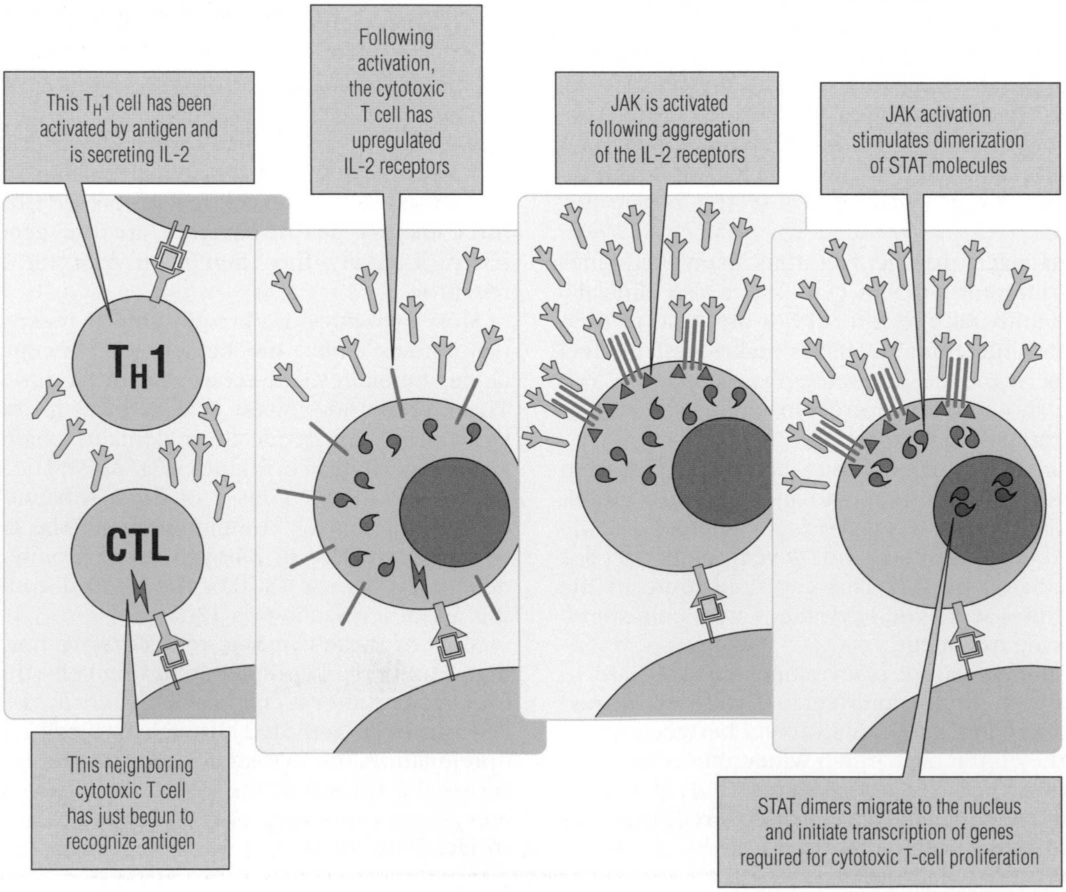

Figure 23.3 This figure shows the key features of hemopoietin family of cytokine receptors and associated signaling molecules. IL, interleukin; T_H1, T-helper cell.

normally loosely associated with the cytoplasmic portion of the cytokine receptors. The JAK enzymes become activated when the receptors are brought together by cytokine binding and then phosphorylate one of several transcription factors called signal transducers and activators (STAT). Once STAT molecules have become phosphorylated, they form a dimer, migrate to the nucleus, and activate transcription of specific genes.

There are several JAK and STAT molecules. For example, when IL-2 binds to receptors on the surface of activated T cells, it activates JAK5, STAT1, and STAT3. When these migrate to the nucleus, they activate genes that initiate T-cell proliferation.

When extracellular levels of cytokines fall, toward the end of the immune response, they cease binding to receptors, and the events leading to gene transcription will come to an end.

Chemokines are a large family of cytokines that have already been mentioned in relation to attracting cells into inflamed tissues (see Chapters 13 and 20). They also have a role in leukocyte homing. For example, chemokines secreted by cells in lymph nodes attract B cells to germinal centers and dendritic cells and T cells to the T-cell areas (see Chapter 13). To achieve these complex signals, there are approximately 50 different chemokines and approximately 20 different receptors. Most of the receptors can bind several different chemokines, and many chemokines can bind different receptors. The chemokine receptors are α helices that span the cytoplasmic membrane seven times (Fig. 23.4). On binding chemokines, the receptors catalyze the replacement of GDP by GTP. One specific chemokine receptor is used as a co receptor for HIV (see Chapter 32).

TNF uses a special family of receptors. TNF is secreted and can be active as a membrane-bound form. It can also be cleaved from the secreting cell membrane and is then free to cause local or remote effects. Both cell-bound and cell-free TNF are present as a trimer and bind to one of two types of receptor, which are also trimers.

There are two other important members of the TNF/TNF receptor family, which you are already familiar with. CD40 and CD40-ligand (CD154) are a pair of costimulatory molecules involved in interactions between T cells and either B cells or antigen-presenting cells (APCs). The other pair is Fas and Fas ligand (Fig. 23.5).

The effects of TNF depend on the target cell it binds to. When TNF binds to infected cells, it induces apoptosis by inducing caspases through death domain engagement, as described Chapter 21. On the other hand, when TNF binds macrophages or endothelial cells, it induces transcription of genes by engaging a special set of adaptor molecules

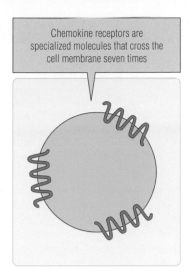

Chemokine receptors are specialized molecules that cross the cell membrane seven times

Figure 23.4 This figure shows a typical chemokine receptor.

that activate nuclear factor κB. Fas /Fas ligand ligation only induces apoptosis in target cells, in a wide range of situations. CD40 / CD154 (CD40 ligand) binding induces gene transcription and has an important role in communication between T cells and either APCs or B cells (Fig. 23.6). In Chapter 16, you also learned that mutations in the *CD154* gene can lead to antibody deficiency.

■ A REVIEW OF SOME OF THE ROLES OF CYTOKINES IN IMMUNE RESPONSES

You should now be familiar with most of the components of the immune system. It is useful at this stage to review how these components fit together, particularly to understand the role of cytokines in communication between the innate and adaptive immune system (Fig. 23.7). You should make sure that you understand the role of cytokines in initiating inflammation, T-cell priming, the development of T-cell specialization, and, finally, the winding down of the immune response.

Acute Inflammation—The Initial Response to Infection

Invading pathogens present danger signals to cells of the innate immune system, which respond by secreting cyto-

FIG 23.5 TNF Family Members & Their Receptors			
TNF-Like Molecule	**TNF Receptor-Like Molecule**	**Induces Apoptosis**	**Induces Gene Transcription**
TNF	TNF receptor	Yes	Yes
CD40 ligand	CD40	No	Yes
Fas ligand	Fas	Yes	No

 MHC II

 Cytokine, Chemokine, etc.

 Complement (C')

 Signaling molecule

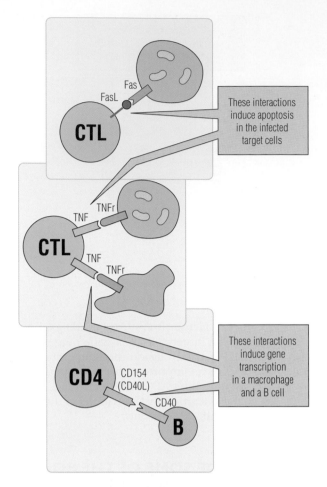

Figure 23.6 This figure shows the different possible effects of TNF family members binding to their receptors. CD40L, CD154 (CD40 ligand); FasL, Fas ligand; TNFr–TNF receptor.

form of surface molecules (CD40, CD80, intercellular adhesion molecule [ICAM]). APCs also secrete costimulatory cytokines, which include IL-1 and type I IFNs, either of which helps initiate T-cell responses.

T-helper cells becoming activated upregulate the IL-2 receptor and begin to secrete IL-2. T-helper cells will not proliferate until IL-2 has bound to its receptor. The IL-2 may have been secreted by the cell itself (autocrine affect) or a neighboring T cell (paracrine effect); either can lead to expansion of T-cell clones. The subsequent events depend on the type of pathogen triggering the response and the site of the response.

Development of Specialized T-Cell Responses

Gut Immunity

Gut-derived T cells secrete a cytokine called transforming growth factor-β (TGF-β). TGF-β induces an immunoglobulin (Ig) class switch from IgM to IgA, which has a major role in mucosal immunity. TGF-β also has potent anti-inflammatory effects and inhibits the effects of most T-cell populations, macrophages, and proinflammatory cytokines. The net result is that, in the gut, most of the immune response is skewed toward the production of IgA.

T_H1 Responses

Intracellular pathogens stimulate APCs to secrete IL-12 and type 1 IFNs. As you can read in detail in Chapter 26, these induce the T-cell transcription factor T-bet, which leads to IFN-γ secretion and a T_H1 phenotype. T_H1 cells favor the production of IgG by B cells, which can then stimulate phagocytosis by activated phagocytes. B-cell IgG production can be supported by IL-6, which acts as a growth factor for B cells. When intracellular pathogens cannot be cleared, there is additional high-level TNF secretion, leading to granuloma production, as you have read in Chapter 22.

T_H2 Responses

Worm infections tend to favor T_H2 responses. It is not clear what inducing signal is produced by APCs in response to worm infection, but the T-cell transcription factor GATA3 is induced, leading to the secretion of IL-4. IL-4 favors B-cell production of IgE, which activates mast cells, which in turn produce more IL-4. In addition, T_H2 cells secrete other cytokines (IL-3, IL-5, and the chemokine eotaxin), which help perpetuate the T_H2 response by stimulating the maturation of mast cells and eosinophils.

The End of the Immune Response

Once a pathogen is cleared, the amount of danger signal received by the innate immune system falls, and levels of cytokines, such as IL-1, type 1 IFNs, and TNF, tend to fall. In addition, there is less antigen for presentation, and T-cell stimulation will decline, leading to lower levels of cytokine production and cytokine-receptor expression. As levels of IL2 in particular fall, T cells produce less Bcl-2 and are prone to undergo apoptosis. These factors tend to wind down the immune response. In addition, inhibitory cytokines,

kines. In the case of bacteria, phagocyte recognition using Toll-like receptor leads to secretion of cytokines including IL-1, TNF, granulocyte-colony stimulating factor (G-CSF), and IL-6. These stimulate local inflammation and may contribute to the development of an acute-phase response. Along with IL-8 and other chemokines, neutrophils are attracted to the site of infection. TNF stimulates local dendritic cells to leave the tissues and migrate to the local lymph node.

The situation is different in the case of viral infections; type I IFN secretion predominates. Type I cytokines have direct antiviral effects, and enhance antigen presentation and the development of T_H1 responses. APCs may themselves be infected with viruses and migrate to local lymph nodes.

T-Cell Priming

The next events take place in the lymph node draining the site of infection. Antigen is presented by dendritic cells and recognized by T cells expressing the appropriate receptor. As you read in Chapter 16, T-helper cells will only become activated if APCs also provide costimulation in the

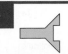 T cell receptor (TCR)

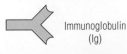 Immunoglobulin (Ig)

 Antigen

 MHC I

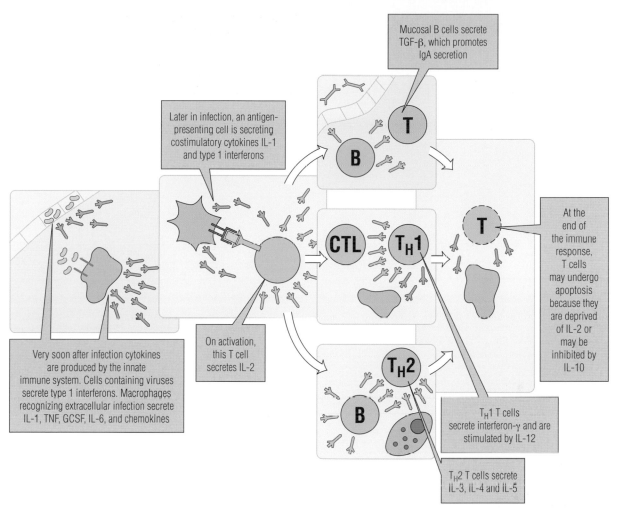

Figure 23.7 This figure summarizes the roles of cytokines in the immune response. Note again how cytokines communicate between the adaptive and innate immune systems. G-CSF, granulocyte-colony stimulating factor; IL, interleukin; T$_H$, T helper; TNF, tumor necrosis factor.

such as IL-10 and TGF-β may play a part in terminating the immune response once a pathogen has been cleared.

Although the numbers of memory T cells are probably maintained by low-level constitutive IL-7 secretion and neutrophil numbers by constitutive G-CSF production, the production of proinflammatory cytokines is switched off in between infections.

LEARNING POINTS   Can You Now ...

1. Define cytokines and explain three of their general principles of action?
2. Predict two different types of clinical problem with using cytokines as treatment?
3. Diagram three different types of cytokine receptor and their associated intracellular signaling pathways?
4. List the roles played by cytokines at different times in the immune response?

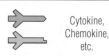 MHC II

 Cytokine, Chemokine, etc.

 Complement (C′)

Signaling molecule

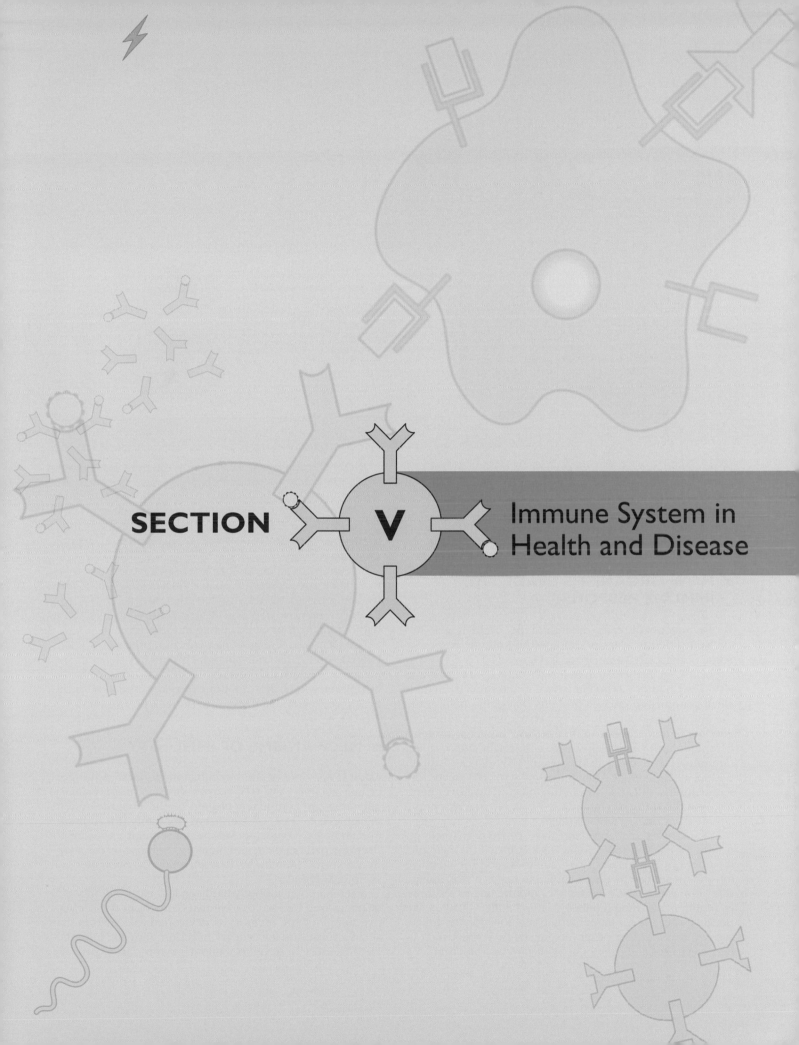

SECTION V

Immune System in Health and Disease

CHAPTER 24

Infections and Vaccines

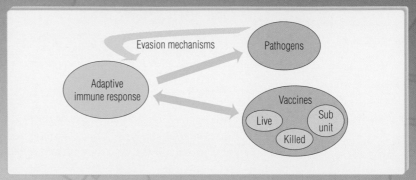

In this chapter, you will review some of the mechanisms pathogens use to evade the immune response. You will then go on to learn about how vaccines, of which there are three main types, can stimulate the immune response. The boxes at the end of the chapter give more details about four different important vaccines.

■ HOW ORGANISMS EVADE THE IMMUNE RESPONSE

To be successful, each different type of pathogen has evolved different ways of evading the immune response. Some of these are summarized in Figure 24.1.

Small RNA viruses, such as influenza (see Box 24.3) and HIV (see Chapter 32) do not have enough capacity in their small genomes to encode proteins that could help evade the immune response. However, a characteristic of the RNA genome is that it tends to mutate, and antigenic proteins belonging to RNA viruses change continually, thus evading immunologic memory. In the case of HIV, this can happen within an individual. After infection with HIV, many different strains will arise within the infected host over just a few months. Influenza mutates more slowly across a population rather than in an individual.

DNA viruses are larger and have capacity in their genomes for evasion tools. Some DNA viruses—for example, members of the herpes virus family—evade the adaptive immune response by downregulating major histocompatibility complex (MHC) expression, and the innate response is required for their control (natural killer [NK] cells). Because there is no immunologic memory for the innate system, it is hard to prime responses to viruses such as herpes viruses and protect individuals from infection.

Bacterial pathogens use a variety of different strategies to evade the immune system. Pneumococcus (*Streptococcus pneumoniae*) and *Haemophilus* sp. evade the innate response (opsonization by complement and phagocytosis) by producing a polysaccharide capsule. These encapsulated organisms are successful pathogens of the respiratory tract.

Mycobacteria, such as *M. tuberculosis*, have waxy coats that block the effects of phagocyte enzymes. They also secrete catalase, which inhibits the effects of the respiratory burst. How macrophages control mycobacteria without killing them is discussed in Chapter 22.

Listeria cause meningitis, particularly in pregnant women. Listeria secrete listeriolysin, which punches holes in the phagolysosome walls. The bacteria can then escape into the cytoplasm, where they are not exposed to the toxic products of the metabolic burst or to proteolytic enzymes.

■ MECHANISMS OF IMMUNITY

Aside from some of the infections mentioned in the preceding section (TB, HIV, herpes viruses), most primary infections are completely cleared by the immune system to achieve a state of sterilizing immunity. In addition, immunologic memory develops: subsequent exposure to the same pathogen elicits a memory response by the adaptive immune system so that infection is prevented or symptoms reduced.

After maternal antibody has been lost, early childhood is characterized by a series of primary infections while effective immunologic memory is developed. Vaccination can act as a substitute for primary infection, allowing immunologic memory to develop without a symptomatic primary

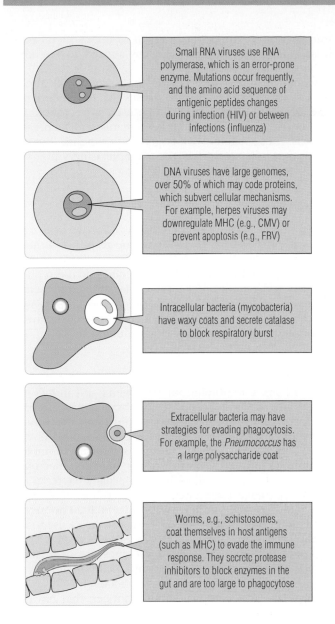

Small RNA viruses use RNA polymerase, which is an error-prone enzyme. Mutations occur frequently, and the amino acid sequence of antigenic peptides changes during infection (HIV) or between infections (influenza)

DNA viruses have large genomes, over 50% of which may code proteins, which subvert cellular mechanisms. For example, herpes viruses may downregulate MHC (e.g., CMV) or prevent apoptosis (e.g., EBV)

Intracellular bacteria (mycobacteria) have waxy coats and secrete catalase to block respiratory burst

Extracellular bacteria may have strategies for evading phagocytosis. For example, the *Pneumococcus* has a large polysaccharide coat

Worms, e.g., schistosomes, coat themselves in host antigens (such as MHC) to evade the immune response. They secrete protease inhibitors to block enzymes in the gut and are too large to phagocytose

Figure 24.1 Strategies to avoid the immune system. CMV, cytomegalovirus; EBV, Epstein-Barr virus; MHC, major histocompatibility complex.

infection. Vaccines are a success story; smallpox is one lethal infection that has been completely eradicated by vaccination. Many other infections (polio, diphtheria, and pertussis) have become relatively rare.

Before we discuss vaccines in detail, we need to mention **passive immunotherapy**. This is the transfer of adaptive immunity—usually antibodies—from one individual to another. Passive immunotherapy is often used to give protective antibodies to an individual who has been exposed to a pathogen. Examples include an individual exposed to rabies (see Box 4.2) or tetanus (see Box 29.2). In these situations, it is possible to give both passive immunotherapy (to reduce the immediate risk of infection) and the vaccine (to induce immunologic memory and reduce the risk for future infection).

Active immunity develops after the immune system has been exposed to antigen in the form of infection or vaccine. Immunologic memory then develops and protects the individual from reinfection. There are various types and compositions of vaccine (Fig. 24.2), each of which has its own advantages and problems. Most vaccines elicit antibodies, and some elicit T-cell responses. Antibodies elicited by vaccines can prevent pathogens from binding onto target cells or prevent the actions of toxins released from pathogens—these are both examples of neutralizing antibodies. Antibodies can also activate complement, and stimulate phagocytosis and NK cell–mediated killing. CD8+ T cells induced by vaccines can inhibit viral replication by secreting interferons or, more often, kill infected cells.

We describe the details of each type of vaccine in this chapter. Boxes 24.1 through 24.4 at the end of the chapter give more specific information about vaccines for smallpox, whooping cough, influenza, and hepatitis B.

■ TYPES OF VACCINE

Live Vaccines

Live vaccines were the first to be discovered, and they are still the most effective; for example, the very successful vaccines against smallpox and polio are live vaccines. Live

FIG. 24.2 Classification Scheme for Vaccines

Types of Vaccine	Component of Vaccine	Examples
Live	Attenuated human pathogen Nonhuman pathogen Recombinant organism	Oral polio, measles, mumps, rubella, influenza* Smallpox vaccine, BCG Experimental; canary pox used as vector for HIV
Killed		Pertussis* Influenza*
Subunit	Purified peptide components Toxoids Polysaccharides Recombinant peptides DNA vaccines	Acellular pertussis* Diphtheria, tetanus Pneumococcus, haemophilus, meningococcus Hepatitis B Experimental, e.g., HIV
*Available in more than one type.		

 MHC II

 Cytokine, Chemokine, etc.

 Complement (C')

 Signaling molecule

vaccines use organisms that are not virulent; although they replicate in healthy vaccine recipients, they do not cause disease. One way of obtaining nonvirulent organisms is to use organisms that have evolved to grow in animals. For example, vaccinia is a virus that causes cow pox and has been used very successfully as a vaccine for smallpox (see the box at the end of this chapter). Other live vaccines use human pathogens that have been **attenuated** (i.e., weakened) so that they are incapable of causing disease. Attenuation has been conventionally carried out by growing the organism in special conditions in vitro. In the future, more live vaccines are likely to be attenuated by direct manipulation of their genomes.

Live vaccines are very effective for three reasons (Fig. 24.3):

- They replicate and thus deliver sustained doses of antigen.
- They replicate intracellularly so they deliver antigenic peptides to major histocompatibility complex (MHC) class I and thus stimulate cytotoxic T cells (CTLs).
- They replicate at the anatomical site of infection, further focusing the immune response. For example, live vaccines given by nose or by mouth elicit immunoglobulin A (IgA) antibodies.

Attenuated live vaccines can cause serious infections in two types of situations. In patients with immunodeficiency, they can cause infection despite attenuation. Occasionally the viruses in live vaccines may spontaneously revert to the virulent wild-type organism. Attenuated polio vaccine differs from the **wild-type** virus in only 10 base pairs. Such small differences make it easy for the virus to mutate back to the virulent form. Polio virus that has reverted from the attenuated to the virulent form has been iden-tified in water supplies. As a result of concerns raised by this finding, the United States has started to use killed polio vaccine once more.

Organisms can also be deliberately genetically altered. For example, viral vectors are viruses that have been made safe for use in humans and can be used as vectors to take the required genes from another organism for expression in cells. These vaccines are largely experimental, but have been used in clinical trials. For example, canary pox virus has been used as a vector for HIV genes.

Killed Organisms

Killed organisms are generally not as effective as live vaccines at eliciting a protective immune response, although they are theoretically much safer. These differences are attributable to the fact that killed vaccines do not replicate in hosts and cannot enter intracellular antigen presenting pathways. At the end of this chapter, we will discuss two vaccines that can be prepared from killed organisms; whooping cough (pertussis), and influenza.

Subunit Vaccines

Subunits are components of pathogens and induce pre-dominantly antibody responses. Subunits can be prepared by destroying virulent organisms, purifying the subunit, and then inactivating it so that it cannot cause disease. Other subunits are prepared using recombinant technology.

Subunits purified from organisms and then inactivated are referred to as toxoids. They are usually bacterial exo-toxins that have been chemically altered to make them safe, although they retain their antigenicity. The neutral-izing antibodies produced block the effects of the toxins. Diphtheria and tetanus toxoid are good examples of this approach. Subunit and toxoid vaccines are generally of low immunogenicity compared with intact organisms, and they may need **adjuvants** to work effectively.

Hepatitis B vaccine is a subunit antigen that has been produced using recombinant techniques (Box 24.4). Hepatitis B vaccine is made up of recombinant virus sur-face peptide. Antibodies raised against surface peptide will prevent the virus attaching to and then entering liver cells. Up to now, hepatitis B vaccine has been very effective. Reasons that peptide vaccines may not remain successful are described in Box 24.4 at the end of this chapter.

Polysaccharides are very poor immunogens, largely because they rely on the response of T-independent B cells (see Chapters 14 and 16) and do not make good vaccines. To overcome this, effective vaccines contain polysaccha-ride that has been chemically conjugated to a peptide antigen: tetanus toxoid is often used. T cells responding to the peptide then provide help for B cells responding to the polysaccharide (see also Box 16.4).

A final type of subunit vaccine is the DNA vaccine. In this experimental approach, the gene for the immuno-genic protein is coated onto gold microspheres and injected directly into cells (e.g., of the skin). In mice, this has resulted in antibody production, indicating that the genes were transcribed (see also Box 10.3).

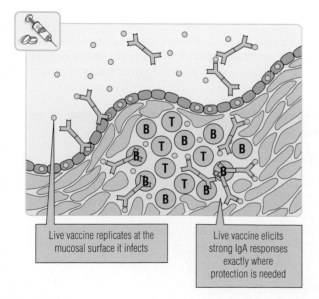

Live vaccine replicates at the mucosal surface it infects

Live vaccine elicits strong IgA responses exactly where protection is needed

Figure 24.3 Live vaccines, such as polio or influenza, replicate at the site of infection.

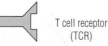 T cell receptor (TCR)

 Immunoglobulin (Ig)

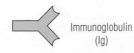 Antigen

 MHC I

Adjuvants

Adjuvants are substances given along with antigen to promote an immune response. Adjuvants appear to provide the danger signal required for the innate immune system to release signals to drive antibody and T-cell responses. Live vaccines generally do not require adjuvants because they are capable of providing danger signals and stimulating Toll-like receptors (TLRs) themselves. For example, bacille Calmette-Guérin (BCG), the live vaccine for tuberculosis, produces large quantities of bacterial sugars, which activate TLRs 2 and 4. Killed whole vaccines also contain substances that activate TLRs and can act as adjuvants.

At the time of this writing, aluminum hydroxide (alum) is the only adjuvant used routinely in humans. It is used to boost the effects of a wide variety of subunit vaccines. Aluminum hydroxide activates macrophages, which then secrete inflammatory cytokines and present antigen to T and B cells. Aluminum is not a powerful adjuvant, and two new approaches are being used to create improved adjuvants.

The first is in vaccine molecules, which activate TLRs. These include molecules such as unmethylated cytokine and guanine sequence (CpG) motifs that have been shown to improve the antigenicity of several subunit vaccines.

A second problem with subunit vaccines is that they do not enter the intracellular antigen processing pathways and so do not elicit cytotoxic T cell (CTL) responses. CTL responses are particularly important in dealing with intracellular infections such as HIV. Immunostimulatory complexes (ISCOMs) are one way that CTL responses can be promoted. ISCOMs are micelles of lipid and subunit antigen that are lipophilic and able to penetrate cell membranes (Fig 24.4). ISCOMS have two special advantages over conventional vaccines:

- The antigen penetrates the cell membrane and is delivered to the antigen-presenting pathways. In this way, subunit antigen can stimulate T cells, including CTL.
- ISCOMs can be used for mucosal vaccines (e.g., through the nose) and induce widespread mucosal immunity in the gut and respiratory tract (see Box 13.3).

Figure 24.5 summarizes some of the experimental vaccine approaches that have been mentioned in this chapter.

■ VACCINE SCHEDULES

Vaccine schedules take into account the clinical implica-

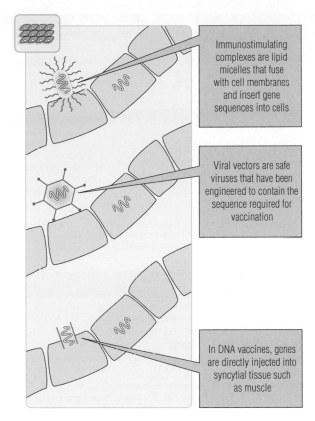

Immunostimulating complexes are lipid micelles that fuse with cell membranes and insert gene sequences into cells

Viral vectors are safe viruses that have been engineered to contain the sequence required for vaccination

In DNA vaccines, genes are directly injected into syncytial tissue such as muscle

Figure 24.4 Technologies that may offer safe vaccines for eliciting cytotoxic T cell responses.

tions of each type of infection. For example, the main purpose of rubella vaccine is to prevent intrauterine infection (which can cause birth deformities), so there is little point in giving it before puberty. On the other hand, it would be desirable to protect very young infants against *Haemophilus*, because this organism causes most damage at this age (see Box 16.5). However, even as conjugate vaccines, polysaccharides do not elicit antibodies in newborn babies.

Vaccine schedules also vary in different parts of the world (Fig. 24.6). For example, in the developing world, measles is a major cause of death in infants and so the vaccine is given as early as possible. In the developed world, measles has become rare and tends to affect school age children, so the vaccine can be given slightly later. The main factor affecting the use of vaccines in the developing world is, however, cost.

FIG. 24.5 How Technologies are Improving Vaccine Effectiveness	
Problem	**Solution in Experimental Vaccines**
Delivery of antigen to intracellular pathways	Live viral vectors; reproduce inside host cells DNA vaccines encode antigens inside cells ISCOMs deliver antigens across cell membrane
Inadequate cytokine stimulation of the adaptive immune system	Toll-like receptor ligands added as adjuvants activate the innate immune system Pro-inflammatory cytokine genes added to DNA vaccine

 MHC II

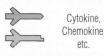 Cytokine, Chemokine, etc.

 Complement (C')

 Signaling molecule

FIG. 24.6   Vaccine Schedules in the Developed and Developing World*

Birth	Developed World	Developing World
2–6 months	Hepatitis B Diphtheria, tetanus, pneumococcal conjugate, Haemophilus conjugate	BCG (TB) Diphtheria, tetanus, hepatitis B, Haemophilus
	Acellular pertussis, inactivated polio	Live polio
6–12 months	Influenza	Measles
1–10 years	Measles, mumps, rubella Varicella	
Early teens	Meningococcus	

*This figure compares vaccine schedules in the developed and the developing worlds and does not include boosters, which are given from time to time. Live vaccines are shown in yellow, killed vaccines in purple, and subunit vaccines in pink. Influenza is available in some countries as a live vaccine.

BOX 24.1   Smallpox Vaccine

Smallpox (variola virus) is a highly contagious viral infection causing a blistering skin reaction and carrying a mortality rate of 10% to 30%. The related cowpox virus (vaccinia) causes a mild, local blistering reaction. It was known for many centuries that cowpox infection could protect against subsequent smallpox infection, but it was not until the end of the 18th century that Edward Jenner formally showed that deliberate inoculation with vaccinia would protect against smallpox. This is where the term vaccination originates.

Global smallpox vaccination was carried out by the World Health Organization, and the last case of smallpox in the community was in 1977. Since 1977, the only cases of smallpox have occurred in laboratory workers. Some supplies of smallpox virus were retained in various laboratories across the world. There is now concern that these supplies of wild smallpox vaccine have been accessed by bioterrorists. Because global vaccination was abandoned at the beginning of the 1980s, most young people are not immune to smallpox and, hence, this virus could be used as a biologic weapon. Some governments have therefore recommended smallpox vaccination, at least for military personnel.

Vaccinia is a live vaccine that is scraped into the surface of the skin. It replicates in the skin and causes considerable local inflammation. In the first week following vaccination, a blister forms, which gradually heals over during the second week. The blister contains viable vaccinia virus and blister fluid can infect other individuals. In patients with defective immune systems, smallpox vaccination leads to widespread dissemination of the vaccinia virus, a generalized rash and the risk of serious illness.

Because vaccinia replicates inside cells in the skin it delivers a high level of antigen to the intracellular antigen presentation pathway and stimulates the development of CTLs. Viruses that have budded off into the extracellular space will be phagocytosed, enter the extracellular antigen pathway, and stimulate helper T cells and antibody production. In the days of the global vaccination scheme, considerable data were established on the longevity of the antibody and CTL responses. Because each individual was vaccinated just once, and because natural vaccinia infection is not endemic, we can pinpoint the exposure to vaccinia vaccination. The absence of environmental vaccinia enables us to be sure that any responses measured are not maintained by re-exposure to this or any cross-reacting organism. Figure 24.7 shows the longevity of the immune response to vaccinia and also the level of protection from infection. The data show that although T-cell responses decline, with a half life of 8 to 10 years, antibody levels and protection from infection last for at least 60 years postvaccination.

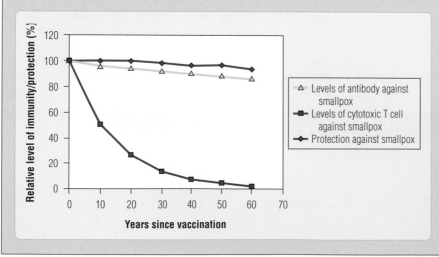

Legend:
- –△– Levels of antibody against smallpox
- –■– Levels of cytotoxic T cell against smallpox
- –◆– Protection against smallpox

X-axis: Years since vaccination
Y-axis: Relative level of immunity/protection (%)

Figure 24.7 Relationship between longevity of antibody and cytotoxic T-cell (CTL) responses and protection from smallpox. The *red columns* are antibody levels and the *blue columns* are levels of cytotoxic T-cell responsiveness. The *black line* with triangles is the degree of protection from smallpox.

 T cell receptor (TCR)   Immunoglobulin (Ig)   Antigen   MHC I

BOX 24.2 Whooping Cough

A 3-year-old boy presents with a 4-week history of coughing attacks. Each coughing attack lasts several minutes, and it is terminated by vomiting. These features are typical of whooping cough (pertussis) and, indeed, because of parental concerns, this child did not receive whooping cough vaccine.

The causative bacterium, *Burdetella pertussis*, kills about 1 in 1000 infected children by damaging the airways. The specific immune response to pertussis is almost entirely antibody mediated. Antibodies prevent the bacteria from attaching to epithelium and neutralize the toxins produced (Fig. 24.8).

Pertussis vaccine does not entirely prevent the infection but it does protect children from the severe complications. The original pertussis vaccine is a killed whole organism. This "cellular" vaccine is very effective and protects more than 90% of those vaccinated from severe complications. However, the vaccine was thought to cause neurologic disease in a tiny proportion of children. The cellular vaccine is still used in the United Kingdom, but not in children with progressive neurologic disorders.

Because of the anxieties about side effects, a subunit vaccine was developed and is in widespread use in the United States. This "acellular" vaccine is made up of pertussis toxins and may be less protective than the killed pertussis vaccine.

Many parents in the United Kingdom and the United States do not allow their children to receive either type of vaccine, because of perceived fears concerning risk. However, there is no good evidence that pertussis causes severe problems in children who have been vaccinated.

The moral of the pertussis story applies to all vaccines used in childhood. It is paradoxic that the success of vaccines in reducing the number of childhood infections means that many parents, clinicians, and the media have forgotten how dangerous these infections can be.

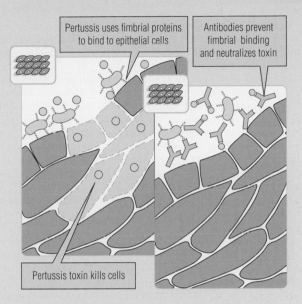

Pertussis uses fimbrial proteins to bind to epithelial cells

Antibodies prevent fimbrial binding and neutralizes toxin

Pertussis toxin kills cells

Figure 24.8 These antibodies against pertussis are typical of neutralizing antibodies. They prevent molecular interactions that are required in disease processes.

 MHC II

 Cytokine, Chemokine, etc.

 Complement (C')

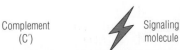 Signaling molecule

BOX 24.3 Influenza

Influenza is a respiratory virus that causes severe infection in the very young and in the elderly. Each year, influenza causes about 36,000 deaths per year in the United States during the influenza season, which lasts from October to February. In 1918, just after the first World War, a new influenza virus emerged and caused the Spanish influenza pandemic. Spanish flu spread around the world in 9 months and caused 40 million deaths. In this box, we explain how this pandemic emerged and how vaccines may be used to prevent it.

Influenza is an RNA virus that uses a protein called hemagglutinin to bind sugars on respiratory epithelial cells. Influenza is cytopathic; it causes damage to the cells it infects. The presence of double-stranded RNA stimulates respiratory tract cells to secrete interferon-α within a few hours of viral infection, which inhibits viral replication (see Chapter 19) and slows the spread of influenza in the lungs.

Dendritic cells migrate to the local lymph node and present antigen to T cells. Under the influence of T-helper type 1 (T_H1) cells, cytotoxic T cells (CTLs) begin to appear after 2 to 3 days. These cells clear the residual infected cells, and, thus, sterilizing immunity is achieved.

Influenza also elicits an antibody response and IgM antibodies begin to appear after about 5 days. These neutralizing antibodies bind to hemagglutinin and prevent virus from infecting cells. The antibody response against influenza develops too late to have a major role in helping to clear established infection and it is most important in preventing reinfection with an identical viral strain.

Influenza is a relatively unstable RNA virus that can undergo spontaneous mutation. Gradual mutations slowly change the viral genome and result in antigenic drift. Because the mutated virus has some antigenic similarity with existing strains, existing immunity is partially protective. This means that there is not a widespread epidemic, and infection is usually mild (Fig. 24.9). More rapid, extensive genetic changes can also occur. These events occur when a host animal is infected with two different strains of flu virus. The two strains exchange segments of genes and a third, new strain is the result. This is referred to as genetic shift and is believed to cause the flu pandemics that occur every few years. Most of these genetic events occur between human and duck flu. There have been some human infections with new strains of duck flu, but at the time of writing, there is no evidence that a new shifted mutant flu virus has emerged from the Far East. If a new shifted virus does emerge, and is capable of human-to-human spread, global infection is very likely to arise within a few weeks because of mass air travel.

Influenza vaccine is effective at preventing infection in individuals at risk for severe complications (e.g., patients with chronic chest problems). The conventional flu vaccine uses killed influenza virus. The flu virus is grown in hen eggs, killed, and then purified. A live vaccine also exists. This is sprayed into the nose and can elicit protective immunoglobulin A (IgA) antibodies in addition to IgG.

To be effective the flu vaccine must contain the most up-to-date strains. The World Health Organization provides guidance for vaccine manufacturers with early warnings of changes in the virus. The vaccine manufacturers select viruses to include in the vaccine in January. During the next 6 months, the selected viruses are grown on eggs until there is enough virus to start manufacturing the vaccine. This process requires virus manufacturers

BOX 24.3 (cont'd)

to obtain tens of millions of eggs during spring each year. By summer, if production has gone to plan, the vaccine (killed or live) is ready for testing. If the vaccine passes its safety tests, it can then be distributed to users.

In most years, there is enough warning of slightly drifted flu virus to enable the production of updated vaccine. However, if a new virus emerges through antigenic shift (after recombination with duck flu), it can take the manufacturers up to 10 months to prepare the new vaccine. In the age of mass air travel, the shifted virus may have spread around the world in this time.

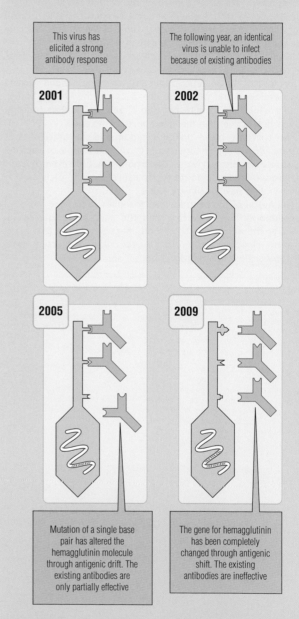

Figure 24.9 Single base pair mutations causing drift are relatively frequent. Shift occurs much less often, probably when human influenza virus exchanges gene sequences with animal viruses (reassortment). Such events overcome immunity on an enormous scale, triggering global pandemics.

 T cell receptor (TCR)　　 Immunoglobulin (Ig)　　 Antigen　　 MHC I

BOX 24.4 Hepatitis B

When the hepatitis B virus invades liver tissue, it can trigger a T-cell response that can result in irreversible liver damage, as you learned in Chapter 22. A long-term complication of viral hepatitis can be liver cancer (hepatoma). In the developing world, many individuals become infected very early in childhood and maintain a carrier status throughout life. The hepatitis B vaccine was the first recombinant subunit vaccine and has been tremendously successful.

In developing countries where hepatitis B is very common, the vaccine has been given to everybody to build up so-called herd immunity. When nearly everyone in a community is immune, the number of carriers falls, thereby protecting the nonimmune. In these countries, hepatitis B vaccination programs have almost eradicated hepatoma—the first example of a vaccine being successful at preventing cancer. In the developed world, the strategy up to now has been to vaccinate only high-risk individuals, for example, people who are at risk through their work, for example, medical students. Increasingly, governments are switching from the selective vaccination strategy to global vaccination, because of the safety, effectiveness, and value of global vaccination.

Hepatitis B vaccine consists of a relatively short peptide derived from the hepatitis B surface antigen, HBsAg, grown in yeast cells. This vaccine stimulates T-helper cells and elicits neutralizing IgG, which prevent the virus from entering hepatocytes in the first place. The recombinant vaccine is very safe and protects 80% to 90% of those vaccinated. Failure to develop protection from hepatitis B following vaccination can be a result of host or viral factors.

Host Factors

The short peptide only contains a few potential T-cell epitopes. Vaccine responses are diminished in individuals who are homozygous at all their major histocompatibility complex (MHC) class II alleles, because these individuals have relatively fewer MHC molecules on which they can display a limited number of antigenic peptides. This is referred to as the "heterozygote advantage" and is explained in detail in Chapter 8.

Viral Factors

Hepatitis B is prone to undergo gradual mutation. In the face of widespread immunity to hepatitis B surface antigen, viral strains with mutations in this protein are at an advantage and can escape vaccine-induced immunity. These strains were very rare when the vaccine was first introduced, but mutations are becoming increasingly common in viral isolates from the very countries where widespread vaccination has been successful.

Possible solutions are to use either a larger peptide or a mixture of peptides. These approaches decrease the chances of particular human leukocyte antigen alleles being unable to bind epitopes and they may reduce the risk of successful viral mutations.

LEARNING POINTS Can You Now ...

1. Describe three different types of vaccine currently in use and how they vary in their safety and efficacy?

2. Explain how we can measure the longevity of immunologic memory from vaccine responses?

3. Describe two different types of whooping cough vaccine and why they are used in different countries?

4. Explain why influenza vaccine may need to be given every year?

5. Describe two newer approaches to vaccination?

 MHC II

 Cytokine, Chemokine, etc.

 Complement (C')

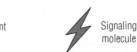 Signaling molecule

CHAPTER 25 Hypersensitivity Reactions

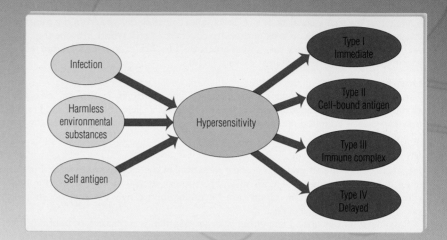

In this chapter, you will learn about how hypersensitivity reactions can be triggered by infections, harmless environmental substances, and autoantigens and can lead to four different types of reactions. Examples of each of the four different hypersensitivity reactions are given in clinical boxes at the end of this chapter, and we go into each of them in much more detail in the next few chapters.

Excessive immune responses that cause damage are called **hypersensitivity reactions**. Hypersensitivity reactions can occur in response to three different types of antigen:

- Infectious agents. We have already discussed how the immune system sometimes overreacts to infections and causes disease; when the immune response contributes to the symptoms of infection, the resultant disease is a type of hypersensitivity.
- Environmental substances. Hypersensitivity can occur in response to innocuous environmental antigens—one example of this is allergy. For example, in hay fever, grass pollens themselves are incapable of causing damage; it is the immune response to the pollen that causes harm.
- Self antigens. Normal host molecules can trigger immune responses, referred to as autoimmunity, and when these cause hypersensitivity **autoimmune disease** is the result.

Hypersensitivity reactions use four different mechanisms for causing disease; these are the topics of Chapters 25 to 30.

■ TYPES OF TRIGGERS FOR HYPERSENSITIVITY

Hypersensitivity to Infectious Agents

Not all infections are capable of causing hypersensitivity reactions. For example, although the common cold elicits a strong immune response, this never appears to cause harm. Other respiratory viruses, for example, influenza can cause hypersensitivity. Influenza virus damages epithelial cells in the respiratory tract, but can sometimes elicit an exaggerated immune responses, which is far more damaging than the virus itself. Influenza can trigger high levels of cytokine secretion—sometimes referred to as a cytokine storm. The cytokines attract leukocytes to the lungs and trigger vascular changes leading to hypotension and coagulation. In severe influenza, inflammatory cytokines also spill out into the systemic circulation, causing ill effects in remote parts of the body, for example, the brain. This is analogous to the cytokine response seen in septic shock, described in Chapter 20, which also leads to a type of cytokine storm.

Infections that are capable of eliciting hypersensitivity do not do so in every case. In Chapter 22, we discussed how hepatitis B virus infection can result in chronic hepatitis in some individuals. The response depends on the infecting dose of virus and the immune response genes of the individual. Another very different example of an infection causing hypersensitivity is immune complex disease caused by streptococci, which is discussed below.

Hypersensitivity to Environmental Substances

For environmental substances to trigger hypersensitivity reactions, they must be fairly small in order to gain access to the immune system. Dusts trigger off a range of responses because they are able to enter the lower extremities of the respiratory tract, an area that is rich in adaptive immune response cells. These dusts can mimic parasites and may stimulate an antibody response. If the dominant antibody is immunoglobulin E (IgE), they may subsequently trigger immediate hypersensitivity, which is manifest as allergies such as **asthma** or **rhinitis**. If the dust stimulates IgG antibodies, it may trigger off a different kind of hypersensitivity, for example, farmer's lung (see Chapter 29).

Smaller molecules sometimes diffuse into the skin, and these may act as haptens, triggering a delayed hypersensitivity reaction. This is the basis of contact dermatitis caused by nickel, discussed in Box 25.4.

Drugs administered orally, by injection, or onto the surface of the body can elicit hypersensitivity reactions mediated by IgE or IgG antibodies or by T cells. Immunologically mediated hypersensitivity reactions to drugs are very common and even very tiny doses of drug can trigger life-threatening reactions. These are all classified as **idiosyncratic adverse drug reactions**. We return to this topic in Chapter 30.

A word of caution is needed here. Lay people, and many clinicians, refer to any hypersensitivity reaction to exogenous substances as **allergy**, and the term originally meant any altered reaction to external substances. A related term, **atopy**, refers to immediate hypersensitivity mediated by IgE antibodies. In this book, this more restrictive definition is also used for allergy because it helps to explain the specific diagnosis and treatment of hypersensitivities mediated by IgE.

Hypersensitivity to Self Antigens

A degree of immune response to self antigens is normal and is present in most people. When these become exaggerated or when tolerance to other antigens breaks down, hypersensitivity reactions can occur. This is autoimmune disease and is discussed in Chapter 27.

■ TYPES OF HYPERSENSITIVITY REACTION

The hypersensitivity classification system used here was first described by Coombs and Gell (Fig. 25.1). The system classifies the different types of hypersensitivity reaction by the types of immune response involved. Each type of hypersensitivity reaction produces characteristic clinical disease whether the trigger is an environmental, infectious, or self antigen. For example, in type III hypersensitivity, the clinical result is similar whether the antigen is streptococcus, a drug, or an autoantigen, such as DNA.

Hypersensitivity reactions are reliant on the adaptive immune system. Previous exposure to antigen is required to prime the adaptive immune response to produce IgE (type I), IgG (types II and III), or T cells (type IV). Because previous exposure is required, hypersensitivity reactions do not take place when an individual is first exposed to antigen. In each type of hypersensitivity reaction, the damage is caused by different aspects of the adaptive and innate systems, each of which should now be familiar to you through discussion of their role in clearing infections.

Type I

Type I hypersensitivity is mediated through the degranulation of mast cells and eosinophils. The effects are felt within minutes of exposure (Box 25.1). This type of hypersensitivity is sometimes referred to as **immediate hypersensitivity** and is also known as allergy (see Chapter 26).

Type II

Type II hypersensitivity is caused by IgG reacting with antigen present on the surface of cells. The bound Ig then interacts with complement or with Fc receptor on

---

FIG. 25.1 Coombs and Gell Classification of Hypersensitivity

	Type I: Immediate Hypersensitivity	Type II: Bound Antigen	Type III: Immune Complex	Type IV: Delayed Hypersensitivity
Onset	Seconds– if IgE preformed	Seconds– if IgG preformed	Hours– if IgG preformed	2-3 days
Infectious trigger	Schistosomiasis	Immune hemolytic anemias	Poststreptococcal glomerulonephritis	Hepatitis B virus
Environmental trigger	House dust mite, peanut, etc.	Immune hemolytic anemias	Farmer's lung	Contact dermatitis
Autoimmunity	Not applicable	Immune hemolytic anemias	Systematic lupus erythematosus	Insulin-dependent diabetes, celiac disease, multiple sclerosis, rheumatoid arthritis
Adaptive immune system mediators	IgE	IgG	IgG	T cells
Innate immune system mediators	Mast cells, eosinophils	Complement, phagocytes	Complement, neutrophils	Macrophages

 MHC II

 Cytokine, Chemokine, etc.

 Complement (C')

Signaling molecule

macrophages. These innate mechanisms then damage the target cells using processes that may take several hours, as in the case of drug-induced hemolysis (Box 25.2).

Type III

Ig is also responsible for type III hypersensitivity. In this case, immune complexes of antigen and antibody form and either cause damage at the site of production or circulate and cause damage elsewhere. Immune complexes take some time to form and to initiate tissue damage. Poststreptococcal glomerulonephritis is a good example of **immune complex disease** (Box 25.3 and see Chapter 29).

Type IV

The slowest form of hypersensitivity is that mediated by T cells (type IV hypersensitivity). This can take 2 to 3 days to develop and is referred to as **delayed hypersensitivity** (Box 25.4 and Chapter 30).

■ DIAGNOSIS AND TREATMENT OF HYPERSENSITIVITY

There are major differences in how the types of hypersensitivity reaction are diagnosed and treated. For example,

although skin tests are used to diagnose both type I and type IV hypersensitivity, the exact type of testing depends on the type of disease suspected. Treatment for each type of hypersensitivity is also very different, as we shall explain in the following chapters.

A criticism of the Coombs and Gell classification system is that it is simplistic; many diseases are caused by an overlap of different types of hypersensitivity. However, some knowledge of the classification system makes it easier to understand how the different disorders come about and how they can be effectively diagnosed and treated.

In this book, we do not provide an exhaustive list of hypersensitivity disorders or work through the different anatomical systems. This is because an understanding of the mechanisms of hypersensitivity enables students to apply this knowledge to other disease settings. There are many more hypersensitivity reactions than we have had an opportunity to discuss in detail.

BOX 25.1   Type I Hypersensitivity: Hay Fever

A 16-year-old boy has had a runny nose and sore eyes since the beginning of July. His symptoms improve indoors, but they return within minutes of going outside. He has never been ill before, although his two sisters both have asthma. A skin prick test is performed (Fig. 25.2), which shows allergy to some common grass pollens. It is almost impossible for him to avoid exposure to pollens, so for the rest of the pollen season, he is treated with nasal steroid spray.

Figure 25.2 Skin prick test. A pollen extract was dropped onto the patient's skin, which was then gently pricked. Within 10 minutes, the area became itchy and a wheal developed, surrounded by erythema. (With permission from the Department of Medical Illustration, St. Bartholomew's Hospital, London.)

BOX 25.2   Type II Hypersensitivity: Drug-Induced Hemolysis

A woman in her thirties presents with acute fatigue and breathlessness. Two days earlier, she was given penicillin antibiotic for a urinary tract infection. She has had the same antibiotic once before without problems. She is found to be pale and mildly jaundiced. The laboratory work shows that her red cells are being destroyed in the circulation. Further testing shows that her serum contains antibodies that react with penicillin to coat her red cells, confirming the diagnosis of penicillin-induced **immune hemolytic anemia**.

Penicillin is a low-molecular-weight compound that is unable to act as an antigen in its own right, but can act as a **hapten** (Fig. 25.3) (see also Box 5.1 and Fig. 5.3). In penicillin-induced hemolysis, previous exposure to penicillin induces immunoglobulin G (IgG) antibodies. On re-exposure, penicillin binds to red cells and becomes a target for IgG. The IgG-coated red cells are taken up and destroyed by the spleen (Fig. 25.4).

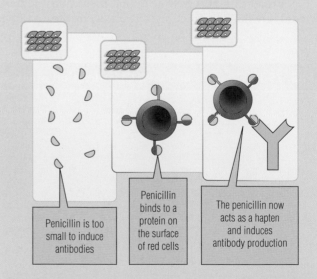

Penicillin is too small to induce antibodies

Penicillin binds to a protein on the surface of red cells

The penicillin now acts as a hapten and induces antibody production

Figure 25.3 Haptens interact with normal proteins from a variety of host tissues.

 T cell receptor (TCR)   Immunoglobulin (Ig)   Antigen   MHC I

BOX 25.2 (cont'd)

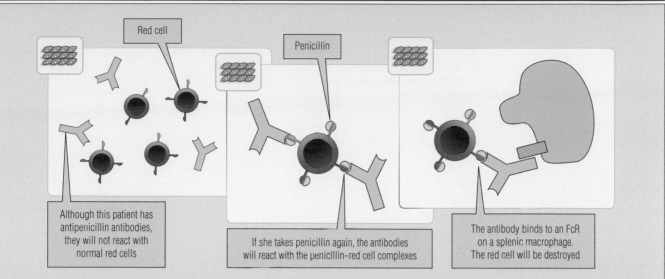

Figure 25.4 Penicillin-induced immune hemolysis. Destruction of red cells takes place within 24 hours of re-exposure to the antigen. FcR, Fc receptor.

BOX 25.3 Type III Hypersensitivity: Poststreptococcal Glomerulonephritis

An 11-year-old boy presents to his family physician with a 3-day history of swelling of the legs and scrotum. He complained of a sore throat about 2 weeks earlier. His urine contains blood and protein. Taken together, these are the findings of acute **glomerulonephritis**. A throat swab is taken and the bacterium *β-hemolytic streptococcus* is grown. He is started on antibiotics for the infection and during the next 3 weeks his edema improves. When he is reviewed at this stage, his urine is normal.

This child had typical poststreptococcal glomerulonephritis. Streptococci induce a potent antibody response. These antibodies interact with antigen, and small circulating immune complexes are produced as a result, especially when antigen is still in excess (Fig. 25.5). These complexes have a tendency to localize in the glomerulus and cause type III hypersensitivity using mechanisms described in detail in Chapter 29.

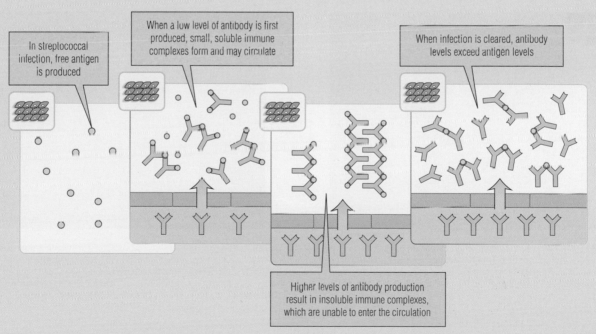

Figure 25.5 Poststreptococcal glomerulonephritis. Acute infections such as streptococcus can trigger circulating immune complexes until the antigen is cleared.

BOX 25.3   (cont'd)

Circulating immune complexes occur during other infections. Some individuals with hepatitis B virus infection are unable to control infection with adequate T-cell responses (see Chapter 22), and there is ongoing viral replication. Although these individuals produce high levels of antibody, there may still be antigen excess and circulating immune complexes may form (Fig. 25.6).

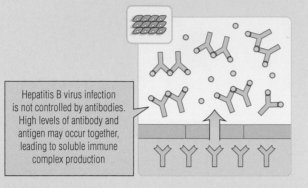

Hepatitis B virus infection is not controlled by antibodies. High levels of antibody and antigen may occur together, leading to soluble immune complex production

Figure 25.6 Chronic infections such as hepatitis B virus cause more long-lasting immune complex disease.

BOX 25.4   Type IV Hypersensitivity: Contact Dermatitis

A 53-year-old man developed an itchy rash on his ankle. He notices that it is worse in the summer and particularly bad if he has been gardening (Fig. 25.7). A dermatologist thinks this is contact dermatitis and organizes a patch test, to various plant extracts (Fig. 25.8). The patch test is read 3 days after the extracts have been applied and confirms sensitivity to dandelion and related weeds.

Contact dermatitis is an example of type IV delayed hypersensitivity. The skin lesions consist of T cells and macrophages and develop 24 to 72 hours after exposure to the antigen. In this way, the lesions of contact dermatitis are very similar to those induced by a tuberculin skin test.

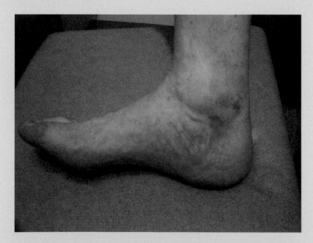

Figure 25.7 The patient has patches of contact dermatitis over his ankle, where fragments of plants have fallen into his gardening boots. (From Helbert M, Flesh and Bones of Immunology. Edinburgh: Mosby, 2006, Figure 32.1.)

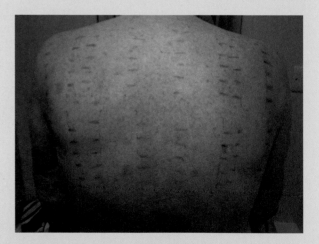

Figure 25.8 In the patch test, possible sensitizing antigens are placed on the skin under a dressing. This photograph shows a typical positive reaction, in this case to extracts of three plants. At the cellular level, the evolution of this test is very similar to a tuberculin skin test. (From Helbert M, Flesh and Bones of Immunology. Edinburgh: Mosby, 2006, Figure 32.2.)

 T cell receptor (TCR)

 Immunoglobulin (Ig)

Antigen

 MHC I

LEARNING POINTS Can You Now ...

1. Explain the Coombs and Gell classification of hypersensitivity reactions?
2. Give two examples of infection causing different types of hypersensitivity?
3. Give three examples of how normally innocuous substances may cause hypersensitivity?

4. Contrast the two different skin tests described in this chapter?

 MHC II

 Cytokine, Chemokine, etc.

 Complement (C')

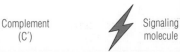 Signaling molecule

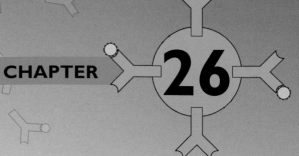

CHAPTER 26

Immediate Hypersensitivity (Type I): Allergy

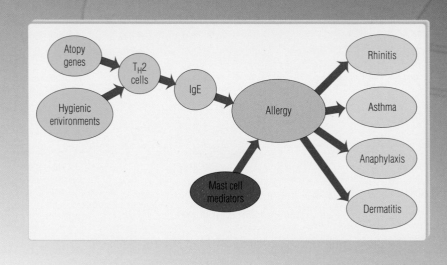

In this chapter, you will read how genes and growing up in a hygienic environment can contribute to the development of an immune system skewed toward T_H2 responses. This leads to excessive immunoglobulin E (IgE) production, which, along with mast cell mediators, leads to the symptoms of allergy. You will learn more about specific allergic disorders.

■ DEFINITIONS

The immunological definition of atopy is an immediate hypersensitivity reaction to environmental antigens, mediated by IgE. Such reactions tend to run in families, and these families are said to have inherited the **atopy** trait. Although the term **allergy** was originally defined as any altered reactivity to exogenous antigens, it is now often used synonymously with atopy. Allergic diseases include anaphylaxis, angioedema, urticaria, rhinitis, asthma, and some types of dermatitis or eczema. The distinction between true allergy and other reactions is important because some of the treatments for allergy would be inappropriate for other types of reaction.

Usually, allergies are very rapid reactions mediated by IgE, and the symptoms develop within minutes of exposure to antigen. However, some allergic reactions continue for a long time (e.g., when the environmental antigen

cannot be easily avoided), and they develop into a late-phase reaction characterized by T-cell infiltrates. This is called the **late-phase response** and is discussed later in this chapter.

The beginning of this chapter explains how allergies develop. Some of this material will be familiar to you, from material in Chapter 15 (T_H1 and T_H2 cells) and Chapter 21 (mast cells). The second half of the chapter describes the clinical features of allergies in more detail.

■ ALLERGEN

Antigens that trigger allergic reactions are referred to as **allergens**. Allergens must find their own way into the body. Some allergens are present in the environment as small particles or low-molecular-weight substances that penetrate the body after being inhaled, eaten, or administered as drugs. Inhaled antigens include pollens, fungal spores, and the feces of the house dust mite. Many allergens, including house dust mite feces, are enzymes. This characteristic may allow them to partially digest innate immune system barriers. Some insect venoms are allergens, and these are injected directly into the skin.

An important part of the treatment of allergy is identification and avoidance of allergens. Careful history taking facilitates identification of allergens. For example, a patient with a runny nose (rhinitis) is likely to be sensitive to aero-allergens. If symptoms occur predominantly in the summer, grass pollen is the likely culprit. If symptoms occur all year round and mainly indoors, sensitivity to house dust mite feces is likely. House dust mite allergy occurs in areas where a cold climate dictates the need for central heating, heavy bedding, and thick carpets—the habitat of this mite.

Additional clues to the identity of allergens can be provided by knowledge of cross-reacting allergens.

- In penicillin allergy, the allergen is the β-lactam core of the penicillin molecule. Patients experience symptoms with different members of the penicillin family—for example, amoxicillin and flucloxacillin. Patients with penicillin allergy can react to other families of antibiotics, such as cephalosporins, which also contain β-lactam ring structures (see Box 5.1).
- Some plant allergens are cross-reactive; for example, patients who have both springtime rhinitis and allergy to foods may be sensitive to cross-reactive proteins present in birch pollen as well as hazelnut, apple, carrot, and potato.

■ DEGRANULATING CELLS

The major cells involved in allergy, mast cells, and eosinophils, are described in Chapter 21, where we explained how these cells evolved to kill parasites. Mast cells are resident in a wide number of tissues (rather like macrophages), whereas eosinophils migrate into tissues where type I hypersensitivity is taking place (rather like neutrophils attracted to sites of inflammation). These cells release the mediators that cause the symptoms of allergy. A third type of degranulating cell is the basophil. These have a similar appearance to mast cells, but they stay in circulation. It is unknown whether they have a special function.

Mast cells are responsible for initiating the symptoms of allergic reactions after allergen and IgE have interacted. Mast cells express receptors for IgE, FcεRI (high-affinity IgE receptor). When allergen cross-links IgE bound to cells by FcεRI, cells release the mediators of the early-phase reaction. However, mast cells, eosinophils, and basophils can also be activated by other stimuli. For example, activated complement generated by infections can activate

mast cells, as can signals transmitted by the nervous system—for example, in response to changes in temperature. It is important to remember that the symptoms described in detail later in this chapter (Fig. 26.1) can be caused by other conditions in addition to allergy.

■ ANTIBODY

IgE is required for type I hypersensitivity reactions. B cells class switch to IgE production when they are costimulated by interleukin-4 (IL-4), secreted by T-helper 2 (T$_H$2) cells. Once IgE is produced, it binds to the high-affinity receptor FcεRI, expressed on resting mast cells resident in tissues and eosinophils that have been activated and migrated into tissues (Fig. 26.2). IgE binds to the FcεRI with such high affinity that although IgE is found at a thousand-fold lower concentration than IgG in serum, mast cells are constantly coated with IgE against different antigens.

Very high levels of IgE are seen in patients infected with parasites—for example, schistosomiasis. Total levels of IgE are also high in people who have inherited the atopy trait. Levels of IgE specific for given allergens can be measured using skin prick testing or enzyme-linked immunosorbent assays (ELISA), when investigating the cause of allergic symptoms.

■ T$_H$2 CELLS

Most adaptive immune system responses in humans produce a mixture of antibodies and cytotoxic T cells. The precise balance of which type of response dominates depends on the type of pathogen the immune system is responding to. In Chapter 22, you read how the immune system responds to chronic intracellular infection, such as TB, with the production of a mainly T$_H$1 response with resulting activation of cytotoxic T cells and macrophages by interferon-γ (IFN-γ). High levels of IgG are also produced in T$_H$1 responses. However, allergy requires the production of large amounts of IgE, which in turn requires help from T$_H$2 cells producing IL-4. In T$_H$2 responses, production of IgG and cytotoxic T cells is inhibited. TB and allergy represent opposite poles of the adaptive

FIG. 26.1 Allergic Diseases

System Affected	Clinical Syndrome	Symptoms
Systemic	Anaphylaxis	Low blood pressure, angiodema and airway obstruction
		May be fatal, for example, allergy to nuts and antibiotics
Airways	Asthma	Reversible airway obstruction in the bronchi
	Rhinitis	Discharge, sneezing and nasal obstruction
		Often coexists with allergic conjunctivitis
Skin	Urticaria	Short-lived, itchy edema of the cutaneous tissues, the lesion is identical to that induced by skin-prick testing.
	Angioedema	Short-lived, non-itchy edema of the subcutaneous tissues.
		Some forms, for example, lip swelling, may be manifestations of food allergy.
	Atopic eczema	Chronic itchy inflammation of the skin. Some cases are caused by food allergy.

All of the above syndromes can be caused by nonallergic mechanisms. For example, infection can also trigger asthma, rhinitis, and urticaria.

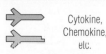 MHC II

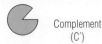 Cytokine, Chemokine, etc.

Complement (C')

 Signaling molecule

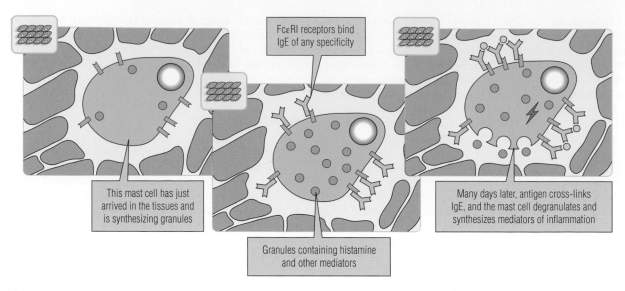

This mast cell has just arrived in the tissues and is synthesizing granules

FcεRI receptors bind IgE of any specificity

Granules containing histamine and other mediators

Many days later, antigen cross-links IgE, and the mast cell degranulates and synthesizes mediators of inflammation

Figure 26.2 Immunoglobulin E (IgE) binds to the FcεR on mast cells. Mast cells become activated when allergen cross-links the IgE molecules.

immune response. Most responses are much less extreme and involve a mix of T_H1 and T_H2 cells.

T_H1-polarized cells are characterized by expressing the transcription factor T-bet, which promotes the secretion of IFN-γ. T_H2 cells express the transcription factor GATA3, which promotes the secretion of IL-4 and associated cytokines IL-5 and IL-13. Both T_H1 and T_H2 T cells arise from developing T cells, which have the capacity to differentiate in either a T_H1 or a T_H2 direction. Whether an immune response differentiates into a T_H1 or T_H2 direction is dictated by whether T-bet or GATA3 becomes the dominant transcription factor (Fig. 26.3).

A third population of T_H cells is the regulatory T cells (Tregs). Tregs play an important role in peripheral tolerance and inhibit both T_H1 and T_H2 cells in an antigen-dependent fashion. Tregs inhibit other T cells by secreting cytokines, such as transforming growth factor-β (TGF-β) and IL-10. Tregs may also have a role during infection; for example, they may prevent overzealous responses that would otherwise lead to hypersensitivity. In most people, Tregs prevent T helper responses from becoming over-polarized toward extremes of either T_H1 or T_H2 cytokine production. For example, in nonallergic individuals, the Tregs are the dominant T-cell type specific for environmental allergens. In other words, in nonallergic individuals, a polarized response to environmental allergens cannot develop because Tregs would inhibit it.

Antigen-presenting cells (APCs) appear to make the decision whether precursor T cells develop toward a T_H1 or T_H2 cytokine profile. In circumstances that are not well understood, an APC favors the production of T_H2 cells. This may be more likely to happen if the antigen is present at a mucosal surface or is associated with molecules that stimulate certain pattern-recognition molecules on the APC. For example, stimulation of Toll-like receptor 2 appears to eventually favor T_H2 responses. Hence, GATA3 is induced, and the stimulated T cell produces small quantities of IL-4. With each successive round of T-cell proliferation, the daughter T cells can become more and more polarized toward a T_H2 phenotype. This can only occur if Tregs do not inhibit the polarization. Additionally, if an APC produces IL-12 (e.g., because of intracellular infection with mycobacteria), a T_H1 response is favored.

Once a T_H2 response is established, high-level IL-4 secretion will stimulate production of IgE by B cells. The IgE produced binds to FcεRI on the surface of mast cells. If antigen cross-links the IgE bound to the FcεRI, mast cells release IL-4. This provides a positive feedback system for the production of more IgE and TH2 cells (see Fig. 26.3). IL-4 also inhibits the production of IFN-γ by T_H1 T cells. Thus, once a T-cell response to an antigen has deviated toward production of T_H2 cytokines, positive feedback sustains and enhances the response. In addition, T_H2 T cells secrete other cytokines (IL-5, IL-13, eotaxin), which help perpetuate the T_H2 response by stimulating the maturation and migration of eosinophils and switching off macrophages (Fig 26.4).

To sum up, APCs make decisions about whether T cells will develop in a T_H1 or T_H2 direction, leading to expression of either IL-4 or IFN-γ. During most responses, a mixture of T_H1 and T_H2 cells are produced, although one type of response will tend to dominate, depending on the triggering infection. T_H1 and T_H2 cells are able to produce positive feedback for their own type of cells, which could lead to extreme polarization of the immune response. Extreme polarization is normally prevented by Tregs. In the absence of Tregs, an immune response may become overpolarized toward T_H2, and allergy may develop.

■ PREDISPOSITION TO ALLERGY

Allergy is very common and is increasing in prevalence in the developed world. Peanut allergy, for example, is both increasing in prevalence (the number of people affected) and severity.

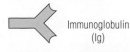 T cell receptor (TCR)

 Immunoglobulin (Ig)

Antigen

MHC I

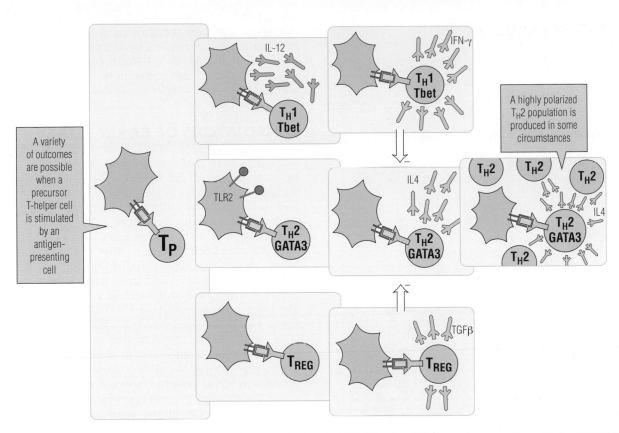

Figure 26.3 In the *top row*, an antigen-presenting cell (APC) is secreting interleukin-12 (IL-12), which favors the production of T$_H$1 cells. In the *bottom row*, a Treg has been produced. In the *middle row*, the APC is being stimulated through Toll-like receptor 2 (TLR2), and a T$_H$2 cell is being produced. As long as this is not inhibited by either T$_H$1 cells or Tregs, a highly polarized T$_H$2 population may be produced. IFN, interferon; TGF, transforming growth factor.

Like all forms of hypersensitivity, predisposition to allergy is caused by genetic and environmental factors. Several genetic factors operating together are the foundation of the atopy trait. The increase in the prevalence of allergy may be explained by environmental factors—the "hygiene hypothesis."

Atopy Trait

In the West, up to 40% of the population have the atopy trait with exaggerated IgE responses to allergens. Allergy tends to run in families; family members either have allergies themselves or are at risk for allergy because they have high levels of IgE against specific allergens. Affected family members may have different allergies—for example asthma, hay fever, or eczema—in response to very different allergens. It is the risk of allergy that is inherited, not the specific allergy.

The genetics of allergy are complex, involving interactions between several genes. For example, polymorphisms in the IL-4 and FcεR1 genes can both increase the risk for allergy. For reasons that are not understood, the FcεR1 inherited from the mother affects the risk for allergy more than the FcεR1 gene inherited from the father. Other unidentified genes are almost certainly also involved.

Hygiene Hypothesis

The increasing incidence of allergies in the developed world is suggestive of the effects of a changing environmental factor. There is little evidence that chemical pollution is responsible for the change in allergy prevalence. However, several strands of evidence support the idea that ecological changes in the environments in which we live have affected exposure to bacterial antigens in early life, and this has increased the risk for allergy:

- Children with allergies tend to live in cleaner houses than those without allergies.
- Growing up on farms and exposure to livestock decreases the risk for allergies.
- Allergy is rare in areas where tuberculosis is common.

The hygiene hypothesis suggests that exposure to organisms, particularly mycobacteria, early in life prevents the highly polarized T$_H$2 responses from developing. The term "hygiene" refers to microbiologic cleanliness. Even developed cities, which might look filthy, can be clean from the microbiologic point of view! Mycobacteria are common environmental organisms, most of which do not cause disease in healthy humans. There are two overlapping ways in which mycobacteria may prevent overpolarized T$_H$2 responses from developing in early life:

 MHC II   Cytokine, Chemokine, etc.   Complement (C')   Signaling molecule

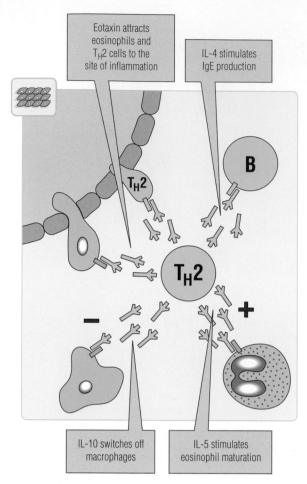

Figure 26.4 Interleukin-4 (IL4), IL10, and eotaxin help sustain the T_H2 response.

- Mycobacteria can survive inside macrophages and provoke a strong T_H1 response. As you read in Chapter 22, mycobacterium tuberculosis has evolved evasion mechanisms that enable it to cause disease in healthy humans. Most mycobacteria are nonvirulent and are unable to overcome the host T_H1 response. According to the hygiene hypothesis, exposure to nonvirulent mycobacteria in rural environments—for example, in animal feces—stimulates T cells to secrete IFN-γ, which inhibits T_H2 responses (Fig. 26.5).
- The second explanation is that nonvirulent mycobacteria may induce conditions that favor the production of Tregs. Instead of producing T_H2 cells, individuals may then produce Tregs that are specific for environmental allergens. As mentioned earlier, it is certainly true that Tregs are the major T cell specific for allergens in non-allergic individuals.

The hygiene hypothesis may be translated into clinical benefits in the future. For example, vaccination with *Mycobacterium vaccae*, a nonvirulent mycobacterium, has been shown to reduce the severity of eczema in allergic children. Drugs can also be used to mimic microorganisms and steer the immune response away from T_H2 polarization. For example, CpG is a nucleotide motif found in viruses that binds to Toll-like receptor 9 and stimulates IL-12 secretion by APCs. Synthetic CpG administered to animals can switch off allergic T_H2 responses.

■ MEDIATORS OF EARLY PHASE

The early phase of allergy is caused by mediators released by mast cells when IgE bound to FcεRI is cross-linked by allergen. Anaphylaxis is the most serious type of allergy and can occur when allergen enters the body from any route. During anaphylaxis, mast cells rapidly synthesize prostaglandins and leukotrienes through the cyclo-oxygenase and lipoxygenase pathways (see Chapter 21). These mediators cause vasodilation and an increase in vascular permeability. Fluid shifts from the vascular to the extravascular space, and there is a fall in vascular tone. The result of widespread mast cell activation is a dramatic fall in blood pressure, which is characteristic of anaphylaxis. Mast cells in the skin, but not the airway, release histamine, which contributes to swelling and fluid shift.

In other forms of allergy, there are more localized changes in blood vessels, restricted to the site of allergen entry. For example, in allergic rhinitis, inhaled allergens stimulate mast cells in the nasal mucosa. There is then vasodilation and edema in the nose, causing nasal stuffiness and sneezing. Leukotrienes (see Chapter 21) increase mucus secretion, which causes the discharge that is characteristic of allergic rhinitis.

Increased mucus secretion in the bronchi also occurs in asthma and contributes to the airflow obstruction. However, in the lungs, leukotrienes cause smooth muscle contraction, which has the most dramatic effects on airflow reduction (Fig. 26.6).

All of these effects can take place within minutes of exposure to allergen. Symptoms persist while exposure to allergen continues. Even if the patient is able to avoid the allergen, late-phase response may occur.

■ MEDIATORS OF LATE PHASE

Type I hypersensitivity reactions are generally characterized by immediate symptoms after exposure to allergens. For example, a patient with asthma who is allergic to cats will develop airway obstruction, characterized by wheeze, seconds after exposure to cat fur. The symptoms improve after an hour or so as the immediate response dies down

Several hours after the acute episode, the airflow in the bronchi may deteriorate again, reflecting the migration of leukocytes, particularly eosinophils, into the bronchi in response to chemokines. The late phase may last several hours (Fig. 26.7).

In some individuals, this process becomes self-perpetuating as T_H2 cells in the bronchial wall secrete cytokines such as IL-4 and attractant chemokines (see Fig. 26.7). The result is chronic allergic inflammation in

 T cell receptor (TCR)

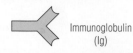 Immunoglobulin (Ig)

 Antigen

 MHC I

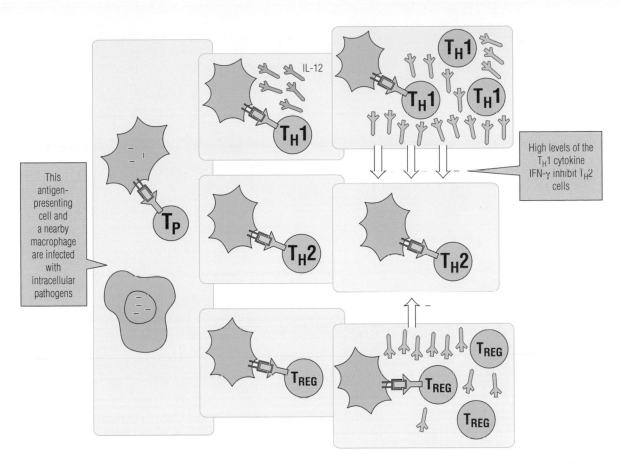

Figure 26.5 The hygiene hypothesis suggests that allergy-promoting T_H2 cells are suppressed by interferon (IFN)-γ released during T_H1 responses. It is possible that Tregs also inhibit T_H2 cells in circumstances where infection is prevalent.

the airways. Mediators released by eosinophils include peroxidase, eosinophil major basic protein, and cationic protein, which all cause direct damage to bronchial tissue. As a result of the chronic allergic inflammation, the bronchial smooth muscle is hypertrophic, and mucus secretion is increased; airflow becomes persistently, rather than intermittently, reduced.

A summary of the types of symptoms caused by allergy is shown in Figure 26.1.

■ TREATMENT

Allergics produce a spectrum of symptoms ranging from mild (e.g., nasal blockage in rhinitis) to life-threatening (e.g., severe asthma or anaphylaxis). The treatment for allergy is tailored to the individual patient's circumstances and symptoms. General measures in the treatment of allergy include identifying and avoiding possible allergens. This is not always possible when the allergen is widespread in the environment, such as with grass pollen. Other treatments involve the use of drugs or desensitization.

Drug Treatments

Some drugs block the end effects of mediator release; for example, β_2-adrenergic agonists, such as salbutamol, mimic the effects of the sympathetic nervous system and work mainly by preventing smooth bronchial muscle contraction in asthma (Fig. 26.8). Epinephrine (adrenaline) is an important drug and can be lifesaving in anaphylaxis. In anaphylaxis, the blood pressure falls dramatically because fluid shifts out of blood vessels and into the tissues when vessel permeability increases. Epinephrine stimulates both α and β adrenergic receptors, decreases vascular permeability, increases blood pressure, and reverses airway obstruction.

Antihistamines block specific histamine receptors and have an important role in allergies affecting the skin, nose, and mucus membranes. Antihistamines are much slower acting than epinephrine in the treatment of anaphylaxis and are not very useful in asthma, because histamine is not an important allergic mediator released by mast cells in the lung.

Specific receptor antagonists block the effects of leukotrienes. Montelukast, for example, reduces the amount of airway inflammation in asthma.

 MHC II

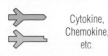 Cytokine, Chemokine, etc.

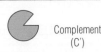 Complement (C')

 Signaling molecule

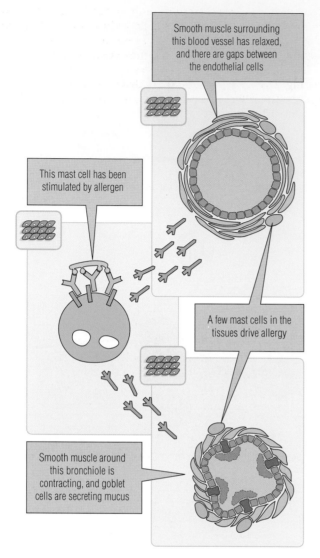

Figure 26.6 contents (speech boxes within image):

- Smooth muscle surrounding this blood vessel has relaxed, and there are gaps between the endothelial cells
- This mast cell has been stimulated by allergen
- A few mast cells in the tissues drive allergy
- Smooth muscle around this bronchiole is contracting, and goblet cells are secreting mucus

Figure 26.6 Mediators of the early phase of allergy have different consequences depending on the target tissue.

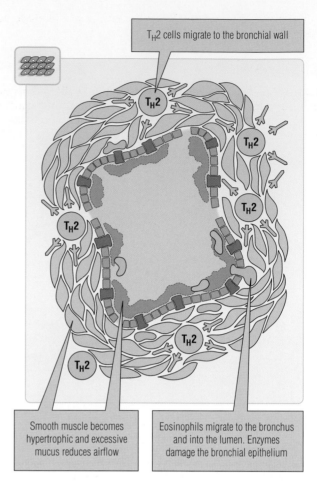

Figure 26.7 contents (speech boxes within image):

- T$_H$2 cells migrate to the bronchial wall
- Smooth muscle becomes hypertrophic and excessive mucus reduces airflow
- Eosinophils migrate to the bronchus and into the lumen. Enzymes damage the bronchial epithelium

Figure 26.7 Chronic allergic inflammation. Compare this with the changes in the bronchus in acute asthma (*lower half* of Figure 26.6).

Corticosteroids are widely used in the prevention of symptoms in patients with allergy. These are discussed in detail in Chapter 30. Corticosteroids can prevent the immediate hypersensitivity reaction, the late phase, and chronic allergic inflammation. To avoid side effects, corticosteroids are often given topically in allergies; for example, inhaled steroids are used in asthma.

Sodium cromoglycate has some effects in preventing allergy attacks. It is thought to work by stabilizing mast cells and reducing degranulation.

Other drugs in development aim to block the T$_H$2 cytokine pathway or prevent IgE binding to the FcεR. There are also interesting approaches to reduce the allergenicity of environmental allergens. For example, one biotechnology company has produced genetically modified cats, which do not produce the cat allergen FelD1. These cats do not provoke allergic symptoms in sensitized

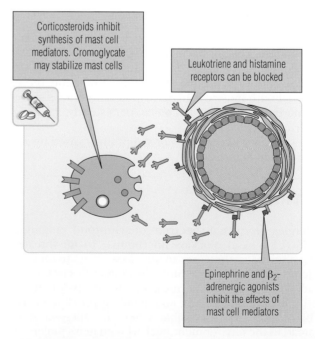

Figure 26.8 contents (speech boxes within image):

- Corticosteroids inhibit synthesis of mast cell mediators. Cromoglycate may stabilize mast cells
- Leukotriene and histamine receptors can be blocked
- Epinephrine and β$_2$-adrenergic agonists inhibit the effects of mast cell mediators

Figure 26.8 Drug treatment for allergy.

 T cell receptor (TCR)

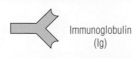 Immunoglobulin (Ig)

 Antigen

 MHC I

patients, but at over $1000 per animal, are not likely to be a popular solution!

Desensitization

Desensitization, or immunotherapy, is a well-established technique that aims to improve allergy symptoms caused by specific allergens. It is most useful when single allergens are involved in the symptoms, and it is often used to prevent anaphylaxis resulting from insect stings. Insect venom is injected subcutaneously in escalating doses. Although treatment starts with very small doses of venom, there is a risk for precipitating a full-blown anaphylactic attack. Therefore, trained staff must perform the desensitization, with access to resuscitation equipment. Over time, the patient is given injections with increasing quantities of venom, eventually corresponding to the amount of venom in an insect sting. At this point, more than 90% of patients will not develop anaphylaxis if they are stung again.

It is not clear whether desensitization works by inducing T_H1 cells, which then drive production of IgG against the allergen or by inducing Tregs, which inhibit polarized T_H2 responses. In either case, once desensitization has been carried out, high levels of allergen-specific IgG will bind venom and prevent it from cross-linking IgE on mast cells (Fig. 26.9). Desensitization illustrates how a different route of administration induces different T-cell populations: T_H1 and/or Treg in the case of subcutaneous administration and T_H2 in the case of a sting on the skin.

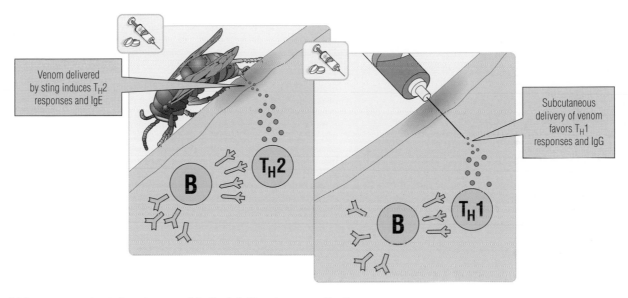

Figure 26.9 Desensitization induces immunoglobulin G (IgG) antivenom antibodies.

 MHC II   Cytokine, Chemokine, etc.   Complement (C')   Signaling molecule

BOX 26.1 Latex Allergy

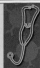

A 25-year-old woman developed tongue and lip swelling a few minutes after the beginning of a dental procedure. She has had similar but less dramatic swelling on several occasions immediately after she has eaten a fruit salad. She has asthma, and her mother and brother both have allergies.

A skin prick test is done to investigate the possibility of allergy to latex and fruits. The skin test results are ready to read in 10 minutes and confirm that she is sensitive to latex, banana, avocado, and kiwi fruit (Fig. 26.10).

Skin prick testing is the preferred method for allergy testing. When the antigen introduced by pricking cross-links IgE on mast cell FcεRI, there is a rapid release of histamine, causing a local flare and wheal reaction. Skin prick tests give immediate results, which the patient can see, and they are cheap and more sensitive than specific IgE testing on blood samples. Although skin prick testing is generally safe, it may be risky when patients have extensive atopic dermatitis or a history of anaphylaxis. Skin prick testing is not possible when patients have taken antihistamines, and in these circumstances, measuring levels of specific IgE is most useful.

The corresponding cartoon (Fig. 26.11) shows how skin swelling rapidly develops.

The rubber, banana, avocado, and kiwi plants are botanically related and contain very similar proteins, to which the patient is allergic. This is an example of cross-reactivity. If she is exposed to these allergens again, it is possible that she could have much more severe reactions, including anaphylaxis. Patient education is important to ensure that she understands how to avoid latex (e.g., during medical and dental procedures and latex condoms) and related fruits in the future.

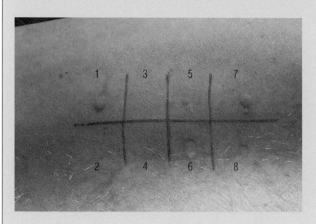

Figure 26.10 Skin prick testing: In order to quality control the test, a histamine solution is applied at position 1 and saline at position 2. These are pricked through the dermis. 10 minutes later, the histamine has given a positive reaction (this would not have happened if the patient had recently taken antihistamines) but the saline has given no reaction (confirming the patient's skin does not simply react to trauma). House dust mite feces and tree pollen were applied at positions 3 and 4; the patient has not reacted to these. Positions 5, 6, 7 and 8 were occupied by fresh juice of avocado, banana, kiwi fruit and latex suspension. The patient has reacted to all four of these, most strongly to kiwi fruit and banana. (With permission from the Department of Medical Illustration, St. Bartholomew's Hospital, London.)

Continued

 T cell receptor (TCR)

 Immunoglobulin (Ig)

Antigen

MHC I

BOX 26.1   Latex Allergy—cont'd

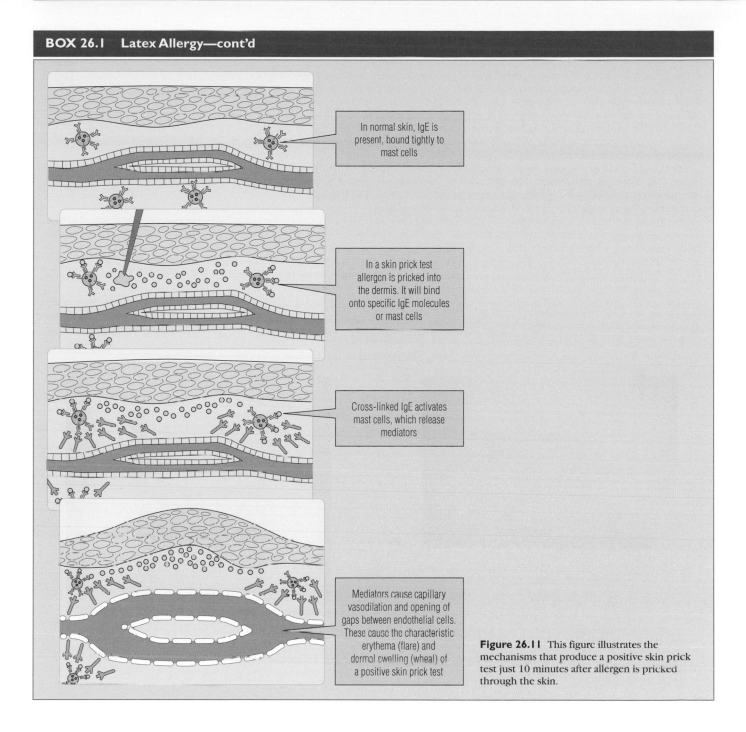

In normal skin, IgE is present, bound tightly to mast cells

In a skin prick test allergen is pricked into the dermis. It will bind onto specific IgE molecules or mast cells

Cross-linked IgE activates mast cells, which release mediators

Mediators cause capillary vasodilation and opening of gaps between endothelial cells. These cause the characteristic erythema (flare) and dermal swelling (wheal) of a positive skin prick test

Figure 26.11   This figure illustrates the mechanisms that produce a positive skin prick test just 10 minutes after allergen is pricked through the skin.

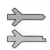 MHC II

 Cytokine, Chemokine, etc.

 Complement (C')

 Signaling molecule

BOX 26.2   Peanut Allergy

A 4-year-old boy has been brought into the emergency department with swelling of the face, generalized itchiness, and drowsiness. The symptoms developed a few minutes after eating a chocolate bar. The emergency department physician finds that he has facial angioedema (Fig 26.12) and urticaria (Fig. 26.13) and that his blood pressure is low. He is given an intramuscular injection of 150 μg of epinephrine, and within minutes he is beginning to recover.

His mother explains that he has had minor reactions to nuts in the past, including lip swelling. The boy also has eczema (Fig. 26.14), and his mother thinks that in the past, this has flared up when he has eaten peanuts. She has concluded that he might be allergic to nuts and has tried to eliminate them from the house. The patient has never had any symptoms from milk.

The patient's mother has kept the chocolate bar wrapper, and this confirms that it "'may contain traces of nut." Highly sensitized individuals can react to tiny quantities of allergen that may contaminate harmless foods during processing. Because this patient appears to be very sensitive to nut allergen, the emergency doctor decides not to refer the patient for skin prick testing. He orders blood samples and arranges for the patient to be seen 2 weeks later in the allergy clinic.

The first blood test shows a high level of mast cell tryptase in the blood. Mast cell tryptase is normally present in the blood at low levels, and its presence at a high level indicates mast cell degranulation has occurred in the 12 hours prior to the blood sample being taken. Taken along with the history, this confirms that anaphylaxis has taken place. The second part of the blood tests results are for specific IgE testing. These show no detectable IgE against cow's milk, which is important because this could possibly have been the allergen in the chocolate bar. The second part of the results show he is allergic to several species of nut. This reactivity to several nuts is quite common because there is cross-reactivity amongst the antigens.

An important part of the management of this boy is to reduce the risk for future exposure to nuts, this involves training patients to avoid foods that may contain hidden nuts. However, repeated exposure is common, and there is a good chance that this patient may then develop life-threatening reactions. He is given an epinephrine intramuscular injector device and trained in its use, in case of future symptoms. Intramuscular epinephrine is an important part of the treatment of anaphylaxis. Epinephrine reverses vasodilatation and closes the gap between endothelial cells. After epinephrine is given, swollen tissues return to normal, and blood pressure is restored.

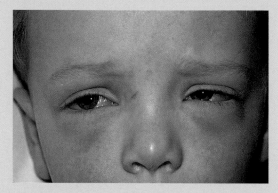

Figure 26.12   This boy has angioedema as a result of exposure to nuts. (With permission from the Department of Medical Illustration, St. Bartholomew's Hospital, London.)

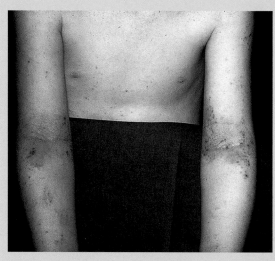

Figure 26.14   Atopic eczema causes a thickened itchy weeping rash, especially affecting the flexures of the knees and the elbows. (With permission from the Department of Medical Illustration, St. Bartholomew's Hospital, London.)

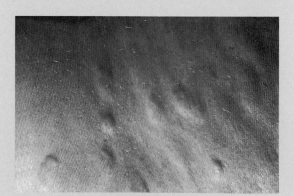

Figure 26.13   Acute urticaria is an itchy rash which can be caused by allergies. When it lasts for more than a few weeks, urticaria rarely has an allergic cause. (With permission from the Department of Medical Illustration, St. Bartholomew's Hospital, London.)

T cell receptor (TCR)   Immunoglobulin (Ig)   Antigen   MHC I

LEARNING POINTS Can You Now ...

1. List the mechanisms of the early and late phases of allergy?

2. Compare the roles of T_H1 and T_H2 cells from the point of view of cytokines?

3. Describe the immunologic factors that predispose to allergy and explain how these may be increasing allergy at a population level?

4. Describe the techniques used to identify allergens involved in immediate hypersensitivity?

5. Describe anaphylaxis and its immediate treatment?

6. List the modes of action of drugs used to treat allergy?

 MHC II

 Cytokine, Chemokine, etc.

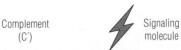 Complement (C')

Signaling molecule

27 How Autoimmune Disease Develops

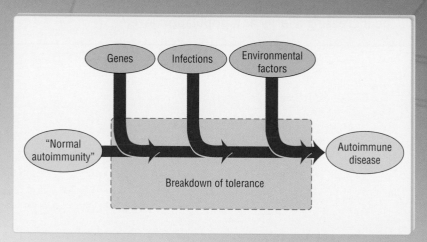

In the main part of this chapter, you will learn how some autoimmunity is a normal finding in healthy individuals, but that more extensive breakdown of tolerance can lead to autoimmune disease. An interplay of genetic factors, infections, and other environmental factors is required for tolerance to break down. At the end of the chapter, you will learn about tests for autoimmunity and the pathogenesis of three autoimmune diseases (insulin-dependent diabetes, celiac disease, and systemic lupus erythematosus) in detail. Chapters 28, 29, and 30 give more detail of the different hypersensitivity reactions leading to several important autoimmune diseases.

■ SOME AUTOIMMUNITY IS NORMAL

Autoimmunity can be defined as adaptive immune responses with specificity for self antigens. Autoimmune responses include both antibodies and T cells and are common in healthy individuals.

Autoantibodies are antibodies directed at normal cellular components, referred to as autoantigens. Most healthy individuals produce some autoantibodies, although these are usually very low level, are of low affinity, and require sensitive tests for their detection. Higher-affinity autoantibodies, detectable with routine clinical tests, are also found in some normal people, especially women and the elderly. For example, low levels of antinuclear antibodies are seen in a fifth of healthy elderly patients.

It has been estimated that after random immunoglobulin (Ig) gene recombination, more than half of the emerging B-cell receptors have specificity for self antigen. The checkpoints in B-cell ontogeny (see Chapter 14) prevent the majority of B cells from producing autoantibodies. Many autoreactive B cells modify their receptors through receptor editing. Those that are unable to do so are either deleted or become nonfunctional. In any case, most autoreactive B cells are unable to secrete Ig in the periphery without help from T-helper cells responding to the same antigen.

This is not the case for B-1 cells, which are able to secrete Ig without T-cell help (see Chapter 14). B-1 cells secrete natural antibodies, which are the major source of autoantibodies in healthy individuals. These B cells break some of the rules that normally apply to B cells and do not alter their Ig genes in response to antigen exposure nor undergo somatic hypermutation. Natural antibody produced by B-1 cells never improves its fit to specific antigen. This means that although natural antibodies bind a wide number of antigens with low affinity, they never have high-affinity binding to specific antigens.

Natural antibodies secreted by B-1 cells have a number of different activities (Fig. 27.1):

- Natural antibodies bind with low affinity to antigens that are present on a large variety of bacteria. This activates complement and helps to clear invading bacteria rapidly. Thus, natural antibodies act like molecules of

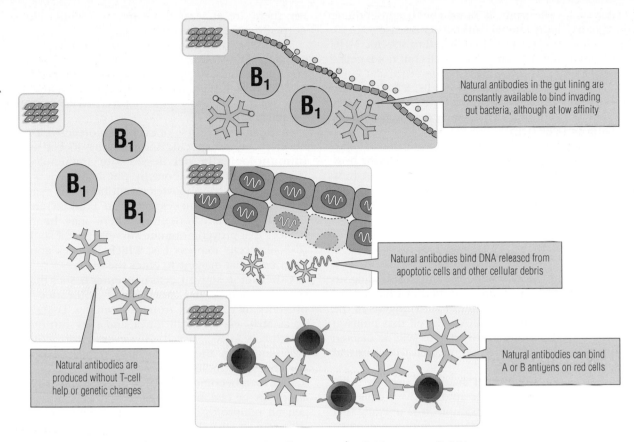

Figure 27.1 Natural antibodies bind a range of antigens with low affinity. Natural antibodies are usually IgM pentamers.

Labels within figure:
- Natural antibodies in the gut lining are constantly available to bind invading gut bacteria, although at low affinity
- Natural antibodies bind DNA released from apoptotic cells and other cellular debris
- Natural antibodies can bind A or B antigens on red cells
- Natural antibodies are produced without T-cell help or genetic changes

the innate immune system —they do not rely on genetic recombination, and they are present before an infection starts.

- Natural antibodies cross-react with the inherited A and B antigens of red cells. Unless they have inherited either A or B antigens, individuals make IgM anti-A and anti-B, even if they have never been exposed to red cells from another person (see Chapter 28). Humans also have natural antibodies against sugars expressed on cells of other animal species. These xenogeneic natural antibodies are discussed further in Chapter 33.

- Another consequence of their low specificity is that natural antibodies can also bind to a series of normal cellular constituents, for example, nuclear proteins and DNA. This explains why some normal people have antinuclear antibodies. The autoantigen-binding ability of natural antibodies may be an accidental consequence of cross-reactivity, but these antibodies may have a role in, for example, clearing up cellular debris.

There are also T cells that break the normal immunological rules. These autoreactive T cells are able to recognize and secrete cytokines in response to autoantigens, such as major histocompatibility complex (MHC), and they are present in most normal individuals in very small numbers. Little is known about these T cells, and there is no clear evidence for a physiologic role. Autoreactive T cells must be closely regulated normally through peripheral tolerance (see Chapter 15) because although most people have them, autoimmune disease only occurs in a minority of people.

■ THE INITIATION OF AUTOIMMUNE DISEASE

Autoimmune disease occurs when autoreactive T cells or autoantibodies cause tissue damage through hypersensitivity reaction types II to IV, defined in Chapter 25. Unlike infectious antigens, autoantigens are almost impossible to clear, despite the immune system's best efforts; consequently, once initiated, autoimmune diseases tend to be active for a long time. Autoimmune diseases are very common and tend to cause chronic diseases, usually lasting months or years. They can affect any organ system and occur at any age. Understanding how autoimmune diseases arise helps us to diagnose, treat, and even prevent these problems.

One possibility is that the natural autoantibodies mentioned above cause autoimmune disease. However, there is evidence that T cells initiate autoimmune disease as follows:

- Even autoimmune diseases caused by IgG-mediated mechanisms (hypersensitivity types II and III) require T-cell help for affinity maturation to produce pathogenic (disease-causing) antibodies.

 MHC II

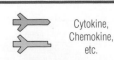 Cytokine, Chemokine, etc.

 Complement (C')

 Signaling molecule

- Transfer of T cells from an animal with autoimmune disease to a healthy animal can transfer disease.
- Autoimmune diseases are often linked to specific MHC genes, which, of course, regulate T cells but not B cells.

There is no evidence that the B-1 cells, which secrete harmless natural antibodies, can also produce the high-affinity, specific antibodies that can cause autoimmune disease without T-cell help.

For T cells to mediate autoimmune disease, they need to overcome tolerance mechanisms. Before we describe how they may do this, we offer a brief reminder about how T cells are tolerized to autoantigen.

■ A REMINDER ABOUT T-CELL TOLERANCE

Tolerance prevents the immune system responding to specific antigens and has been described in Chapters 14 and 15. T cells are initially tolerant of autoantigens in the thymus; this is central tolerance. Any T cell that binds at high affinity to self peptide in the thymus will be deleted by negative selection in a process referred to as **central tolerance**.

However, it is not possible for every self peptide to be expressed in the thymus, so some autoreactive T cells may escape negative selection. For example, it is unlikely that every possible peptide from a remote, complex organ like the brain is expressed in the thymus, and, therefore, some brain-specific T cells may reach the periphery. For potentially autoreactive T cells that have escaped to the periph-

ery, there are at least three more potential blocks that normally prevent stimulation (Fig. 27.2).

The first way of preventing autoreactive T cells from becoming stimulated is to sequester (hide) the self antigen. Some molecules, such as DNA, are normally hidden inside healthy cells. If they leak out of cells, for example, during cell death, they are rapidly cleared by complement or natural antibodies.

In the normal course of events, autoreactive T cells may never encounter specific antigen if it is locked away in an **immunologically privileged site**. Immunologic privilege can be brought about by physical barriers that prevent access to lymphocytes or antibody. For example, the blood-brain barrier makes the brain a "no go" area for the immune system. Alternatively, there may be molecular devices that prevent immune surveillance of some tissues; testicular cells express Fas, which induces apoptosis in any T cells that manage to enter the testis.

Other autoreactive T cells may enter tissues that express specific antigen and **peripheral tolerance** normally prevents these T cells from responding. Tissue cells express MHC class I at all times, and they can be induced to express MHC class II. However, autoreactive T cells emerging from the thymus also require expression of costimulatory molecules such as CD80 (B7) or CD40. Rather than become stimulated, naive T cells will undergo apoptosis or become anergic when they recognize antigen on nonprofessional antigen-presenting cells. Anergic cells remain alive, but are prevented from responding to antigen.

Autoreactive T cells that have escaped to the periphery can also be prevented from responding by regulatory

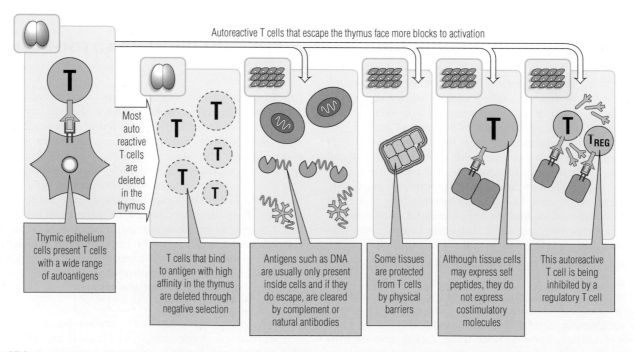

Autoreactive T cells that escape the thymus face more blocks to activation

Most auto reactive T cells are deleted in the thymus

Thymic epithelium cells present T cells with a wide range of autoantigens

T cells that bind to antigen with high affinity in the thymus are deleted through negative selection

Antigens such as DNA are usually only present inside cells and if they do escape, are cleared by complement or natural antibodies

Some tissues are protected from T cells by physical barriers

Although tissue cells may express self peptides, they do not express costimulatory molecules

This autoreactive T cell is being inhibited by a regulatory T cell

Figure 27.2 T-cell tolerance. The majority of autoreactive T cells are killed in the thymus. Peripheral tolerance, sequestration of antigens, and T-regulatory cells prevent T cells reacting with autoantigens in the periphery.

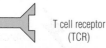
T cell receptor (TCR)

Immunoglobulin (Ig)

Antigen

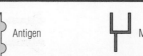
MHC I

T cells. Regulatory T cells appear to be specific for the identical antigen as the T cell they are inhibiting. They inhibit effector T cells by a number of mechanisms, including secretion of inhibitory cytokines such as interleukin-10 (IL-10) and transforming growth factor-β (TGF-β).

■ THE BREAKDOWN OF T-CELL TOLERANCE

Tolerance can break down centrally or peripherally. Each of the tolerance mechanisms mentioned in the previous section can break down. Central tolerance can break down following inheritance of two different types of genetic polymorphisms.

First, self peptides can be expressed at variable levels in the thymus. For example, insulin is expressed in the normal thymus, where it tolerizes T cells through negative selection. The level of insulin expression in the thymus is genetically determined. Some individuals inherit insulin genes, which are transcribed at lower levels than normal, so less insulin is expressed in the thymus and insulin-reactive T cells are less likely to be deleted (Fig. 27.3). Additionally, inheritance of certain MHC alleles, which are less efficient at presenting self peptides to T cells, can increase the risk for acquiring autoimmune diseases, including type I diabetes.

There are a number of ways in which peripheral tolerance can break down. For example, hidden ("cryptic") antigens may become exposed to the immune system. Molecules that are normally rapidly removed from the extracellular environment, for example, DNA released by dying cells is normally removed by molecules such as mannan-binding lectin and complement component C1. If DNA cannot be removed by these mechanisms, it may provoke an immune response, which may be the first step in the development of the autoimmune disease systemic lupus erythematosus (see Box 27.3 at the end of this chapter).

Some antigens are normally kept physically separated from the immune system. The testis is an example of a tissue that is not usually patrolled by T cells. Following vasectomy, sperm antigens may leak out of the genital system. These antigens can cause the production of auto-antibodies against sperm in some patients. Such patients remain infertile, even if the vasectomy is reversed, because of the antisperm antibodies.

Peripheral tolerance can also break down if tissue cells acquire the ability to present self peptides. This can happen when professional antigen-presenting cells, such as monocytes and macrophages, are recruited to sites of infection. These cells express costimulatory molecules and cytokines that enable naive T cells to respond to self peptides expressed by tissue cells. In this situation, an appropriate inflammatory response to infection spreads to include inappropriate responses to self antigens.

Another possible mechanism leading to the breakdown of peripheral tolerance is when an immune response to an infection elicits antibodies or T cells that cross-react with host tissues, so-called "**molecular mimicry**." An example of this is acute rheumatic fever, which can occur rarely following infection with the bacterium β-hemolytic streptococcus. Patients develop a complex of symptoms including rash, heart, and nervous system involvement. In

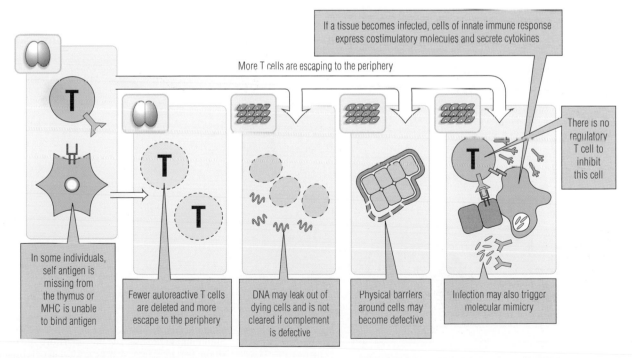

Figure 27.3 How T-cell tolerance breaks down. Tolerance needs to break down at several of the points illustrated here in order for autoimmune disease to develop.

 MHC II   Cytokine, Chemokine, etc.   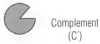 Complement (C')   Signaling molecule these individuals, streptococcal infection induces antibodies that cross-react with heart tissue and trigger type II hypersensitivity. In this instance, streptococcal antigens mimic heart antigen. The infection is able to overcome the tolerance mechanisms that normally prevent the production of autoreactive antibodies because streptococcus activates the innate immune response, through its pattern-recognition molecules. Rheumatic fever is a transient illness and does not cause the chronic disease that is typical of most autoimmune disease. Similar bacteria can cause poststreptococcal glomerulonephritis (see Chapter 25) through a very different mechanism.

There are a handful of other rare examples of infections triggering off short-lived autoimmune disease using molecular mimicry. However, none of the autoimmune diseases persists for more than a few weeks. The current view is that infections may sometimes initiate autoimmune disease using molecular mimicry, but that other genetic and environmental factors are required for its maintenance.

In Chapter 26 you learned how regulatory T cells (Tregs) can prevent overpolarized T_H2 responses and the development of allergy. The same may be true of autoimmune disease, which may be more likely to develop if regulatory T cells are unable to inhibit autoreactive T cells. Failure of regulatory T cells may lead to exaggerated autoimmunity and disease. This happens in a rare genetic disease called IPEX, in which the main transcriptional factor for Tregs, Foxp3, is mutated. Though very rare, this syndrome provides evidence that Tregs normally inhibit the development of autoimmune disease in humans.

Individuals who have inherited identical genetic predispositions to autoimmunity (e.g., identical twins) do not always develop the same autoimmune disease. If they develop autoimmune disease at all, they may do so at very different times. This is because environmental factors usually play a dominant role in establishing autoimmunity. It is likely that several environmental triggers, operating in

sequence, are required for disease to develop. This complexity (Fig. 27.4) explains why it has been difficult to unravel the pathogenesis of autoimmune disease. As you will read in Chapter 34, similar "multihit" mechanisms, combinations of genetic and environmental factors, are required to produce malignancies.

■ TESTS FOR AUTOIMMUNE DISEASE

All of the tests for autoimmune disease rely on detecting evidence of autoantibodies and, as a practicing physician, you will frequently ask for these tests to be carried out. In Chapter 5, you learned that there are two main types of test for antibody specificity. The first is direct immunofluorescence, which is used to find evidence of autoimmune processes in tissues. This is only possible in accessible tissues, such as skin, as in the example of the patient in Box 27.3 at the end of this chapter. The technique of direct immunofluorescence is briefly reviewed in Fig. 27.5.

In most cases, it is much simpler to test a blood sample for autoantibodies. There are three different types of autoantibody test in routine use. All three tests rely on antibody in the patients serum binding on to antigen mounted on a solid phase. The bound antibody is then detected with different types of detection system. The development of these tests illustrates how technology has changed over the years. The three different types of autoantibody test are as follows:

• The original autoantibody test was indirect immunofluorescence. In this case, the antigen is cells or tissue mounted on a glass slide. The detection system is anti-human IgG conjugated to a fluorescent tag, which is detected in an ultraviolet microscope (Fig. 27.5B). Islet cell and endomysial antibodies and antinuclear anti-

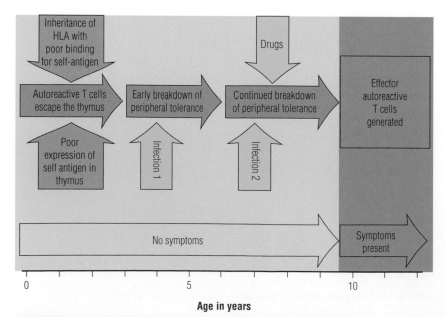

Figure 27.4 This figure illustrates how a series of different factors may be required to initiate an autoimmune process. The precise nature and timings of the two infections may be critical in determining the type of autoimmunity that results. Genetic factors are shown in pink and nongenetic factors in blue.

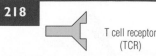
T cell receptor (TCR)

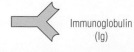
Immunoglobulin (Ig)

Antigen

MHC I

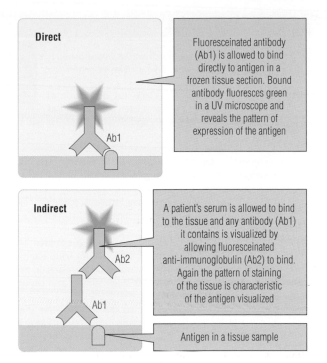

Direct

Fluoresceinated antibody (Ab1) is allowed to bind directly to antigen in a frozen tissue section. Bound antibody fluoresces green in a UV microscope and reveals the pattern of expression of the antigen

Ab1

Indirect

A patient's serum is allowed to bind to the tissue and any antibody (Ab1) it contains is visualized by allowing fluoresceinated anti-immunoglobulin (Ab2) to bind. Again the pattern of staining of the tissue is characteristic of the antigen visualized

Ab2

Ab1

Antigen in a tissue sample

Figure 27.5 This figure shows the principles of direct and indirect immunofluorescence.

bodies are used to illustrate indirect immunofluorescence in Boxes 27.1 through 27.3.

- The next type of test to be developed was enzyme-linked immunosorbent assay (ELISA). ELISA uses purified antigen fixed onto a plastic surface. The plastic surface (usually the bottom of a "well") is incubated with serum. The detection system in ELISA is an anti-human IgG antibody conjugated to an enzyme. The enzyme is able to generate either a color change or fluorescence. The amount of color or fluorescence is proportional to the level of autoantibody present in the sample. The advantages of ELISA are that antigens can be purified (in principle giving more specific results), there is higher sensitivity to lower levels of antibody, and there is the ability to quantify antibody levels.

- The most recent version of solid-phase testing uses mixtures of microscopic colored beads coated in antigen. The beads are manufactured so that the specific antigen that coats each bead is indicated by the color of the bead. The beads are incubated with serum, and the detection system is an antihuman IgG labeled with a fluorescent molecule. The beads are fed through a device that operates in a similar fashion to a flow cytometer. The device identifies the antigen coating each bead and calculates the amount of antibody in serum (proportional to the degree of fluorescence). Bead-based platforms have the advantages of ELISA but are also capable of detecting several different antibodies at once.

Although autoantibodies can be very helpful in diagnosing autoimmune diseases, there is one important pitfall to understand. As explained earlier, some autoantibodies can be found at low level in perfectly healthy individuals. For example, antinuclear antibodies, which are found at high levels in patients with systemic lupus erythematosus, can be found at low levels in many normal individuals, particularly women, and more often with increasing age. Other individuals tend to produce autoantibodies transiently following infections, presumably as a result of nonspecific activation of the immune system. These **false positives** contribute to the **low specificity** of some of these tests.

 MHC II

 Cytokine, Chemokine, etc.

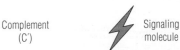 Complement (C')

Signaling molecule

BOX 27.1 Insulin-Dependent Diabetes Mellitus

A 9-year-old boy has been performing poorly at school for several weeks. He is drinking large amounts of water. His mother is concerned because his older sister was diagnosed as having diabetes after having the same symptoms, 4 years earlier, when she was 8 years old.

The boy has a moderately raised fasting glucose but there are no ketones in his urine; these findings are not diagnostic of diabetes. His serum is tested by indirect immunofluorescence for autoantibodies, and it is shown to contain islet cell antibodies (Fig. 27.6), which are very suggestive of insulin-dependent diabetes mellitis (IDDM). He starts taking insulin and, 5 years later, has had no complications of diabetes.

The islet cell antibodies seen in IDDM are generally not required for the diagnosis in individuals who have high blood glucose and ketones in the urine. The presence of islet cell antibodies may help to make the diagnosis in patients with less clear features, as in this case. In IDDM, pancreatic islets' β cells are damaged by T cells. The islet cell antibodies are a marker of this process and do not have any role in inducing islet cell damage.

IDDM is an example of type IV hypersensitivity. T cells invade the pancreatic islets and specifically destroy the insulin-secreting β cells. Once autoreactive T cells have entered the pancreatic islets, β cells are destroyed over a few weeks. There appears to be little chance of regenerating β cells once they have been destroyed, and patients must start life-long insulin replacement.

If an identical twin develops IDDM, there is a 50% chance his or her twin will also do so; this is called the **concordance rate**. The most important genetic factor, conferring about 90% of the genetic risk, is the HLA type. In Caucasians, IDDM occurs frequently in people who inherit the HLA allele *DQ2*. In most *HLA-DQ* alleles, position 57 in the HLA-DQ β-chain is occupied by an aspartic acid residue. With HLA-DQ2, this position is replaced by another amino acid residue. Figure 27.7 shows how this single amino acid residue change in the β-chain of HLA-DQ2 affects the risk for developing IDDM.

Several other genetic polymorphisms also affect the risk for diabetes. For example, polymorphisms near to the insulin gene affect insulin expression in the thymus. Individuals who inherit a polymorphism leading to lower levels of insulin secretion in the thymus have an increased risk for diabetes. This presumably happens because low expression allows insulin-reactive T cells to reach the periphery.

Even in identical twins, the risk for concordance with diabetes is only 50%, and, therefore, environmental factors must be very important. One possible environmental culprit is infection, which may cause low-grade inflammation in the pancreatic islets. The inflammatory signals attract innate immune system cells, which express costimulatory molecules and secrete cytokines. These allow tissue antigens to be presented to autoreactive T cells.

However, although IDDM is a common autoimmune disease, no single infection has been identified that consistently acts as a trigger. Furthermore, the prevalence of IDDM is increasing at about 3% per annum at a time when childhood infections are decreasing in intensity in the developed world. This has led some researchers to suggest that it may be either absence of infection or experiencing infections at a different age that triggers IDDM. This is analogous to the hygiene hypothesis that is proposed to explain the increase in allergy prevalence in genetically predisposed individuals (see Chapter 26). It may be that in "hygienic" circumstances, regulatory T cells are not generated, and autoreactive T cells are not prevented from destroying pancreatic islet β cells.

Figure 27.8 illustrates these views about IDDM pathogenesis. The precise timing of infections may be more important than whether or not an infection takes place in this kind of model.

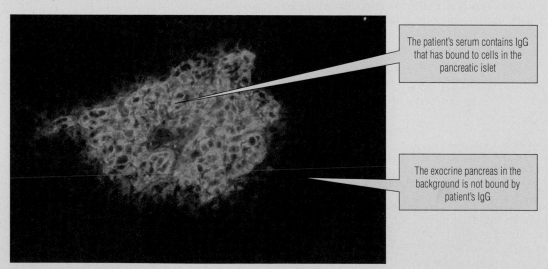

The patient's serum contains IgG that has bound to cells in the pancreatic islet

The exocrine pancreas in the background is not bound by patient's IgG

Figure 27.6 This slide shows antibodies against pancreatic islet beta cells. A section of animal pancreas has been placed on a slide. The patient's serum is incubated on the slide. Patient's immunoglobulin, which has not bound to the tissue, is washed off. Patient's IgG, which has bound to tissue, is detected with antihuman IgG labeled with a fluorescent dye.

Continued

 T cell receptor (TCR)

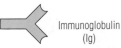 Immunoglobulin (Ig)

 Antigen

 MHC I

BOX 27.1 Insulin-Dependent Diabetes Mellitus—cont'd

IDDM is common and can reduce life expectancy considerably. In families in which one child has been affected, it is possible to periodically screen the other siblings for islet cell antibodies. In children who develop islet cell antibodies, immunosuppressive drugs, such as ciclosporin (see Chapter 11) can delay the onset of diabetes. These drugs work by inhibiting T cells, but soon after the drugs are stopped (they are too toxic to be used for long periods of time), the disease becomes apparent.

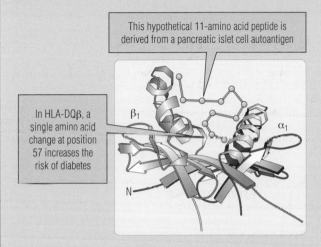

This hypothetical 11-amino acid peptide is derived from a pancreatic islet cell autoantigen

In HLA-DQβ, a single amino acid change at position 57 increases the risk of diabetes

Figure 27.7 Current thinking is that HLA-DQ2 has reduced binding for a pancreatic islet cell antigen. Consequently, T cells which recognise islet cell antigen cannot be deleted in the thymus, and the potential for autoimmunity is increased.

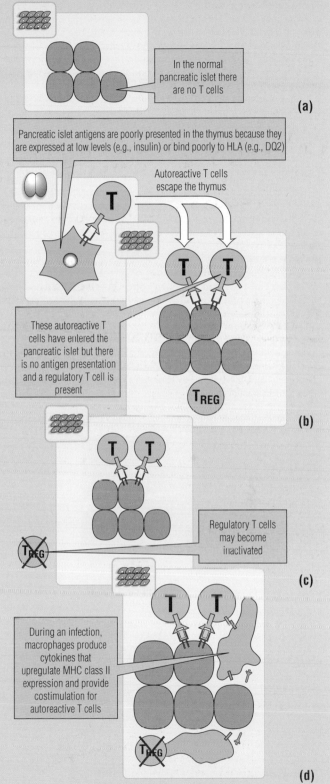

In the normal pancreatic islet there are no T cells

(a)

Pancreatic islet antigens are poorly presented in the thymus because they are expressed at low levels (e.g., insulin) or bind poorly to HLA (e.g., DQ2)

Autoreactive T cells escape the thymus

These autoreactive T cells have entered the pancreatic islet but there is no antigen presentation and a regulatory T cell is present

(b)

Regulatory T cells may become inactivated

(c)

During an infection, macrophages produce cytokines that upregulate MHC class II expression and provide costimulation for autoreactive T cells

(d)

Figure 27.8 Pathogenesis of insulin-dependent diabetes. In the normal pancreatic islet, there are no autoreactive T cells (**A**). The genetic factors that allow autoreactive T cells to escape the thymus are well understood (**B**). The exact significance of regulatory T cells in IDDM (**C**) is unclear. Infection is thought to have a role in increasing major histocompatibility (MHC) expression (**D**).

 MHC II

 Cytokine, Chemokine, etc.

Complement (C')

 Signaling molecule

BOX 27.2 Celiac Disease

The younger sister of the diabetic patient discussed in Box 27.1 develops diarrhea and weight loss. She is shown to have mild malabsorption. Her serum is tested by indirect immunofluorescence and is found to contain IgA autoantibodies against endomysium (Fig. 27.9). ELISA testing shows that she has antibodies against tissue transglutaminase. These findings are suggestive of celiac disease, and a jejunal biopsy shows she has atrophy of the villi, also consistent with this. The patient is started on a gluten-free diet, and her symptoms improve dramatically. The endomysial antibodies are no longer present 6 months later.

Celiac disease is the most common cause of small bowel disease in the developed world, causing a spectrum of clinical problems ranging from mild anemia to severe malnutrition.

Celiac disease is an autoimmune disease in which lymphocytes and macrophages infiltrate the jejunum. Celiac disease is, therefore, a type IV delayed hypersensitivity reaction against an exogenous antigen, gliadin, and an autoantigen, tissue transglutaminase.

• Wheat, rye, and barley contain a protein called gluten, which in turn contains a polypeptide, gliadin. When gliadin is removed from the diet, the symptoms of celiac disease and jejunal histology improve.
• Tissue transglutaminase is an enzyme that converts the amino acid glutamine to glutamic acid. It can irreversibly bind to substrate peptides. Endomysial antibodies are an indirect way of detecting antibodies to tissue transglutaminase.

Identical twins have a high concordance rate (75%) for celiac disease. Most patients with this disease have inherited the HLA-DQ2 allele. In celiac disease, jejunal T cells recognize gliadin peptides bound to HLA-DQ2 (Fig. 27.10). However, pockets on the side of the peptide-binding groove on HLA-DQ2 only bind charged amino acids; gliadin will not bind unless glutamine residues have been converted to glutamic acid by tissue transglutaminase. As a result of binding to gliadin, tissue transglutaminase itself becomes a target of autoantibodies (Fig. 27.11).

Tissue transglutaminase is present at high quantities in endomyseum, the connective tissue between smooth muscle cells. Endomyseal antibody testing using indirect immunofluorescence performs as well as ELISA for tissue transglutaminase in testing for celiac disease.

Members of the same family will often develop IDDM and celiac disease. Family members may also be at higher risk for developing autoimmune thyroid or adrenal disease or gastritis. These diseases frequently coexist in the same individuals, and they are called organ-specific autoimmune diseases.

The HLA genes are all closely situated on chromosome 6, and they tend to be inherited as a block, called a haplotype (see Chapter 8). One relatively common haplotype consists of HLA alleles *B8*, *DR3*, and *DQ2*. It is the inheritance of this haplotype that explains why organ-specific autoimmune disease occurs in families. The *HLA-DQ2* allele increases the risk for IDDM and celiac disease. It is not clear which genes in the MHC are associated with the other organ-specific autoimmune diseases, and there are many possible candidate genes (see Fig. 8.10). Different family members tend to have different autoimmune disease, presumably because slightly different environmental factors trigger each different disease.

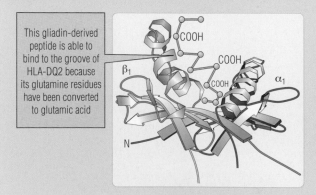

Endomysium is the connective tissue between smooth muscle cells

The black dots are smooth muscle cells cut in cross section. They do not bind patient's IgG

Figure 27.9 Patients with celiac disease have autoantibodies against endomysium, connective tissue surrounding bundles of smooth muscle fibers. In the test illustrated here, a section of animal tissue has been placed on a slide. This is incubated with patient serum, and the IgG is detected with a fluorescent anti-IgG antibody. Endomysium is a good source of tissue transglutaminase, the autoantigen in celiac disease.

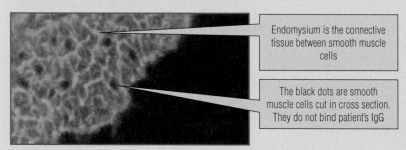

This gliadin-derived peptide is able to bind to the groove of HLA-DQ2 because its glutamine residues have been converted to glutamic acid

Figure 27.10 Gliadin peptides bound to HLA-DQ2.

Continued

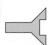 T cell receptor (TCR)

 Immunoglobulin (Ig)

 Antigen

 MHC I

BOX 27.2 Celiac Disease—con'td

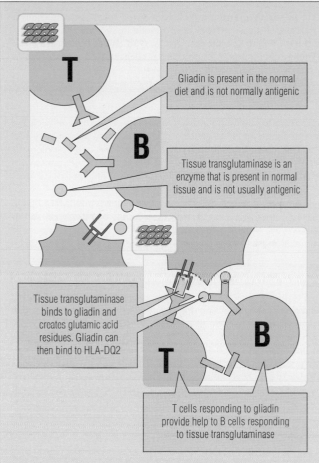

Gliadin is present in the normal diet and is not normally antigenic

Tissue transglutaminase is an enzyme that is present in normal tissue and is not usually antigenic

Tissue transglutaminase binds to gliadin and creates glutamic acid residues. Gliadin can then bind to HLA-DQ2

T cells responding to gliadin provide help to B cells responding to tissue transglutaminase

Figure 27.11 The pathogenesis of celiac disease. Jejunal damage in celiac disease is mediated by T cells responding to deaminated gliadin, bound to HLA-DQ2. These T cells produce cytokines, such as interferon-γ, which may damage villi. The pathogenic role of the antibodies produced against gliadin and tissue transglutaminase is unclear, although both antibodies are useful diagnostically.

BOX 27.3 Systemic Lupus Erythematosus

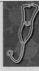

A young woman develops a rash in a sun-exposed area—her face (Fig. 27.12A). She has also developed painful lesions in the pulps of her toes (Fig 27.12B). A skin biopsy is taken for direct immunofluorescence and shows her skin contains deposits of IgG and complement (Fig. 27.13). She was also found to have some abnormalities on blood testing. These included an antinuclear antibody (done by indirect immunofluorescence, Fig. 27.14) and anti DNA antibodies (by ELISA). These findings are strongly suggestive of

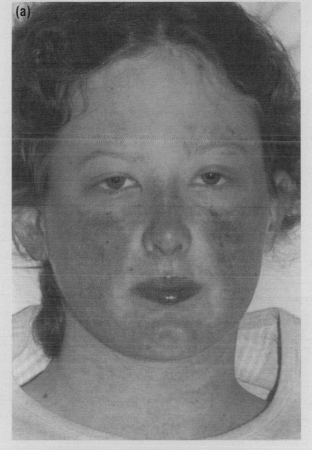

(a)

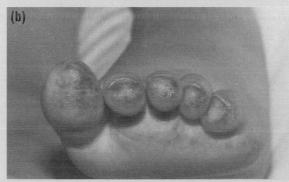

(b)

Figure 27.12 This woman has a facial rash typical of systemic lupus erythematosus (**A**). The lesions on her toes reflect underlying vasculitis—blood vessel inflammation (**B**).

Continued

 MHC II

 Cytokine, Chemokine, etc.

 Complement (C')

 Signaling molecule

BOX 27.3 Systemic Lupus Erythematosus—cont'd

systemic lupus erythematosus. Note that the DNA antibodies found in the blood sample do not bind nuclei in vivo. This is because the IgG antibodies form immune complexes with DNA that has been released from cells. This case history is continued in Chapter 29.

Systemic lupus erythematosus (SLE) is an autoimmune disease mediated by immune complexes, that is, type III hypersensitivity. The hypersensitivity reaction in SLE is mediated by antibodies against DNA and other nuclear components, such as ribonucleoproteins (Fig. 27.15).

There is a detailed description of how SLE causes disease in Chapter 29. In this chapter, we are concerned with how high levels of antibodies against DNA and ribonucleoproteins are generated. Although SLE is an antibody-mediated disease, the key step in its pathogenesis is the loss of T-cell tolerance to DNA.

Genes play an important role in the pathogenesis of SLE; the concordance rate for SLE in identical twins is approximately 60%. SLE is more frequent in individuals who inherit the HLA allele DR2. In addition, polymorphisms in the genes for debris-clearing proteins are also important. Some proteins of the innate immune system are involved in clearing up cellular debris. For example, MBL and complement component C1q can recognize and bind fragments of DNA. These fragments are then cleared, perhaps through phagocytosis. Patients with low levels of C1q, or MBL, are at higher risk for SLE, presumably because DNA produced as a result of cell death is able to trigger production of anti-DNA antibodies.

Toll-like receptor 9, expressed on B cells and dendritic cells, has a physiologic role in recognizing bacteria by binding unmethylated CpG motifs. Normally, recognition of bacterial CpG DNA motifs leads to increased immunoglobulin secretion by B cells or interferon secretion by dendritic cells. In patients with SLE, immune complexes containing DNA are capable of stimulating Toll-like receptor 9. This leads to increased secretion of type I interferons and may provide additional stimulation for B cells to perpetuate the secretion of anti-DNA antibodies (Fig. 27.15).

Infections may promote the process by increasing the apoptosis of cells and triggering additional secretion of type I interferons.

Two additional factors affect the development of SLE. In general, autoimmune diseases are more common in women, although SLE is an extreme example, affecting women 20 times more frequently than men. The higher incidence of autoimmunity in women is probably related to higher levels of the sex hormone estrogen. SLE can sometimes develop shortly after starting estrogen-containing contraceptive pills, and it often gets worse during pregnancy, when estrogen levels are high. Estrogen has the physiologic effect of increasing antibody production, and it may thus increase autoantibody secretion. Some autoimmune diseases (e.g., IDDM) affect men and women equally. These autoimmune diseases tend to be caused by T cells rather than antibody.

Exposure to ultraviolet light (UV) has a role in triggering SLE, and sun-exposed skin is often affected by a characteristic rash. It is not yet clear how UV has these effects. One possible mechanism is that UV induces apoptosis in cells in the skin. An alternative is that UV induced skin damage triggers the release of proinflammatory cytokines, such as TNF or type I interferons, which either costimulate B cells or add to local tissue damage.

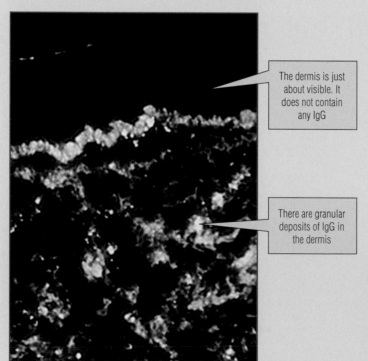

The dermis is just about visible. It does not contain any IgG

There are granular deposits of IgG in the dermis

Figure 27.13 A section from a fresh skin biopsy is incubated with antihuman IgG tagged with a fluorescent label. When viewed under an ultraviolet light microscope, IgG in the tissue produces green fluorescence. Just how these deposits are formed is discussed in Chapter 29. (Courtesy of Dr. R. Cerio, Royal London Hospital, UK.)

Continued

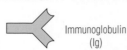 T cell receptor (TCR)

Immunoglobulin (Ig)

Antigen

MHC I

BOX 27.3 Systemic Lupus Erythematosus—cont'd

Figure 27.16 illustrates the series of events that may be required to trigger SLE. Low levels of antinuclear antibody are present in many healthy individuals. It is known that several years before the development of SLE symptoms, antinuclear antibody levels can increase. In addition, the production of antibodies specifically against double-stranded DNA commences. The factors that switch patients from symptom-free to symptomatic SLE are not well documented but probably include infections, UV exposure, and estrogens.

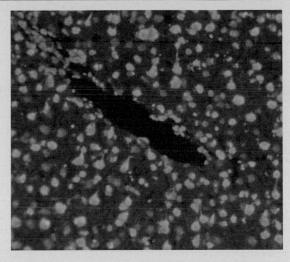

Figure 27.14 The slide shows antinuclear antibody by indirect immunofluorescence. A piece of animal tissue is mounted on a slide, and the patient's IgG is bound to nuclei in the tissue.

(a)

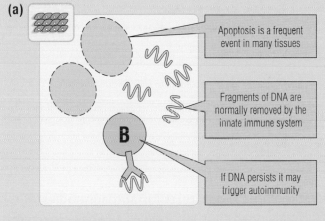

Apoptosis is a frequent event in many tissues

Fragments of DNA are normally removed by the innate immune system

If DNA persists it may trigger autoimmunity

(b)

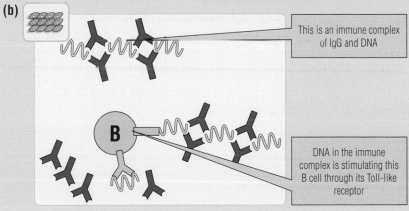

This is an immune complex of IgG and DNA

DNA in the immune complex is stimulating this B cell through its Toll-like receptor

Figure 27.15 Impaired clearance of DNA may initially prime production of anti DNA antibodies (**A**). Immune complexes containing DNA may then stimulate Toll-like receptors and perpetuate antibody secretion (**B**).

Continued

 MHC II

 Cytokine, Chemokine, etc.

Complement (C')

Signaling molecule

BOX 27.3 Systemic Lupus Erythematosus—cont'd

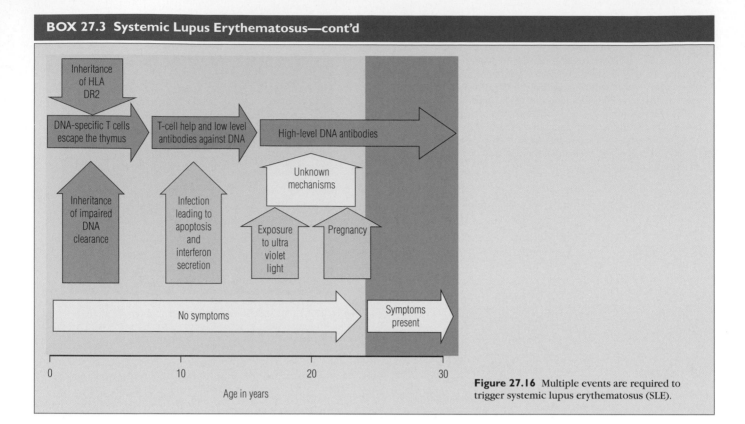

Figure 27.16 Multiple events are required to trigger systemic lupus erythematosus (SLE).

LEARNING POINTS Can You Now ...

1. List what evidence there is for autoimmunity in normal, healthy individuals?
2. Describe the origin and function of natural antibodies?
3. Describe how the immune system tolerates most autoantigens and how tolerance can break down?
4. Describe how immunofluorescence tests and ELISAs are used to detect autoantibodies?
5. Contrast direct and indirect immunofluorescence?
6. List three blood tests for autoantibodies?
7. Explain why autoantibodies can have low specificity in the diagnosis of autoimmune disease?
8. Using the examples of insulin-dependent diabetes, celiac disease, and systemic lupus erythematosus, describe how genes and environmental factors work together to cause autoimmune disease?

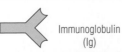 T cell receptor (TCR)

 Immunoglobulin (Ig)

Antigen

 MHC I

28 Antibody-Mediated Hypersensitivity (Type II)

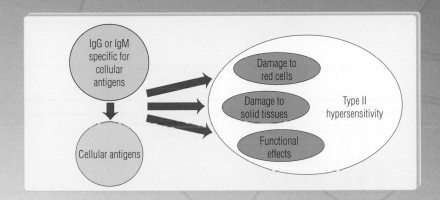

Type II hypersensitivity reactions are a consequence of immunoglobulin G (IgG) or IgM binding to the surface of cells. Antibody binding frequently damages red blood cells, either through activation of complement or because the antibodies opsonize the target erythrocytes. This is referred to as immune-mediated hemolysis. Antibody binding may also damage solid tissues, where the antigen may be cellular or part of the extracellular matrix (e.g., basement membrane). Less often, antibodies may modify the function of cells by binding on to receptors for hormones, which we illustrate with autoimmune thyroid disease and Wegener's granulomatosis. Hyperacute graft rejection is also a version of type II hypersensitivity, and this is discussed in Chapter 33.

■ IMMUNE-MEDIATED HEMOLYSIS

Red Cell Antigens

Red cells express a variety of antigens, some of which are alleles inherited in a mendelian fashion (Fig. 28.1).

The rhesus blood group system consists of three loci—C, D, and E—of which D is the most important. Most individuals express a D locus antigen, and therefore they are **rhesus positive**. About one in six people are homozygous for a null D allele; they express no D antigen and therefore they are **rhesus negative**. D is a conventional protein antigen, and rhesus negative individuals make IgG anti-D after exposure to the antigen.

The A and B blood group antigens are oligosaccharide molecules produced on the surface of red cells. These

sugars are inherited in a codominant fashion: an individual can inherit the A antigen (blood group A), the B antigen (blood group B), both A and B (blood group AB), or a null allele (blood group O). The A and B antigens are similar to oligosaccharide expressed on bacteria. Anti-A and anti-B are IgM natural antibodies (see Chapter 27), physiologically produced as a defense against bacteria and capable of cross-reacting with A or B red cell antigens. Hence, individuals who are blood group O, and have inherited neither A nor B antigen, will produce IgM against A and B, whether or not they have been exposed to these antigens.

Other antigens are nonallelic—the same molecule is expressed by everyone. For example, the I antigen is expressed by adults on the surface of red cells. I behaves as a regular self-antigen and should not normally elicit anti-I antibodies.

Antigens of the ABO and rhesus systems are alloantigens—they differ from person to person. The antibodies produced against these antigens can cause type II hypersensitivity when cells are transferred from one individual to another, for example, in blood transfusion or during pregnancy.

Antigens of the rhesus and I systems can also act as autoantigens. They can cause type II hypersensitivity when they become targets of autoimmunity.

Anti–Red Cell Antibodies

IgM antibodies against red cell antigens are produced as natural antibodies against A and B or as auto-antibodies against I in some types of autoimmune hemolytic anemia (AIHA; see later). IgM antibodies are very effective at

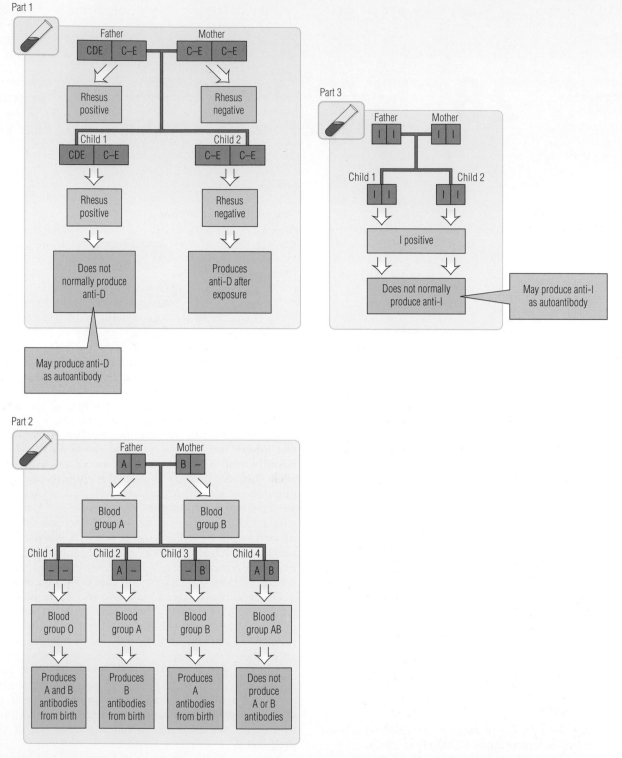

Figure 28.1 Genes (*orange*), antigens (*yellow*), and alloantibodies (*blue*) involved in the blood group systems. Alloantibodies are produced spontaneously against A and B and after exposure to D. As shown, D and I may sometimes become targets for autoantigens.

 T cell receptor (TCR)

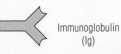 Immunoglobulin (Ig)

 Antigen

 MHC I

activating complement, causing damage through activation of the membrane attack complex (Fig. 28.2).

IgG antibodies are produced against rhesus antigens, either as a response to allogeneic stimulation (Box 28.1) or in some types of AIHA (see later). IgG is not very effective in activating complement and does not cause hemolysis in the circulation. Instead, IgG-coated red cells are recognized by Fc receptors on resident macrophages in the liver and spleen. These macrophages are stimulated by bound cells to phagocytose fragments of the red cells, which are damaged in the process.

Types of Immune-Mediated Hemolysis

Alloimmune Hemolysis

The rhesus antigens behave like a conventional antigen—exposure is required to produce IgG antibody. This most frequently occurs in pregnancy when IgG antibodies against rhesus antigens cross the placenta and cause hemolytic disease of the newborn. As described in the clinical box at the end of this chapter, these IgG antibodies cause fairly gradual destruction of red cells. This is because the IgG-coated red cells are only slowly recognized by macrophages in the spleen, which have Fc receptors for IgG.

Incompatibility in the ABO system is the most common cause of serious blood transfusion reactions. For example, an A-positive individual requiring a transfusion possesses natural antibodies against B-positive cells. If B-positive cells are inadvertently transfused, they will be rapidly hemolyzed in the circulation. The hypersensitivity reaction can take place within seconds of the donor cells entering the recipient. IgM reactions are very fast because

pentameric IgM is able to very efficiently activate complement. This is because each IgM molecule is able to aggregate antigen more effectively and because of the greater numbers of Fc components (which activate the early classic complement cascade).

Units of blood for transfusion contain mainly red cells and very little antibody-containing plasma. The recipient's antibodies and the donor's red cell antigens must be checked for compatibility prior to transfusion. In emergencies, when the laboratory does not have time to determine the recipient's blood group, O cells, which have neither A nor B antigens, can be used for transfusion into any type of recipient.

Autoimmune Hemolysis

AIHA can be triggered by infections or drugs (see the clinical box in Chapter 25) or it can be part of generalized autoimmune diseases such as systemic lupus erythematosus (see Chapter 29). Autoantibodies can also be produced by malignant clones of B cells in diseases such as chronic lymphatic leukemia or lymphoma. However, most cases of AIHA are not explained. Red cell antigens can become targets for IgG and IgM autoantibodies.

The most common type of AIHA is caused by IgG autoantibodies against rhesus antigens. The antibody-coated red cells are only slowly removed by the spleen, and the onset of anemia is gradual.

The I antigen is generally the target when IgM antibodies cause AIHA. Much more rapid and dangerous intravascular hemolysis occurs as a result of complement activation. Another feature of IgM antibodies is that they often bind red cells best at temperatures below 37°C. These cold hemagglutinins can cause red cells to aggregate

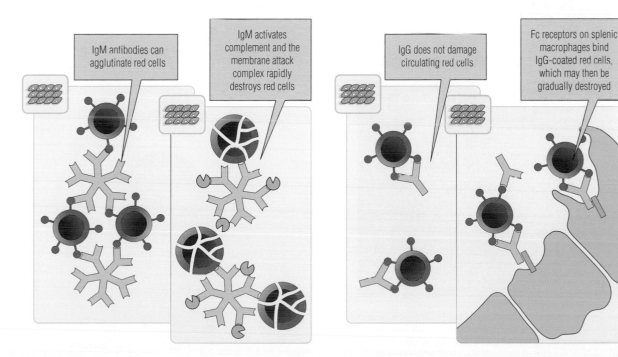

Figure 28.2 Mechanisms of immune hemolysis. IgM antibodies are more dangerous than IgG antibodies in immune hemolysis. Ig, immunoglobulin.

 MHC II   Cytokine, Chemokine, etc.   Complement (C')   Signaling molecule

in vessels in the hands and feet, which may cause ischemic damage.

Similar alloimmune and autoimmune processes can affect platelets and neutrophils.

Type II Autoimmune Hypersensitivity Against Solid Tissue

Autoantibodies can also attack and damage components of solid tissues. For example, in Goodpasture's syndrome, IgG autoantibodies bind a glycoprotein in the basement membrane of the lung and glomeruli. Antibasement membrane antibody activates complement, which can trigger an inflammatory response. Goodpasture's syndrome can be diagnosed by finding antibodies to glomerular basement membrane in patient's serum on indirect immunofluorescence (Fig. 28.3). In a variety of other comparable conditions, IgG antibodies bind to other cells or tissue components. For example, in the blistering skin condition, pemphigus, antibodies bind on the intercellular cement protein desmoglein. In another example, myasthenia gravis, IgG binds on to the acetylcholine receptor in skeletal muscle, causing widespread weakness. A characteristic that this group of diseases shares—along with autoimmune hemolytic anemia—is that the diagnosis can be made by detecting the autoantibody in blood samples. Treatment is aimed at removing or blocking the autoantibody.

■ TYPE II HYPERSENSITIVITY AND ANTIBODIES THAT AFFECT CELL FUNCTION

In other situations, antibodies bind to cells and affect their function. These antibodies can simply stimulate the target

organ function without causing much target organ damage, which we illustrate with Graves' disease. In other situations, stimulation of cells by autoantibody leads to tissue damage, for example, in Wegener's granulomatosis.

Graves' Disease

Graves' disease is the most common cause of hyperthyroidism, often affecting young women (Box 28.2) with a family history. Graves' disease is linked to the human leukocyte antigen (HLA) allele *DR3*. In Graves' disease, the thyroid is stimulated by an autoantibody that binds onto the thyroid-stimulating hormone (TSH) receptor (Fig. 28.4). The anti-TSH receptor antibody mimics the effects of the hormone. Graves' disease is, thus, a special type of type II hypersensitivity. In pregnant women with Graves' disease, IgG thyroid-stimulating antibody can cross the placenta and cause transient neonatal hyperthyroidism. Graves' disease is associated with exophthalmos (protruding eyes) resulting from T cells infiltrating the orbit of the eye. Exophthalmos is thought to be caused by an orbital antigen that cross-reacts with a thyroid antigen.

Wegener's Granulomatosis

A much rarer disease is Wegener's granulomatosis, a type of blood vessel inflammation (vasculitis) affecting the nose, lungs, and glomeruli. Patients with Wegener's granulomatosis have autoantibodies that react with proteinase 3, a proteolytic enzyme present in neutrophils (Box 28.3). These autoantibodies are referred to as classic antineutrophil cytoplasmic antibodies (cANCA). Proteinase 3 is normally present in the cytoplasm, but when neutro-

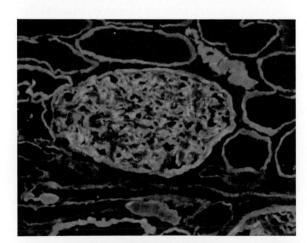

Figure 28.3 Indirect immunofluorescence has been used to detect autoantibodies in this patient with Goodpasture's syndrome. Kidney tissue is used as the target antigen for this test. There is linear staining along the glomerular basement membrane, which appears to be "lit up" in comparison with the renal tubules in the background.

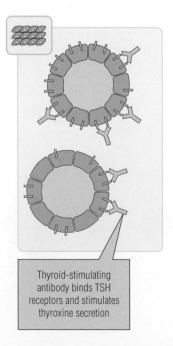

Thyroid-stimulating antibody binds TSH receptors and stimulates thyroxine secretion

Figure 28.4 Graves' disease. The autoantibodies against the thyroid-stimulating hormone (TSH) receptor mimic the effects of the hormone.

 T cell receptor (TCR)　　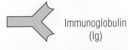 Immunoglobulin (Ig)　　 Antigen　　 MHC I phils are activated—for example, by cytokines released during infections—it is expressed on the cell surface. Proteinase 3 then becomes accessible to cANCA antibodies, which bind neutrophils, inhibit migration, and stimulate the oxidative burst, and cytokine and enzyme release (Fig. 28.5). Neutrophils damage vessels in Wegener's granulomatosis by being immobilized in vessel walls and then triggering inflammation. Why the nose, lungs, and glomeruli are particularly affected is not clear.

Prevention and Treatment of Type II Hypersensitivity

Allogeneic hemolytic reactions are preventable. Transfusion reactions can be prevented by carefully checking that the donor and recipient are compatible and that the recipient has no antibodies that could react with donor red cells (cross-matching). Hemolytic disease of the newborn is preventable by ensuring that rhesus-negative women receive anti-D antibodies after miscarriage or labor.

When type II hypersensitivity is mediated by IgM, such as during an ABO-incompatible blood transfusion, it is very hard to block the effector mechanism. This is because complement activation takes place very rapidly, and there are no safe, effective complement-blocking drugs.

Treatment of IgG-mediated type II hypersensitivity aims to reduce autoantibody levels or prevent effector cells from causing damage.

Immunosuppressive drugs can reduce B-cell autoantibody secretion, although the benefits only take place gradually, over several weeks. This is because immunoglobulin has a half-life of several weeks, and therefore autoantibody that has already been secreted takes several weeks to disappear. In more urgent situations, plasmapheresis reduces autoantibody levels, but is uncomfortable and time consuming for patients and is reserved for situations in which antibody needs to be rapidly removed, such as Wegener's granulomatosis and Goodpasture's syndrome.

A characteristic of some of the autoimmune disease associated with IgG autoantibodies (autoimmune hemolytic anemia, myasthenia gravis, Graves' disease) is that they also cause disease in the fetus when autoantibodies cross the placenta.

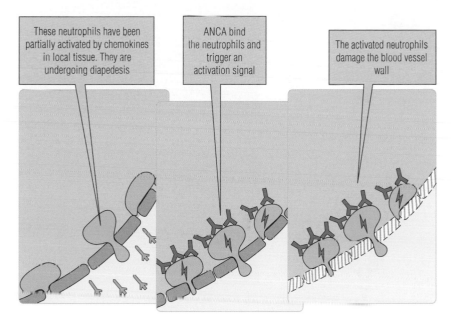

These neutrophils have been partially activated by chemokines in local tissue. They are undergoing diapedesis

ANCA bind the neutrophils and trigger an activation signal

The activated neutrophils damage the blood vessel wall

Figure 28.5 This figure shows how Wegener's granulomatosis may develop. In this example, the neutrophils have been partially activated during the response to an infection and then are stimulated further by ANCA antibodies. ANCA, anti-neutrophil cytoplasmic antibodies.

 MHC II

 Cytokine, Chemokine, etc.

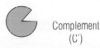 Complement (C')

 Signaling molecule

BOX 28.1 Hemolytic Disease of the Newborn

A woman presents to the antenatal clinic in week 28 of her pregnancy. She is a refugee from a developing country. In the past, she has had one healthy child, born without complications. Over the next few weeks, the pregnancy runs smoothly, but the woman is found to be rhesus blood group negative. Further tests show that she has antibodies to the rhesus D antigen. At 34 weeks of pregnancy, an ultrasound scan shows signs of fetal distress. Labor is induced, and a baby girl is born. She is profoundly anemic. A Coombs' test on the baby's blood is positive, confirming the diagnosis of hemolytic disease of the newborn (Fig. 28.6).

If a rhesus-negative woman carries a rhesus-positive fetus, she will produce antibodies if fetal cells leak into the maternal circulation. This can occur during pregnancy and, especially, during labor (Fig. 28.7). Rhesus antigens act as conventional antigens, and, therefore, IgG antibody levels increase with each successive pregnancy with a rhesus-positive child. The IgG antibodies produced crossed the placenta and bound fetal red cells, which were then destroyed in the fetal spleen and liver.

The treatment for hemolytic disease of the newborn is exchange transfusion, a technique that replaces fetal red cells with donor rhesus-negative cells.

Hemolytic disease of the newborn is entirely preventable through the use of anti-D antibody injections (Fig. 28.8). Anti-A or anti-B antibodies only very rarely cause hemolytic disease of the newborn, because IgM natural antibodies are not actively transported across the placenta.

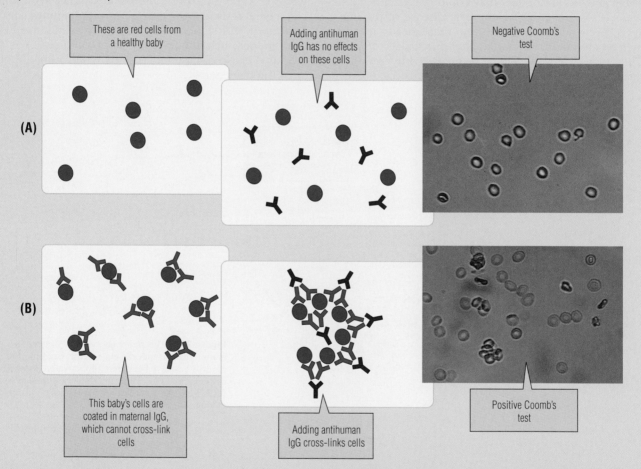

Figure 28.6 The Coombs test detects cells coated with antibody. In a healthy child (**A**), addition of antihuman IgG has no effects, whereas in a child with hemolytic disease of the newborn (**B**), antihuman IgG cross-links red cells, leading to agglutination. Ig, immunoglobulin.

Continued

 T cell receptor (TCR)

 Immunoglobulin (Ig)

 Antigen

 MHC I

BOX 28.1   Hemolytic Disease of the Newborn—cont'd

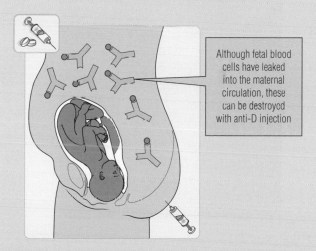

During labor fetal red cells leak into the mother

The maternal anti-D antibodies cross the placenta and attack fetal red cells

Labor

First pregnancy

Post partum

Second pregnancy

This rhesus-negative woman has conceived a rhesus-positive fetus

The fetal red cells survive long enough to elicit an IgG response

Figure 28.7 Hemolytic disease of the newborn.

Although fetal blood cells have leaked into the maternal circulation, these can be destroyed with anti-D injection

Figure 28.8 Anti-D antibody should be given to rhesus-negative women pregnant with a rhesus-positive child. Anti-D destroys rhesus-positive fetal cells in the maternal bloodstream before she has an opportunity to make her own anti-D, which can affect the next pregnancy. Anti-D is a type of passive immunotherapy, and it can prevent hemolytic disease of the newborn when used appropriately.

 MHC II

 Cytokine, Chemokine, etc.

 Complement (C')

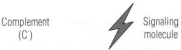 Signaling molecule

BOX 28.2 Graves' Disease

A 62-year-old woman complains of increasing anxiety and restlessness. Her doctor notices that she has an enlarged thyroid gland and fast pulse: both signs of hyperthyroidism. In addition, she has exophthalmos (Fig. 28.9). Blood tests show that her thyroid gland is overactive, and she has autoantibodies to thyroid peroxidase and the thyroid-stimulating hormone receptor. These are diagnostic of Graves' disease. She is treated with antithyroid drugs, and her symptoms improve.

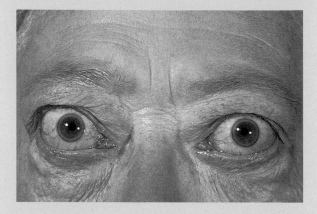

Figure 28.9 This patient with Graves' disease has exophthalmos (protruding eyes) because of swelling of the orbital soft tissue. (With permission from the Department of Medical Illustration, St. Bartholomew's Hospital, London.)

BOX 28.3 Wegener's Granulomatosis

A 40-year-old lady presents with extreme fatigue and dark-colored urine. These symptoms have developed over the last few weeks but have become much worse over the past 3 days. She also has a history of nasal stuffiness and nosebleeds over several weeks. Ulcerated lesions are present in the nose. Her urine is shown to contain erythrocytes. The family doctor is suspicious that she may be developing renal failure and orders urgent renal biochemistry on a blood sample from the patient. This shows a markedly elevated creatinine and urea, consistent with renal failure. The patient's potassium level is dangerously high (accounting for her weakness), and the family doctor arranges the patient to be admitted to hospital for urgent treatment.

The hospital team corrects the high potassium level and arranges tests to identify the cause of the renal failure. A blood sample is sent to the laboratory and tested urgently for autoantibodies that are associated with diseases causing renal impairment. The laboratory work shows that antiglomerular basement and antinuclear antibodies are both negative (ruling out Goodpasture's syndrome and systemic lupus erythematosus, respectively). The patient does have a positive cANCA by indirect immunofluorescence, suggestive of Wegener's granulomatosis (Fig. 28.10). Her serum is tested for antibodies to proteinase 3 by enzyme-linked immunosorbent assay (ELISA). This test is also positive. These results are very suggestive of Wegener's granulomatosis, and the renal medicine team starts specific treatments. The first of these is plasmapheresis, aimed at reducing

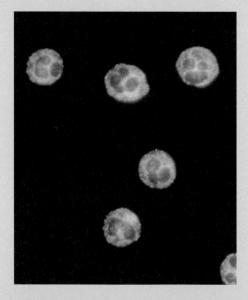

Figure 28.10 Antineutrophil cytoplasmic antibodies (cANCA). These images show indirect immunofluorescence using patient serum on normal neutrophils. The patient's IgG is reacting with neutrophil cytoplasm (which fluoresces) but not nuclei (which remain dark).

Continued

 T cell receptor (TCR)

 Immunoglobulin (Ig)

 Antigen

 MHC I

BOX 28.3 Wegener's Granulomatosis—cont'd

the level of circulating autoantibodies (Fig. 28.11). This treatment is not widely available, but is sometimes used to quickly remove disease-causing antibodies. She is also started on corticosteroids, which inhibit the activity of the neutrophils in the inflamed blood vessels. In addition, she is started on cyclophosphamide, an immunosuppressive drug with particular activity against B cells. Cyclophosphamide gradually reduces autoantibody secretion.

Just before these treatments are started, a confirmatory renal biopsy is taken. Unlike the autoantibody blood tests, the results of these are not available for 3 days. The renal biopsy shows glomerulonephritis, confirming the diagnosis of Wegener's granulomatosis.

Over the next 4 weeks, the patient's kidney function improved. Her nasal symptoms also improved considerably. At the same time, the autoantibodies disappeared from her blood. Because Wegener's granulomatosis can relapse, the patient is monitored from the point of view of her kidney function and by checking her serum for ANCA.

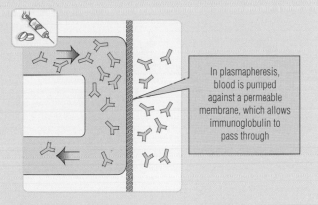

In plasmapheresis, blood is pumped against a permeable membrane, which allows immunoglobulin to pass through

Figure 28.11 Treatment of type II hypersensitivity by plasmapheresis.

LEARNING POINTS Can You Now ...

1. List the antigens involved in autoimmune and alloimmune hemolysis?

2. Explain how IgG and IgM antibodies can cause hemolysis?

3. Describe how autoantibodies cause hyperthyroidism?

4. Explain how autoantibodies cause the symptoms of Wegener's granulomatosis?

5. List which tests are used to diagnose these autoimmune diseases?

6. List preventive actions and treatments for type II hypersensitivity diseases?

 MHC II   Cytokine, Chemokine, etc.   Complement (C')   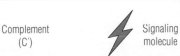 Signaling molecule

29 Immune Complex Disease (Type III Hypersensitivity)

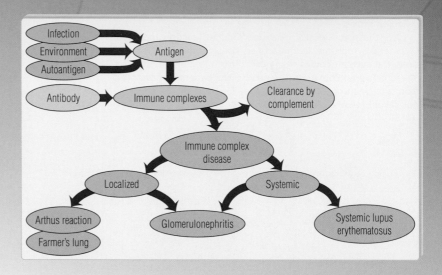

In this chapter you will learn how immune complexes can form in certain circumstances, when antibodies combine with antigen. The antigens can be derived from infection, innocuous environmental substances, or autoantigen. Immune complexes are usually cleared by the complement system, but when this does not happen, immune complex diseases may arise. Farmer's lung and the Arthus reaction are given as examples of local immune complex disease. Poststreptococcal glomerulonephritis is an example of circulating immune complex disease and is described in Chapter 25. In this chapter, you will learn more about another systemic immune complex disease—systemic lupus erythematosus (SLE).

Immune complexes are lattices of antigen and antibody; they may be localized to the site of antigen production or circulate in the blood. They are produced as part of the normal immune response and are usually cleared by mechanisms involving complement, as described later. Immune complexes cause disease in a number of situations.

■ ANTIGENS IN IMMUNE COMPLEXES

Antigens that can form immune complexes must be **polyvalent**; each antigen molecule must be able to bind more than one antibody molecule. For immune complexes to develop, antigen must be present for long enough to elicit

an antibody response. Immune complexes usually form when antigen is in slight excess of antibody (Fig. 29.1). Immune complexes may form when antigen is produced from one of three sources:

- Infectious antigens
- Innocuous environmental antigens
- Autoantigens

Infectious Antigens

Most infections are short-lived and controlled by the immune response. Even in such rapidly controlled infections, immune complexes may cause hypersensitivity—for example, after streptococcal infection (see Chapter 25). Infections such as hepatitis B are not always controlled and can cause sustained high levels of antigen in blood (**antigenemia**), resulting in more chronic disease.

Innocuous Environmental Antigens

Harmless environmental antigens can elicit an immunoglobulin G (IgG) response if they are small enough to enter the tissues. A good example is fungal spores, which cause the localized immune complex disease farmer's lung (Box 29.1). Drugs are also environmental antigens and sometimes cause localized immune complexes, for example, the **Arthus reaction** (Box 29.2).

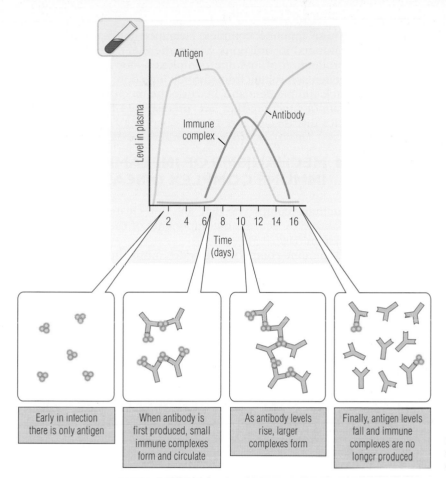

Figure 29.1 The largest immune complexes form at a time during infection when antibody levels slightly exceed antigen levels.

Drugs can also cause circulating immune complexes. This leads to a disorder referred to as **serum sickness**. The name was coined in the period before antibiotics were available, when patients with infections were given immune horse serum. Nowadays, serum sickness most often happens as a result of the occasional use of mouse monoclonal antibodies to treat cancer or autoimmune disease (see Chapter 35). Repeated exposure leads to production of antimouse antibodies and circulating immune complexes. Serum sickness then causes fever, rash, and joint pain. This problem can be overcome by genetically manipulating the mouse antibodies to humanize them.

Autoantigens

Autoantigens can only cause immune complex disease in the presence of autoantibodies. DNA is an antigen in SLE (Box 29.3). SLE is the most prevalent immune complex disease. DNA is released into the circulation when cells die, especially if innate immune system mechanisms usually responsible for clearing DNA are defective (see Chapter 27). DNA that is not rapidly cleared can elicit an antibody response.

■ ANTIBODIES IN IMMUNE COMPLEXES

Immune complexes will only form when the ratio between antigen and antibody is exactly right. At low levels of antibody, each antigen molecule binds several immunoglobulin molecules (see Fig. 29.1). When antibody and antigen levels are approximately equal, or antibody levels are slightly in excess, large complexes can form. When antibody exceeds antigen, small complexes form.

During an infection, this means that immune complexes will be produced very transiently, at the point where antibody levels are increasing. Immune complexes rarely become persistent during infections and do so only when the infection cannot be cleared by antibodies (e.g., hepatitis virus infections).

■ CLEARANCE OF IMMUNE COMPLEXES

Immune complexes can form in normal individuals when antibodies are produced during infections. The immune

 MHC II

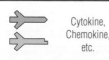 Cytokine, Chemokine, etc.

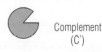 Complement (C')

 Signaling molecule

complexes must be cleared or they will cause disease through the mechanisms described later. Two mechanisms involving complement can clear immune complexes (see also Chapter 19).

Complement Breaks Down Large Soluble Complexes

Immune complexes of antigen and immunoglobulin contain high numbers of immunoglobulin Fc in close proximity, which activates complement through the classic pathway (Fig. 29.2). Small molecular components, especially activated C3, are produced through activation of the complement pathway. These molecules insert themselves into, and break up, the lattice of the immune complex.

Complement Receptor 1 Transfers Complexes to Phagocytes

Red cells transfer circulating immune complexes from tissues and blood to the phagocytes of the liver and spleen. Red cells express complement receptor 1 (CR1), the receptor for activated C3. Immune complexes bind to the complement receptor CR1 on red cells, which then circulate through the liver and spleen. In the liver and spleen, receptors take up the immune complexes and, in doing so, stimulate the macrophages to phagocytose them (see Fig. 29.2). This mechanism is very efficient and can entirely remove immune complexes from the circulation in a few minutes. Furthermore, because the spleen is home to a large population of B cells, antigens originally present in the periphery are rapidly presented to B cells to boost antibody production.

Failure of Clearance

These immune complex clearance mechanisms can be saturated in situations where there is excessive, ongoing production of immune complexes—for example, in antigenemia resulting from chronic infection. Some individuals lack complement and, because the mechanisms described cannot function, they are predisposed to immune complex disease (see Box 19.2 in Chapter 19).

■ MECHANISMS OF INFLAMMATION IN IMMUNE COMPLEX DISEASE

Immune complexes that are not cleared rapidly cause damage by activating components of the innate immune system (Fig. 29.3).

Immune complexes activate complement. Although this process helps to clear complexes, low-molecular-weight anaphylatoxins are produced, which increase permeability of blood vessels and are chemotactic for leukocytes.

Complexes bind onto, and activate, cells such as neutrophils, mast cells, and platelets. Neutrophils and mast cells release proteolytic enzymes, which damage blood vessels and initiate inflammation. Activated platelets bind to the endothelium and form thrombi.

If antigen is present predominantly at one site, immune complexes cause localized damage—for example, the Arthus reaction (see Box 29.2) and farmer's lung (see Box 29.1). Small complexes, produced when antigen is in excess, enter the circulation and form circulating immune complexes. Circulating complexes cause damage to blood vessels, ranging from inflammation of the vessel walls to occlusion of the vessel and ischemic damage. Immune

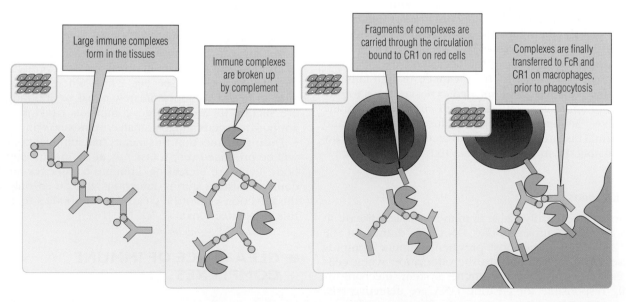

Figure 29.2 Clearance of immune complexes. Red cells are not damaged when immune complexes are transferred to macrophages. CR1, complement receptor 1; FcR, Fc receptor.

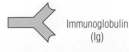 T cell receptor (TCR)

 Immunoglobulin (Ig)

Antigen

 MHC I

complex disease is one cause of vessel inflammation (**vasculitis**). Circulating immune complexes cause damage at specific sites, especially the kidney, skin, and joints.

■ IMMUNE COMPLEX DISEASE IN THE KIDNEY

Involvement of the kidney in type III hypersensitivity is a common cause of renal failure. The kidney is often affected because blood pressure in the glomerulus is four times higher than that in the systemic circulation. High blood pressure increases immune complex deposition in vessel walls. Glomerular cells express the complement receptor CR1, which may predispose to immune complex deposition at this site. Synovial cells also express CR1, which may explain why joints are also often involved in circulating immune complex disease.

Immune complex disease in the kidney can result in two clinically defined syndromes:

- **Nephrotic syndrome**, in which protein leaks into the urine and there is gradual-onset renal failure
- **Nephritis**, in which there is rapid-onset renal failure, blood and protein in the urine, and hypertension

Both types of disease are produced by inflammation in the glomeruli (**glomerulonephritis**). In the nephrotic syndrome, immune complexes are deposited in the glomerular basement membrane where they activate complement (Fig. 29.4). This usually causes subtle damage to the basement membrane, which allows proteins to leak into the urine. In nephritis, by comparison, there is a cellular infiltrate in addition to complement activation. Neutrophils are attracted into the glomeruli, and the resulting inflammation causes blood and protein to leak into the urine, impairing the ability of the kidney to excrete toxic metabolites. Which type of glomerular lesion is produced depends on several factors, including the size of immune complexes, the rate at which they are produced, and the duration of immune complex production.

In poststreptococcal glomerulonephritis (see Box 25.3), the renal disease is dramatic but short-lived because infection is brought under control by the immune response. When drugs cause immune complex–mediated kidney disease, stopping the drug improves kidney function. In SLE, the immune complexes contain autoantigens and, therefore, the renal disease has gradual onset but is not self-limiting (see Box 29.3).

Immune complexes are not the only immunologic cause of glomerulonephritis. Renal damage can also occur in Wegener's granulomatosis and Goodpasture's syndrome (see Chapter 28) and when immunoglobulin light chains damage the kidney in multiple myeloma (see Chapter 34).

Laboratory tests are crucial in the investigation of nephritis and the nephrotic syndrome. Indirect immunofluorescence is used to find antibodies implicated in immune complex disease (e.g., anti-DNA antibodies) or other types of autoantibody (e.g., antineutrophil cytoplasmic antibody (cANCA) and antiglomerular basement membrane antibody). Sometimes it is necessary to do direct immunofluorescence on a renal biopsy specimen to determine what type of process is causing damage.

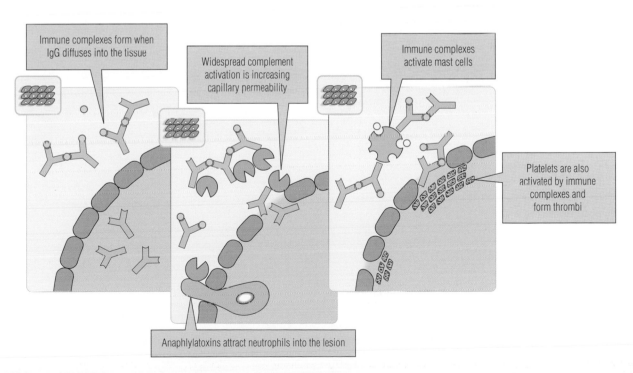

Figure 29.3 Immune complexes cause damage by activating the innate immune system.

 MHC II

Cytokine, Chemokine, etc.

 Complement (C')

 Signaling molecule

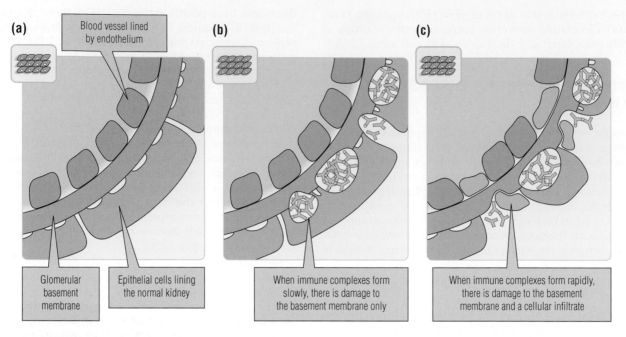

Figure 29.4 Nephrotic syndrome. **A**, A normal glomerulus. **B**, Slow complex formation, for example in hepatitis B virus infection. **C**, Rapid complex formation, for example, following streptococcal infection.

■ TREATMENT OF IMMUNE COMPLEX DISEASE

Antigen avoidance is possible in some cases of type III hypersensitivity—for example, farmer's lung or some drugs and vaccines. In the case of autoantigens, however (e.g., DNA), avoidance is clearly not possible.

In autoimmune causes of immune complex disease, corticosteroids block some of the damage caused by effector cells—for example, neutrophils. Cyclophosphamide is an alkylating agent that impairs DNA synthesis and prevents rapid proliferation of cells, such as lymphocytes. Although cyclophosphamide has some effects on T cells, its main benefit is in reducing B-cell proliferation and hence autoantibody levels. Cyclophosphamide is often used in severe SLE.

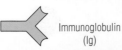 T cell receptor (TCR)

 Immunoglobulin (Ig)

 Antigen

MHC I

BOX 29.1 Farmer's Lung

A 23-year-old farmer complains of breathlessness, cough, malaise, and fever on several occasions after feeding his cattle. The symptoms develop several hours after exposure to hay and last about 2 days. A blood sample shows he has immunoglobulin G (IgG) antibodies against mold extract. In addition, his symptoms are reproduced 5 hours after deliberate challenge with mold spores in hospital, confirming a diagnosis of farmer's lung. He is instructed to breathe through a filter mask when handling hay, and his symptoms do not recur.

Patients with farmer's lung produce IgG antibodies against proteins in mold spores. Immune complexes form in the lungs after exposure to spores. Over several hours, these immune complexes trigger inflammation in the alveoli (Fig. 29.5). The process is very different from IgE-mediated hypersensitivity, which produces immediate symptoms on exposure to antigen and does not produce fever or symptoms outside the lungs.

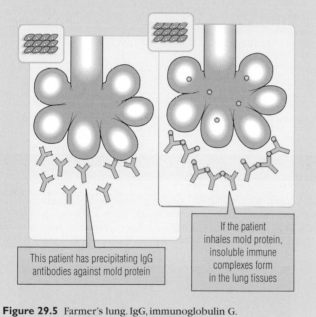

This patient has precipitating IgG antibodies against mold protein

If the patient inhales mold protein, insoluble immune complexes form in the lung tissues

Figure 29.5 Farmer's lung. IgG, immunoglobulin G.

BOX 29.2 The Arthus Reaction

A drunk medical student has lacerated his leg, and he is in the emergency department to have the wound sutured. His last tetanus vaccine was just over 5 years ago. In accordance with hospital policy, a booster tetanus vaccination is given, although, in the resulting struggle, this is inadvertently given intradermally. Twelve hours later, a painful lesion at the site of the vaccination wakes the patient from his sleep (Fig. 29.6). This is an Arthus reaction.

Vaccines are usually given intramuscularly so that the antigen can diffuse into the lymphoid system. Antigens injected intradermally cannot diffuse out rapidly. The purpose of tetanus booster vaccination is to maintain high antibody levels in individuals who repeatedly injure themselves. Our medical student, therefore, had a local depot of antigen and preexisting antibodies. Immune complexes formed in situ and activated complement, mast cells, and neutrophils, triggering a very localized type III hypersensitivity reaction (Fig. 29.7).

The Arthus reaction develops more slowly than the immediate type I hypersensitivity reaction, but faster than the delayed type IV hypersensitivity reaction. Thus, the delay in onset of a skin reaction to exogenous antigens gives important clues to the nature of the mediators. IgE-mediated reactions occur within 5 minutes, immune complexes cause symptoms after 12 hours or so, and T-cell lesions develop 2 to 3 days after exposure.

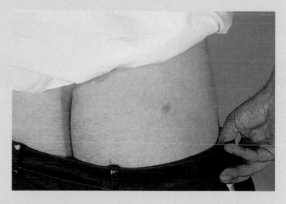

Figure 29.6 The Arthus reaction takes 12 hours to develop because immune complexes must form in situ and then activate mast cells and neutrophils. (With permission from the Department of Medical Illustration, St. Bartholomew's Hospital, London.)

Continued

 MHC II    Cytokine, Chemokine, etc.   Complement (C')   Signaling molecule

BOX 29.2   The Arthus Reaction—cont'd

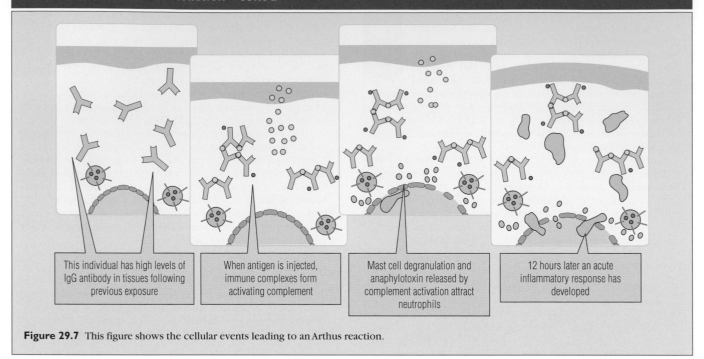

This individual has high levels of IgG antibody in tissues following previous exposure

When antigen is injected, immune complexes form activating complement

Mast cell degranulation and anaphylotoxin released by complement activation attract neutrophils

12 hours later an acute inflammatory response has developed

Figure 29.7 This figure shows the cellular events leading to an Arthus reaction.

BOX 29.3 Systemic Lupus Erythematosus

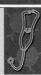

A woman in her early twenties with joint pains and a rash has been diagnosed with systemic lupus erythematosus (SLE; see Box 27.3). As you read in Chapter 17, indirect immunofluorescence shows her blood contains an antinuclear antibody (see Fig. 27.14) and ELISA (enzyme-linked immunosorbent assay) testing shows she has a high level of antibodies against DNA. Her joint pains initially respond well to nonsteroidal anti-inflammatory drugs, and her rash improves when she avoids strong sunlight.

One year later, at the rheumatology clinic, she mentions that her joint pain is now much worse. Routine urine testing shows a high level of protein, and her renal function is deteriorating. Because SLE can cause a range of different renal problems, a biopsy is carried out. Direct immunofluorescence shows deposits of complement and IgG in the glomeruli, consistent with immune complex disease (Fig. 29.8). The findings are similar to those from the skin biopsy carried out earlier (see Fig. 27.13). Conventional microscopy shows that she has a cellular inflammatory infiltrate in the glomerulus. The prognosis for this kind of renal disease in SLE is poor if no treatment is given. The patient was treated with several intravenous courses of the immunosuppressive drug cyclophosphamide, and her renal function and joint problems improved considerably.

The joint, skin, and kidney involvement is very typical of circulating immune complex disease. In addition to joint, skin, and kidney involvement, SLE can affect the central nervous system and placenta, the latter causing miscarriage.

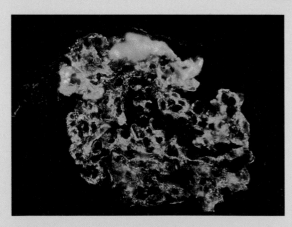

Figure 29.8 This is a direct immunofluorescence slide showing IgG deposited in the kidney of a patient with systemic lupus erythematosus. For direct immunofluorescence, tissue from the patient is required.

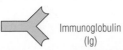 T cell receptor (TCR)

 Immunoglobulin (Ig)

Antigen

 MHC I

LEARNING POINTS — Can You Now ...

1. Describe the antigens and antibodies that most frequently cause immune complexes?
2. Explain how immune complexes are normally cleared?
3. Describe the pathogenesis of farmer's lung, as an example of local immune complex disease?
4. Describe the pathogenesis of SLE as an example of systemic autoimmune disease?

5. Compare direct and indirect immunofluorescence in the diagnosis of SLE?
6. Explain why the kidney is frequently involved in immune complex disease?
7. Describe two clinical outcomes of immune complex disease involving the kidney?

 MHC II

 Cytokine, Chemokine, etc.

 Complement (C')

 Signaling molecule

30 Delayed Hypersensitivity (Type IV)

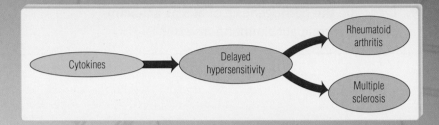

In this chapter, you will read how T cells mediate delayed hypersensitivity reactions. Multiple sclerosis and rheumatoid arthritis are two important autoimmune diseases mediated by delayed hypersensitivity reactions. You will learn about the types of anti-inflammatory drug used to treat these conditions and how modifying the actions of cytokines can affect delayed hypersensitivity. At the end of this chapter, you will read about how all four different types of hypersensitivity reaction can cause reactions to drugs.

Delayed hypersensitivity was originally defined as reactions taking place 2 to 3 days after exposure to antigen—for example, tuberculin skin testing (see Box 22.4). We now know that delayed hypersensitivity is characterized by T helper 1 (T_H1) cells driving inflammatory responses mediated by macrophages.

Delayed hypersensitivity can be a physiologic reaction to pathogens that are hard to clear—for example, *Hepatitis B virus* and *Mycobacterium tuberculosis*. Mycobacterial infections trigger the most extreme delayed hypersensitivity reactions, which are characterized by granuloma formation, extensive cell death, and the appearance of caseous necrosis (see Chapter 22).

Delayed hypersensitivity can also occur in response to innocuous environmental antigens, such as nickel, in some cases of contact dermatitis. These antigens must have a low molecular weight in order to enter the body. The very small size of these substances means that they must act as **haptens** to become antigenic. Contact dermatitis occurs as a result of exposure to a wide range of other chemicals, including cosmetics and, normally harmless, plant extracts (e.g., poison ivy).

Delayed hypersensitivity reactions also take place against autoantigens. For example, in insulin-dependent diabetes mellitus (see Chapter 27), T cells respond to pancreatic islet cell antigens, damaging the islets and eventually preventing insulin secretion.

■ DELAYED HYPERSENSITIVITY REACTIONS ARE DRIVEN BY T_H1 CELLS

In Chapter 20, we described how delayed hypersensitivity reactions are initiated when tissue macrophages recognize the presence of danger signals and initiate the inflammatory response. Dendritic cells, loaded with antigen, migrate to local lymph nodes where they present antigen to T cells. Specific T-cell clones proliferate in response to antigens, and these migrate to the site of inflammation. T cells and macrophages stimulate one another through the cytokine network (see Chapter 22). Tumor necrosis factor (TNF) is secreted by both macrophages and T cells and stimulates much of the damage in delayed hypersensitivity (Fig. 30.1).

Because of the need for antigen presentation by T cells, delayed hypersensitivity reactions are often associated with very specific human leukocyte antigen (HLA) alleles, as in insulin-dependent diabetes and celiac disease (see Chapter 27).

■ TYPE IV HYPERSENSITIVITY DISEASE

In this chapter, we discuss two other common autoimmune diseases caused by delayed hypersensitivity: rheumatoid arthritis (RA) and multiple sclerosis (MS). Celiac disease and insulin-dependent diabetes are discussed in Chapter 27.

Rheumatoid Arthritis

RA is a common disabling condition. In RA, the synovial membrane lining both joints and tendon sheaths is swollen up to 100 times its normal size. The synovium is infiltrated by chronic inflammatory cells, including T cells and macrophages (Box 30.1). The inflammatory process is driven by the T cells, although it is not yet proven what antigen these are responding to. There is some evidence that the synovial T cells are responding to **heat shock proteins** (HSP). HSPs were first discovered in bacteria, where they are produced in response to heat and other stress. Very similar HSPs are found in human cells, and it is possible that infection triggers a response against bacterial HSP, which then directs T cells against human HSP. This mechanism would represent a type of molecular mimicry (see Chapter 27).

Cytokines secreted by T cells and macrophages in the synovium cause the majority of symptoms in RA (Fig. 30.2). Although more than 100 cytokines have been found in synovium from patients with RA, the cytokine pattern shows skewing toward a T_H1 pattern. For example, despite the presence of so many cytokines, no interleukin-4 (IL-4) is detected. There is also plentiful secretion of pro-inflammatory cytokine secretion, with high levels of TNF, IL-1, and IL-6. TNF is a particularly pleomorphic cytokine and affects many different cells. For example, in RA, TNF activates the following cell types:

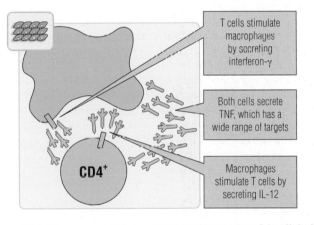

T cells stimulate macrophages by secreting interferon-γ

Both cells secrete TNF, which has a wide range of targets

CD4+

Macrophages stimulate T cells by secreting IL-12

Figure 30.1 Tumor necrosis factor (TNF) mediates many of the clinical features of delayed hypersensitivity reactions, for example, rheumatoid arthritis. IL, interleukin.

- Endothelium upregulates adhesion molecules, attracting neutrophils to the synovium.
- Neutrophils are activated to produce metalloproteinases, which digest synovial matrix proteins.
- Osteoclasts are activated to destroy bone at the joint margins, creating **erosions**.

Although RA is predominantly a delayed hypersensitivity reaction, T-cell cytokines stimulate B cells in the synovium to produce rheumatoid factor. Rheumatoid factor is frequently produced during chronic infections, presumably as a bystander effect of T-cell cytokines. Hence, rheumatoid factor is not specific for RA. In RA, rheumatoid factor may produce immune complexes within the joint, adding to the inflammation.

Multiple Sclerosis

MS is generally a severe disease; 50% of patients are disabled within 15 years of onset. Early in MS, there are recurrent bouts of inflammation, producing demyelinating plaques in different parts of the central nervous system (CNS). Later in MS, there is chronically progressive disease in which extensive axonal loss occurs.

MS affects about 1 in 1000 people in Northern Europe and central North America. In more tropical areas, the prevalence is much lower. Individuals who move from lower- to higher-risk areas have an increased risk for developing MS, suggesting that environmental factors are more important than genes for the geographic variation in prevalence. Two strands of evidence support infections as being an environmental trigger for MS:

- Demyelination that superficially resembles MS is very occasionally seen following documented infections, such as measles.
- In patients with MS, infections can precipitate relapses.

Genes are involved to a lesser extent in MS; the concordance rate among identical twins is only 30%. The disease, therefore, most likely results from the interplay between susceptibility genes and the microbial environment.

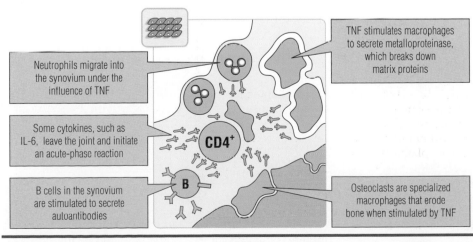

Neutrophils migrate into the synovium under the influence of TNF

Some cytokines, such as IL-6, leave the joint and initiate an acute-phase reaction

B cells in the synovium are stimulated to secrete autoantibodies

CD4+

B

TNF stimulates macrophages to secrete metalloproteinase, which breaks down matrix proteins

Osteoclasts are specialized macrophages that erode bone when stimulated by TNF

Figure 30.2 Most of the features of rheumatoid arthritis are attributable to the effects of cytokines. IL, interleukin; TNF, tumor necrosis factor.

 MHC II

 Cytokine, Chemokine, etc.

 Complement (C')

 Signaling molecule

Initially in MS, there are acute attacks in which inflammatory lesions consisting of T cells and macrophages develop in the affected nervous tissue. The inflammatory lesions cause the reversible, relapsing disability typical of early MS (Fig. 30.3). Although there is active inflammation in the vicinity, myelin loss impairs the ability of neurons to conduct impulses, resulting in neurologic symptoms. Once the inflammation settles, the disability improves. Between attacks, there is usually good recovery of function, at least early in the disease. The chronic disability that usually occurs later in MS is the result of another process—axonal loss. Although demyelinated nerve cells can remyelinate to some extent, axon loss from the nerve cell is irreversible.

Although T cells are thought to initiate much of the damage in MS, there are also B cells in the CNS that secrete antibodies against a wide variety of brain components, including myelin basic protein. These antibodies may participate in inflammation and also provide a marker of antibody production in the CNS, which can sometimes help to make a diagnosis of MS.

Treatment

In delayed hypersensitivity, it is sometimes possible to avoid the relevant environmental antigens. For example, some types of contact dermatitis are improved by avoiding exposure to nickel. In celiac disease, avoiding dietary gluten improves symptoms and reduces levels of antiendomysium antibodies. In these examples, an exogenous antigen is driving an autoimmune disease. Where the cause is an endogenous antigen, treatment is more complex. Options currently used are anti-inflammatory drugs (which mainly have effects on effectors of delayed hypersensitivity, especially macrophages) and immunosuppressive drugs (which have effects on T cells).

Anti-Inflammatory Drugs

Anti-inflammatory drugs work by cutting down the mediators released during inflammation, usually by cells of the innate system. For example, nonsteroidal anti-inflammatory drugs (such as aspirin, ibuprofen, and indomethacin) inhibit arachidonic acid metabolism (see Chapter 21).

Endogenous corticosteroids suppress the immune response during physiologic stress. Corticosteroids are often used as immunosuppressive drugs during the treatment of autoimmunity and allergy, and following transplantation. Their effects are mediated by affecting gene transcription when used at low-to-moderate doses. Corticosteroids bind specific receptors, which transport them to the nucleus and are responsible for binding to regulatory gene sequences. At higher doses, they affect cell signaling directly.

Although corticosteroids are thought to affect the transcription of 1% of all genes in a wide range of cells, their dominant therapeutic effects are on phagocytes. Effects on lymphocytes may be largely a result of poor antigen processing and costimulation provided by phagocytes.

The side effects of corticosteroids are well known. From the immunologic point of view, immunosuppression is a particular concern, and it may result in reactivation of infections normally controlled by macrophages—for example, tuberculosis.

Corticosteroids have some effects in MS, but only at high, intravenous doses. Corticosteroids probably work in MS by reducing the actions of macrophages (Box 30.2). Corticosteroids are of some value in RA but are too toxic for long-term use.

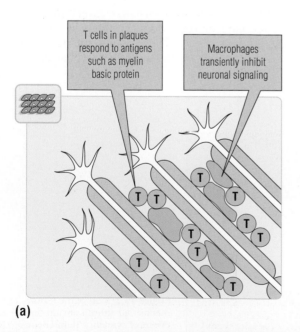

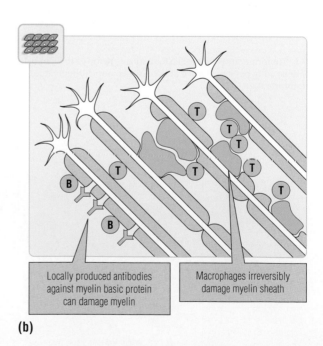

(a) (b)

Figure 30.3 Multiple sclerosis. The lesions in acute relapsing (**A**) and chronic progressive (**B**) multiple sclerosis are different.

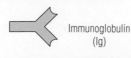 T cell receptor (TCR)

 Immunoglobulin (Ig)

Antigen

MHC I

Newer approaches introduced in the past 10 years exploit our increasing knowledge of cytokines in inflammation. TNF is a key cytokine in delayed hypersensitivity reactions—for example, RA. Three strategies have been developed to prevent TNF binding to receptors on cells involved in the inflammatory response (Fig. 30.4).

- Mouse monoclonal antibodies can prevent TNF binding to its receptor. However, patients produce antibodies against the mouse-specific epitopes on the immunoglobulin. These neutralizing antibodies prevent the anti-TNF from working, which can cause serum sickness-like reactions (see Chapter 29).
- Chimeric antibodies are engineered to combine mouse and human fragments; chimeric anti-TNF antibodies are very effective—up to 80% of patients with RA have clinical improvements. Fully humanized monoclonal antibodies are not produced in humans, but contain no molecules of mouse or other nonhuman origin.
- A different strategy has been to make recombinant TNF receptor/Fc molecules, to mop up TNF. These are constructed using human protein sequences to overcome problems with neutralizing antibodies. These molecules are also effective in RA.

Each of these approaches has been successful in RA, but none of the anti-TNF drugs completely switches off RA. This is because of the redundancy of cytokines, in other words, the fact that in most situations several cytokines are involved in immunologic processes. An anti–IL-1 drug (anakinra) has been developed and is also successful in some patients with RA. It may be that combinations of anticytokine drugs will ultimately be used in these situations.

TNF has a physiologic role in combating infections. One concern over drugs that block the effects of TNF is that they may predispose to infections. Some patients have developed tuberculosis following TNF-blocking drugs. These drugs are also very expensive and unfortunately are not available for many patients with RA. There is a fuller discussion on therapeutic monoclonal antibodies in Chapter 35.

Recombinant interferon (IFN)-β has benefits in some patients with MS and delays the development of acute attacks of nervous system inflammation. There is some evidence to suggest that IFN-β has long-term benefits and can prevent the chronic disability associated with demyelination.

You will remember from Chapter 19 that the type I interferons (IFN-α and IFN-β) have potent antiviral effects and weaker immunostimulatory effects (increasing antigen presentation and activating natural-killer cells). It is, therefore, surprising that IFN-β is effective in MS, where anti-inflammatory effects would be expected to be more beneficial. One possibility is that IFN-β reduces the migration of T cells across the blood–brain barrier. This illustrates the pleomorphism of cytokines—that is, that any one cytokine can have multiple effects on many different cell types.

No matter how it works, there are some important drawbacks with IFN-β treatment for MS. First, IFN-β activates the acute-phase response, and patients often complain of fever. Second, if patients produce anti-IFN-β antibodies, treatment stops being effective. IFN-β is produced using recombinant technology in nonhuman cells; because these cells do not add sugar molecules to the IFN-β molecule in the same way as human cells, recombinant IFN-β is antigenic. When technology is used to make the recombinant IFN-β molecule resemble the human molecule, the risk for developing neutralizing antibodies is reduced by 50%. Finally, like most recombinant proteins, IFN-β is very expensive.

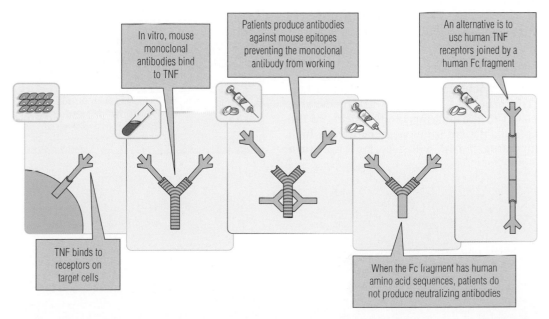

In vitro, mouse monoclonal antibodies bind to TNF

Patients produce antibodies against mouse epitopes preventing the monoclonal antibody from working

An alternative is to use human TNF receptors joined by a human Fc fragment

TNF binds to receptors on target cells

When the Fc fragment has human amino acid sequences, patients do not produce neutralizing antibodies

Figure 30.4 Monoclonal antibodies can block the effects of tumor necrosis factor (TNF) in rheumatoid arthritis; for example, the formation of new erosions is prevented.

 MHC II

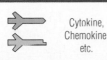 Cytokine, Chemokine, etc.

 Complement (C')

 Signaling molecule

Immunosuppressive Drugs

Immunosuppressive drugs inhibit the specific immune response that drives delayed hypersensitivity and are most relevant in autoimmune delayed hypersensitivity, when antigen cannot be avoided. Immunosuppressive drugs are dealt with in Chapter 33 as they are most often used in transplant recipients. The benefits of immunosuppressive drugs must be balanced against their dangerous side effects, particularly increasing the risk for infection. For example, in insulin-dependent diabetes, pancreatic islet cell function can be maintained while patients receive immunosuppressive drugs. However, the drugs would have to be given for life and the side effects are unacceptable; insulin replacement is a safer option. Immunosuppressive drugs have not been widely tested in MS.

Some Hypersensitivity Reactions are Driven by Mixed Mechanisms

The Gell and Coombs classification of hypersensitivity (see Chapter 25) is an oversimplification and many diseases overlap the different types. For example:

- The late phases of the type I reactions in asthma and atopic dermatitis are characterized by T-cell infiltrates, more typical of type IV reactions.
- Although MS and RA are both type IV reactions, autoantibodies (antimyelin basic protein and rheumatoid factor) play an important role.

Other diseases mix hypersensitivity to environmental antigens and autoantigens.

In celiac disease, there is a hypersensitivity reaction to an environmental antigen but also features of autoimmunity, such as antibodies to tissue transglutaminase.

Understanding the different types of hypersensitivity gives clues to the diagnosis and treatment of these important conditions. For example, diagnosis by finding autoantibodies and therapeutic use of plasmapheresis is appropriate in Wegener's granulomatosis but not in RA.

Immunologically Mediated Drug Reactions

Drug reactions are common, affecting up to 15% of hospital patients. The majority of reactions are predictable and directly related to the pharmacologic effects of the drug. For example, if a patient is given an incorrectly high dose of a sedative drug, he/she will sleep for longer than expected. Other side effects are less predictable, and these are described as being **idiosyncratic**. Some of these reactions may occur when a patient lacks an enzyme that is responsible for metabolizing a drug. For example, a patient who has low levels of the appropriate metabolizing enzyme will experience excessive sleepiness, even after the correct dose of sedative.

Idiosyncratic drug reactions also commonly have an immunologic basis. Some of these effects are mediated by the innate immune system; for example, morphine can stimulate mast cell degranulation, leading to histamine release and the development of the itchy rash urticaria. Reactions can also involve the adaptive system, and they can cause any type of hypersensitivity (Fig. 30.5). These reactions only occur after a patient has previously been exposed to a drug so that antibodies or reactive T cells can develop.

It is important to diagnose the cause of these reactions, because repeat exposure can lead to life-threatening reactions. Laboratory tests can provide indirect evidence of immunologic hypersensitivity. For example, elevated blood mast cell tryptase levels suggest mast cell involvement through innate mechanisms or type I hypersensitivity. Direct tests such as specific immunoglobulin E testing (see Chapter 26) are not often helpful, because the patient may be reacting to one of several metabolites rather than the drug itself.

FIG. 30.5   Immunologically Mediated Drug Reactions

Hypersensitivity Type	Reaction	Useful Test
I	Anaphylaxis	Specific IgE test (Ch. 27) Skin prick testing (with caution!)
II	Drug-induced hemolysis	Coomb's test (Ch. 28)
III: Localized	Arthus reaction to vaccines	Antibody levels (Ch. 29)
III: Circulating complexes	Serum sickness with monoclonal antibodies	
IV	Contact dermatitis to antibiotic-containing cream	Patch testing (Ch. 25)

 T cell receptor (TCR)   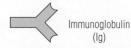 Immunoglobulin (Ig)   Antigen   MHC I

BOX 30.1 Rheumatoid Arthritis

A 50-year-old man complains of a 6-month history of pain in his hands, wrists, and feet. The pain is worse in the morning, when his joints are stiff for an hour or so. The metacarpophalangeal and proximal interphalangeal joints in both of his hands are swollen and tender (Fig. 30.6). He also has reduced movement in his wrists and elbows. Blood tests show he is having an acute-phase response with an elevated sedimentation rate and C-reactive protein. A radiograph of his hands shows erosions (Fig. 30.7), typical of rheumatoid arthritis. His blood also contains rheumatoid factor: IgM anti-IgG autoantibodies. These are not diagnostic of rheumatoid arthritis, but they do indicate a poor prognosis.

The patient is started on a nonsteroidal anti-inflammatory drug and feels somewhat better, with decreased pain and stiffness. However, a year later, examination shows more joint involvement, and there has been a progression of the changes on radiograph. Once he is started on an antitumor necrosis factor drug, his symptoms improve considerably, and there is no progression of his disease over the next year.

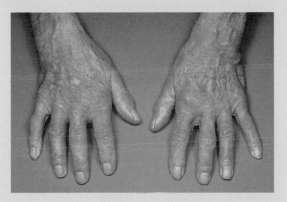

Figure 30.6 Swelling of the metacarpophalangeal and proximal interphalangeal joints is characteristic of rheumatoid arthritis. (With permission from the Department of Medical Illustration, St. Bartholomew's Hospital, London.)

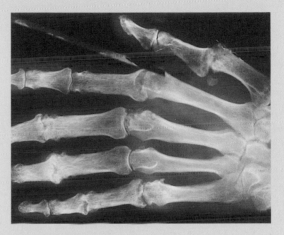

Figure 30.7 This radiograph shows erosions—areas of "bitten out" bone along the joint margins of the metacarpophalangeal joints—in rheumatoid arthritis. (With permission from the Department of Medical Illustration, St. Bartholomew's Hospital, London.)

 MHC II

 Cytokine, Chemokine, etc.

 Complement (C')

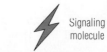 Signaling molecule

BOX 30.2 Multiple Sclerosis

A 22-year-old woman complains of visual impairment in her left eye. On two occasions, 4 years and 1 year earlier, she had noticed numbness and tingling in both legs for several weeks. She did not go to see a doctor about these symptoms. On both occasions, she became pregnant, and the symptoms improved. About 2 months ago, she had some unsteadiness on her feet. These symptoms also improved after 2 weeks or so, and again she did not seek medical advice.

On examination, she has signs of optic neuritis in her left eye. A magnetic resonance imaging (MRI) brain scan is performed, which shows many lesions in the white matter (Fig. 30.8). The diffuse, asymmetric lesions are consistent with the patchy inflammation that is seen in MS. She also has a lumbar puncture, and examination of cerebrospinal fluid (CSF) shows oligoclonal bands (Fig. 30.9), consistent with active inflammation in the CNS.

The history of different types of neurologic symptoms over time in this patient is typical of multiple sclerosis. Symptoms in multiple sclerosis often improve during pregnancy, possibly because estrogens inhibit the activity of T_H1 cells. Together, the clinical, MRI, and CSF findings are diagnostic of MS. Over the next few weeks, her vision improves on high-dose corticosteroid treatment.

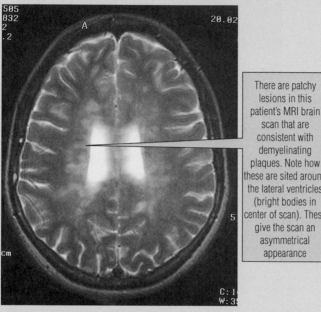

There are patchy lesions in this patient's MRI brain scan that are consistent with demyelinating plaques. Note how these are sited around the lateral ventricles (bright bodies in center of scan). These give the scan an asymmetrical appearance

Figure 30.8 This magnetic resonance brain scan shows plaques of demyelination. (Courtesy of Dr. J. Evanson, Royal London Hospital, UK.)

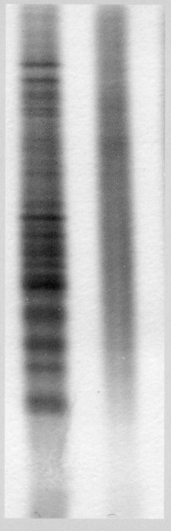

Figure 30.9 This figure shows high-resolution electrophoresis of the patient's CSF (*strip on left*) and serum (*strip on right*) stained for IgG antibody. The CSF shows 20 or so bands, each corresponding to IgG antibody produced by a small population of different B cells resident in the central nervous system. The same oligoclonal B-cell populations are not present outside the CNS, and there are thus no bands in the serum sample. (CSF electrophoresis courtesy of Prof. H. Willison, University of Glasgow.)

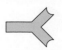 T cell receptor (TCR)

 Immunoglobulin (Ig)

 Antigen

⊥ MHC I

LEARNING POINTS Can You Now ...

1. Recall how delayed hypersensitivity reactions rely on the cytokine network?

2. Describe the pathogenesis, diagnosis, and treatment of the common disorders multiple sclerosis and rheumatoid arthritis?

3. Describe the benefits and problems of recombinant proteins, such as interferon-β and antitumor necrosis factor monoclonal antibodies, being used in delayed hypersensitivity?

4. Describe the benefits and limitations of corticosteroids in delayed hypersensitivity?

5. Describe the clinical implications of cytokine redundancy and pleomorphism in anti inflammatory treatments?

6. Describe how the Gell and Coombs classification of hypersensitivity is used to diagnose and treat a wide range of disorders?

 MHC II

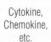 Cytokine, Chemokine, etc.

 Complement (C')

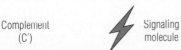 Signaling molecule

31 Primary Immunodeficiency

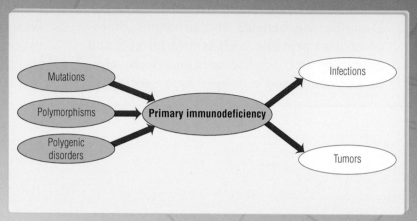

Genetic mutations, polymorphisms, and polygenic factors can cause primary immunodeficiency. You will have encountered several of these individual disorders in previous chapters and may need to review these sections at this stage. Primary immunodeficiency predisposes patients to infections and tumors. In this chapter, we explain how different types of infections can suggest the presence and severity of different types of immune deficiency. You will also read how primary immunodeficiency is diagnosed and treated.

■ SIGNIFICANCE OF IMMUNODEFICIENCY

Immunodeficiency results in an increased risk for opportunistic infections and tumors. Two types are recognized:

1. **Primary immunodeficiency** has a genetic basis and is relatively rare.
2. **Secondary immunodeficiency** is more common and is caused by lesions outside the immune system; in these cases, treating the external problem, for example, chronic lymphocytic leukemia, will improve the immune response.

■ INFECTIONS PROVIDE CLUES TO THE TYPE OF IMMUNODEFICIENCY

Healthy individuals experience infections, too. This is particularly true in early life when immunity to common pathogens has not developed. It is normal, therefore, for a 6-year-old child to have three or four upper respiratory tract infections over the winter period. However, it would be unusual for a child to have continuous, recurrent upper respiratory tract infections or to experience bouts of pneumonia.

Repeated or unusual infection is an important sign of immunodeficiency. The type of infection gives clues to the cause and degree of immunodeficiency (Fig. 31.1).

Repeated infection with encapsulated bacteria is a sign of defective antibody production, as antibody is a key player in the eradication of these extracellular organisms. Antibody (immunoglobulin G [IgG] and IgA) is the main defense against respiratory tract infection, and antibody deficiency causes recurrent respiratory infection caused by *Pneumococcus* or *Haemophilus* spp., which leads to irreversible damage to the bronchi: bronchiectasis. However, infections with staphylococci, gram-negative bacteria, and fungi are more characteristic of a reduced number or abnormal function of phagocytes. For unknown reasons, some complement defects predispose to meningitis caused by *Neisseria meningitidis* (see Chapter 19).

T cells and macrophages have a particular role in recognizing and eradicating intracellular infection. Defects in T cells or macrophages predispose to infection with intracellular organisms such as protozoa, viruses, and intracellular bacteria, including mycobacteria (Fig. 31.1). Reactivation of latent herpes virus infection is particularly linked to T-cell immunodeficiency. Recurrent attacks of cold sores (*Herpes simplex*) or shingles (*Herpes varicella zoster*) may suggest mild immunodeficiency. Herpesvirus-induced tumors, notably Kaposi's sarcoma (*Human*

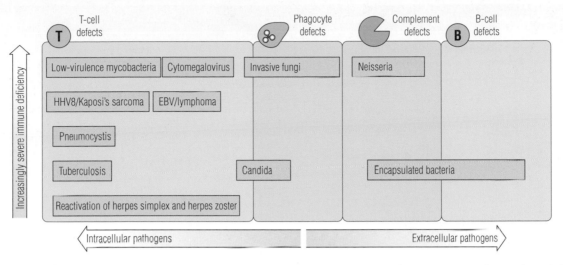

Figure 31.1 The type of opportunist infection also gives clues to the degree and cause of immunodeficiency. For example, mycobacteria indicate defects in T-cell immunity, whereas extracellular encapsulated bacteria indicate defects in antibody or complement. Note also that the severity of the immune deficiency is also reflected in the type of infection. Candida can cause infection in very mild immune deficiency (and even sometimes in healthy people), whereas invasive fungal infections nearly always indicate severe immune deficiency. EBV, Epstein-Barr virus; HHV, human herpesvirus.

herpes virus 8) and non-Hodgkin's lymphoma (*Epstein-Barr virus*), are characteristic of T-cell dysfunction. These are discussed further in Chapter 34.

The severity of T-cell immunodeficiency is also reflected in patterns of mycobacterial infection (see Fig. 31.1). *Mycobacterium tuberculosis* is a virulent organism causing lung infection in immunocompetent people. In mild T-cell immunodeficiency, the same organism spreads outside the lungs. More severe immunodeficiency predisposes to widespread infection with mycobacteria of low virulence normally found in the environment (e.g., *Mycobacterium avium intracellulare* complex).

■ CAUSES OF PRIMARY IMMUNODEFICIENCY

The causes of primary immunodeficiencies can be classified as:

- Mutations: rare, affect any part of the immune system and cause severe disease
- Polymorphisms: very common traits, affect any part of the immune system and cause a moderate increased risk for infection
- Polygenic disorders: relatively common, affect mainly antibodies and cause severe disease

You will have come across many of these conditions in earlier chapters. To aid your learning of these conditions, we have summarized them in a table (Fig. 31.2).

Mutations and Immunodeficiency

More than 100 mutations leading to immune deficiency are known. In this book, we have described a dozen or so important mutations in genes for the adaptive immune systems that cause immunodeficiency (Fig. 31.3). Many mutations result in **severe combined immunodeficiency** (SCID), which refers to a group of disorders affecting both T and B cells. SCID is the most severe type of primary immunodeficiency and can be caused by cytokine γ chain receptor defects, *Rag* mutations, and mutations in Zap-70. Some of these disorders are autosomally inherited (e.g., RAG deficiency; see Box 7.1), and there may be a family history of consanguinity (marriage of related individuals). Others are X-linked (e.g., γ-chain deficiency) (see Box 12.3) and the hyper-IgM syndrome (see Box 16.3), and there may be a history of early deaths in maternal uncles. The DiGeorge syndrome (see Box 15.1) is caused by a large part of chromosome 22 being translocated to other chromosomes and is not inherited.

Polymorphisms and Immunodeficiency

Genetic polymorphisms are alleles (different forms) of the same gene occurring at a single locus in at least 1% of the population. Eye color is a good example of genetic polymorphism. Human leukocyte antigen (HLA) alleles are polymorphic and affect the outcome of infections, including hepatitis B, hepatitis C, and HIV (see Box 3.1). Individuals with HLA alleles that are unable to bind viral peptides have a worse outcome. Polymorphisms of chemokines and their receptors associated with risk of HIV (see Chapter 32) are discussed elsewhere.

Mannan-binding lectin (MBL) is a collagen-like protein that binds sugars in bacterial cell walls and activates the classic complement pathway (see Chapter 19). Polymorphisms in MBL and complement affect the risk for infections (Fig. 31.4). The effects of polymorphisms on individuals are small and may only be discovered in studies on populations.

Polymorphisms persist in different frequencies in different populations, affected by prevalent infections. The best

 MHC II   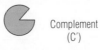 Cytokine, Chemokine, etc.   Complement (C′)   Signaling molecule

FIG. 31.2 Disorders Causing Primary Immunodeficiency

	Part of Immune System	Name of Disorder	Defect	Main Type of Infection	Chapter
Monogenic	Innate	Chronic granulomatous disease	Defective respiratory burst	Staphylococcus and fungi	20
		Complement deficiency	Defects in complement proteins	Bacteria, especially *Neisseria*	19
	Adaptive	Autosomal-recessive SCID	Recombinase (*Rag*) mutations	All pathogens	7
		Wiskott-Aldrich syndrome	Actin cytoskeleton		31
		X-linked SCID	Defective cytokine receptor common γ chain		12 / 15
		DiGeorge	Absent thymus	Intracellular pathogens	11
		Zap 70	Defects in T-cell signaling		10
		TAP defects	Impaired peptide expression on MHC		
		Hyper-IgM syndrome	Mutations in CD154	*Pneumococcus and Haemophilus*	16
		X-linked antibody deficiency	Mutations in *btk*		11
Polygenic	Adaptive	Common variable immunodeficiency	Not known		31
		IgG$_2$ deficiency			31
		Specific antibody deficiency			
		IgA deficiency		Most patients do not have infections	31
Polymorphisms	Innate	HLA	Affects antigen presentation	Viruses	31
		Mannan-binding lectin	Complement component	Many pathogens	31

known example lies outside the immune system. The hemoglobin S polymorphism (sickle cell anemia) protects against malaria and is more common in populations living in, or with origin in, malarious zones.

Polygenic Disorders

Polygenic disorders are caused by the interaction of several genes, with a contribution from environmental factors. **Common variable immunodeficiency** (CVID) and IgA, IgG2, and specific antibody deficiency are relatively common polygenic disorders affecting mainly antibody production. **IgA deficiency** affects about 1 in 600 people, although why infections are only seen in about one third of patients is unclear. Celiac disease (see Chapter 27) is more common in patients with IgA deficiency.

CVID (see Box 31.1) occurs in about 1 in 20,000 young people, affecting men and women equally. CVID is the most common primary immunodeficiency requiring treatment. Patients have low levels of total IgG, although other findings (e.g., levels of IgA and IgM, and numbers of B and T cells) are variable. CVID is a convenient label for what will probably emerge as a heterogeneous group of diseases. CVID causes recurrent bouts of infection of the respiratory tract, starting in early adult life. Infections involving the gut, skin, and nervous system also occur (Box 31.2). Autoimmunity is common in CVID and frequently includes pernicious anemia and thyroid disease, arthritis, and immune thrombocytopenia.

The genetic loci in IgA deficiency and CVID are not known, but they may include the HLA genes. Although 25% of patients have a family history of either CVID or IgA deficiency, environmental factors are also important. Antirheumatic and anticonvulsant drugs have been implicated in precipitating both IgA deficiency and CVID.

Two types of related but milder primary immunodeficiency exist in patients with a tendency to develop recurrent infections with *Pneumococcus* or *Haemophilus* spp. despite normal total IgG. These patients may have a **deficiency of IgG$_2$**, a subclass of IgG produced in response to polysaccharide antigens by B cells in the spleen (B-1 cells) without T-cell help. In other patients, levels of IgG$_2$ are normal, but there is a failure to respond to polysaccharide antigens, with poor titers of antibodies to pneumococcal antigens, even after vaccination. **Specific antibody deficiency** is often seen transiently during infancy and permanently following splenectomy (Box 13.1), but does exist as a disease entity in its own right.

■ DIAGNOSIS

Because children with SCID have defective T cells and B cells, they develop infections in the first few weeks of life. Children with SCID often have unusual or recurrent infection, failure to thrive, diarrhea, unusual rashes, a family history of neonatal death or of consanguinity, and a very low total lymphocyte count (below 1×10^9/L [10^6/ml]). In

 T cell receptor (TCR)

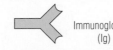 Immunoglobulin (Ig)

 Antigen

 MHC I

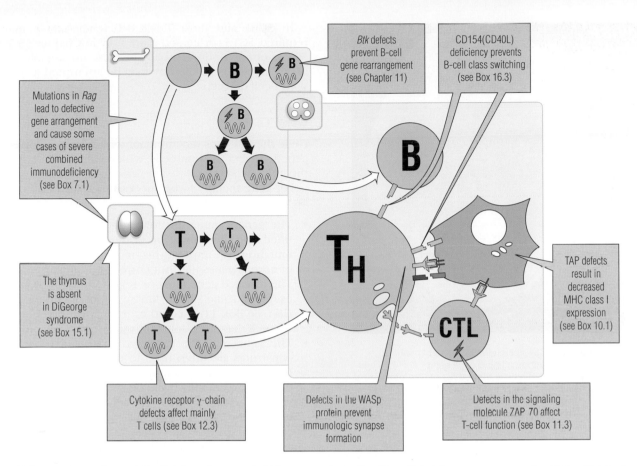

Figure 31.3 Disorders with mainly T-cell defects, for example, DiGeorge syndrome, Zap-70, and Jak defects, present soon after birth with infections with intracellular pathogens. B-cell disorders, for example, X-linked agammaglobulinemia, present at age around 6 months, when maternal antibody levels have fallen. Btk, Bruton's tyrosine kinase; CTL, cytotoxic T lymphocytes; TAP, transporter associated with antigen presentation.

such infants with suspected T-cell immunodeficiency, lymphocyte numbers should be measured by flow cytometry (see Chapter 5).

Antibody deficiency presents later in life because babies are born with maternal Ig transferred across the placenta. This protects the patient for the first few months of life. Some forms of antibody deficiency (e.g., CVID) does not present until adulthood. The most common indication for testing for antibody deficiency is chronic or recurrent bacterial respiratory infection. IgG, IgA, and IgM should be measured. In patients with low levels of Igs, causes of secondary immunodeficiency, such as protein loss from the gut or kidneys, should be excluded. If total Igs are normal, IgG subclasses and specific antibodies against *Haemophilus* and *Pneumococcus* spp. should be measured. If these tests are all normal, it is important to check that there are no problems with complement or neutrophil function (e.g., chronic granulomatous disease, see Chapter 20) before concluding that there is no immunodeficiency.

Genetic Testing

Testing for mutations is difficult because each affected family can carry a unique sequence. For example, there are

several hundred mutations identified in the gene *Btk* in families affected by X-linked agammaglobulinemia.

However, once a preliminary diagnosis of a disease caused by mutation is made, it can be confirmed by genetic testing. Genetic testing also determines whether family members are carriers, and it can be used to carry out antenatal diagnosis in subsequent pregnancies.

■ TREATMENT

The aim of treatment is to prevent infection. In cases of mild immunodeficiency, such as IgG$_2$ deficiency, prophylactic antibiotics may be adequate.

In more severe antibody deficiency, immunoglobulin replacement therapy is required. Administration of immunoglobulin is a type of *passive* immunotherapy (see Chapter 4 and Box 4.2). Antibodies against a wide range of pathogens are needed, and, therefore, Ig pooled from several thousand normal donors is used. Ig replacement can be given intravenously or subcutaneously. Replacement therapy is very different from high-dose Ig replacement therapy, which is immunosuppressive.

Plasma donors are screened for HIV and hepatitis B and C antibodies. Manufacturing processes to purify IgG will

 MHC II

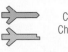 Cytokine, Chemokine, etc.

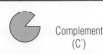 Complement (C')

 Signaling molecule

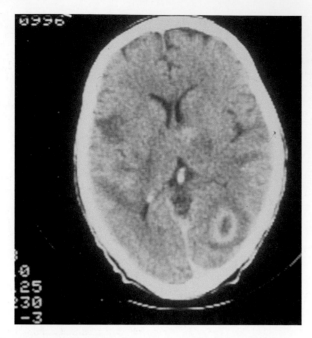

Figure 31.4 This patient has been unlucky enough to inherit polymorphisms in the genes encoding complement C2 and C4 and mannan-binding lectin. These reduce the activity of the complement cascade and predispose the patient to unusual infections. The ring-enhancing lesion seen in the cerebral cortex in this computed tomographic brain scan is typical of a brain abscess. (With permission from the Department of Medical Illustration, St. Bartholomew's Hospital, London.)

destroy many pathogens, but further steps are usually taken to reduce the risk for hepatitis C carriage—for example, pasteurization (heating to 56°C) or adding detergents. None of these steps is guaranteed to remove **prions**, the agents responsible for "mad cow disease" and variant Creutzfeldt-Jakob disease. At the time of writing, plasma from the UK is not used in Ig manufacture because of the theoretic risk for transmission of prions.

If SCID is suspected, and HIV infection has been excluded, the infant should be referred to a specialist center where the diagnosis will be confirmed and definitive treatment given (often stem cell transplant [SCT]). Until this can be done, simple steps are taken to avoid serious infection. These include avoiding live vaccines (e.g., measles, mumps, rubella, and polio) and using prophylaxis against opportunist infections, such as *Pneumocystis carinii* pneumonia.

In SCID and most T-cell deficiencies, SCT may be required. SCT is discussed more fully in Chapter 33. When SCT is not an option (usually because no suitable donors are available), gene therapy may be attempted in patients with T-cell defects.

Gene Therapy

Gene therapy uses recombinant technology to correct the genetic defect in stem cells, which can then reconstitute the immune system.

For gene therapy to be successful, several criteria must be met.

- The genetic mutation for each patient must be identified, and there must be evidence that correcting the mutation will improve his or her conditions. Insertion of normal genes may not correct a dominant mutation.
- The inserted gene must be regulated appropriately. For example, some of the kinase genes mentioned (*Jak*, *Btk*; see Box 11.4) could cause inappropriate cell activation if they were constitutively active in recipient cells.
- The gene must be delivered to the cell safely. Viral constructs are often used to deliver the normal gene. Healthy humans contain many harmless retroviruses that may recombine genetic sequences with the viral vector. The new viruses produced may be able to cause disease.
- Gene therapy must not cause malignancy. If a gene with an active promoter is inserted next to an oncogene, the latter may become constitutively active and cause cancer. This is known as **insertional mutagenesis**, and it remains a major cause for concern.

As discussed in Chapter 12, gene therapy has been used successfully in a handful of patients with γ-chain deficiency, a type of X-linked SCID. Stem cells are transfected with the γ-chain gene and give rise to large numbers of normal daughter cells. These cells proliferate and replace the abnormal cells because the transfected γ-chain gene allows them to proliferate in response to cytokines; these cells have a strong **survival advantage**. The normal cytokine gene is transfected at random into anywhere in the genome. There have been two major problems with gene therapy for X-linked SCID. The first is that the procedure does not work for older children, perhaps because of loss of thymic function. The second problem is that the normal gene may be inserted next to an oncogene. This can immortalize the transfected cells and has given rise to leukemia in a small number of children given gene therapy. In the future, gene therapy is likely to be applied to other types of primary immunodeficiency caused by mutations.

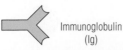 T cell receptor (TCR)   Immunoglobulin (Ig)   Antigen   MHC I

BOX 31.1 A Delayed Diagnosis

A 25-year-old woman has been referred with daily sputum production and worsening shortness of breath. She had recurrent chest infections whilet a college student, and she was unable to complete her studies and graduate. Over the past 3 years, her chest symptoms have become continuous. She has chronic sinusitis and has had three (unsuccessful) sinus drainage operations. She is a nonsmoker with an unremarkable family history.

On examination, she has clinical signs of bronchiectasis, which is confirmed on computed tomography of her lungs (Fig. 31.5). Bronchiectasis is irreversible damage to the airways caused by repeated bouts of infection. *Haemophilus* bacteria are present in her sputum.

Her immunologic investigations are shown in Figure 31.6.

Causes of secondary immunodeficiency were excluded. She is given a test vaccination with a vaccine containing pneumococcal polysaccharide. Further testing shows that she does not respond to the vaccine, and she now meets diagnostic criteria for common variable immunodeficiency (CVID). Her symptoms improved on intravenous immunoglobulin, and she has subsequently graduated as a mature student.

CVID often develops in the late teens and early twenties. Once immunoglobulin is started, the frequency and severity of respiratory infections diminishes. However, when the diagnosis is delayed, as in this case, irreversible complications may have already developed. Checking immunoglobulin levels in patients with recurrent or unusual infections can prevent the development of this scenario.

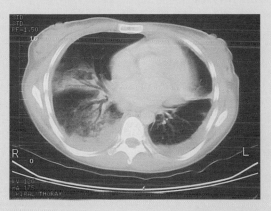

Figure 31.5 This lung scan shows bronchiectasis and patchy pneumonia in a woman with common variable immunodeficiency. In the right lung the bronchi are visible because of the consolidation in the surrounding lungs. The bronchi are somewhat dilated and their lumens are not smooth. (With permission from the Department of Medical Illustration, St. Bartholomew's Hospital, London.)

FIG. 31.6 Immunologic Investigations in This Patient with Common Variable Immunodeficiency

Component	Patient Values	Normal Range
IgG (g/L)	0.2	7.0–18.0
IgA (g/L)	0.1	0.8–4.0
IgM (g/L)	0.2	0.4–2.5
CD3$^+$ T cells (cells $\times$ 10^6/L)	420	820–2100
CD19$^+$ B cells (cells $\times$ 10^6/L)	230	760–4200

 MHC II

  Cytokine, Chemokine, etc.

Complement (C′)

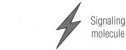 Signaling molecule

BOX 31.2 Wiskott-Aldrich Syndrome

The patient in Figures 31.7 and 31.8 presented as a young child with bruising and bleeding, which were found to be due to a reduction in the number of circulating platelets. He also had severe eczema and unusual viral infections. In Figure 31.7, multiple warty lesions can be seen on his face. These lesions are molluscum contagiosum and are caused by a member of the *poxvirus* family. In children with normal immune systems, molluscum contagiosum causes a transient infection, usually with only one or two lesions, which are cleared within a few weeks by cytotoxic T cells. The unusually extensive and persistent infection seen in the patient described in this clinical box is typical of an opportunist infection.

The patient also had a type of malignancy known as B-cell lymphoma. As discussed in Chapter 34, lymphoma in patients with immune deficiencies is often caused by the *Epstein-Barr virus*.

The patient's clinical characteristics (low platelet count, eczema, infection, and malignancy) led his pediatrician to suspect Wiskott Aldrich syndrome, a primary immunodeficiency. A DNA sample was obtained from the patient, and the Wiskott Aldrich syndrome protein (*WASP*) gene was sequenced. The patient's *WASP* gene was found to contain a mutation, confirming the diagnosis.

Wiskott-Aldrich syndrome is an X-linked disorder, but in this particular family, there was no history of affected male relatives and his mutation was thought to have occurred *de novo*.

The patient's lymphoma was brought under control and he underwent stem cell transplant (see Chapter 33). Two years later, he has recovered from his transplant and leads a normal life (Fig. 31.8).

Wiskott-Aldrich syndrome protein (WASp) regulates the actin cytoskeleton. In ways that are not well understood, defects in WASp prevent the normal development of platelets. How WASp defects affect the immune system is much more clearly understood. After normal T-cell activation, Zap 70 (see Chapter 11) activates WASp molecules leading to changes in the cytoskeleton, which appear to culminate in the formation of an immunologic synapse (see Chapter 16) and, in cytotoxic T cells, delivery of perforin and granzyme into target cells (Fig. 31.9). With defects in these T-cell functions, it should come as no surprise that intracellular viral pathogens cannot be cleared in patients with Wiskott-Aldrich syndrome. In addition, these patients have defects in B-cell and dendritic cell function, resulting in impaired antibody production.

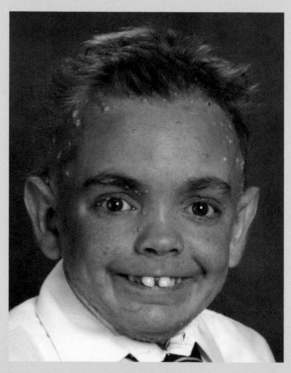

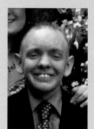

Figure 31.8 The same patient shown in Figure 31.7 2 years after stem cell transplantation.

Figure 31.7 This photograph shows the patient with Wiskott-Aldrich syndrome who is described in the clinical box. The wart lesions on his face are molluscum contagiosum.

Continued

 T cell receptor (TCR)

 Immunoglobulin (Ig)

 Antigen

 MHC I

BOX 31.2 Wiskott-Aldrich Syndrome—cont'd

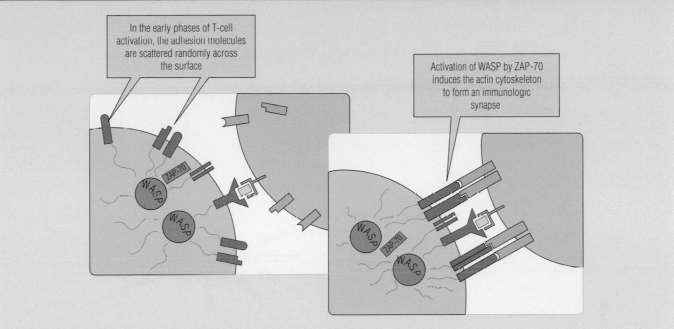

Figure 31.9 WASp has a role in organizing the actin cytoskeleton after T-cell activation. In Wiskott-Aldrich syndrome, these events do not take place normally because of mutations in the *WASp* gene.

LEARNING POINTS — Can You Now ...

1. List the clinical features that would make you suspect primary immunodeficiency?
2. Construct lists of the types of infection affecting patients with T-cell and B-cell disorders?
3. List the primary immunodeficiencies caused by mutations, polymorphisms, and polygenic factors?
4. Write short notes on immunoglobulin replacement and gene therapy?

 MHC II

 Cytokine, Chemokine, etc.

 Complement (C')

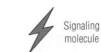 Signaling molecule

32 Secondary Immunodeficiency

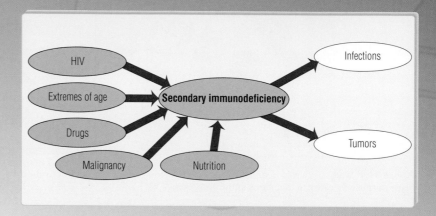

In this chapter, you will learn about several secondary immunodeficiencies. Of these, HIV is the most important, because it is common and causes severe immunodeficiency. Secondary immunodeficiency causes the same infections and tumors as primary immunodeficiency. The exact type of infection depends on what part of the immune system the secondary immunodeficiency affects.

■ HIV INFECTION

More than 40 million people are infected with HIV. Each year, 3 million people die of HIV infection, including half a million children. Whatever type of physician you become, you will encounter HIV-infected patients and will need to understand the natural history of HIV disease. Understanding how HIV interacts with the immune system will help you understand how anti-HIV drugs work and why vaccines have been difficult to develop.

Entry of HIV into Host Cells

HIV is a very simple virus (Fig 32.1A). Its genome only contains three genes, although through RNA splicing and peptide processing, it encodes about nine different proteins. HIV is a **retrovirus**, and its RNA genome is reverse transcribed into a DNA template in host cells. The genome, along with some enzymes, is surrounded by an envelope, which consists of two glycoproteins, gp120 and gp41, used to bind and enter host cells (Fig. 32.1B–E):

1. gp120 initially binds CD4 molecules. HIV binds the long, flexible CD4 molecule easily, but this interaction does not bring the virus close to the host cell surface. The presence of CD4 on cells is a prerequisite for HIV, which, therefore, only infects CD4$^+$ T cells, monocytes (and monocyte derived macrophages), and dendritic cells (Fig. 32.1B).
2. gp120 then binds onto one of two chemokine receptors (Fig. 32.1C), either CCR5 (expressed mainly on macrophages, dendritic cells, and mucosal T cells) or CXCR4 (expressed on most T cells). The gp120 molecules in different strains of HIV preferentially bind on to one or other chemokine receptor. Thus, some HIV strains preferentially infect monocytes or dendritic cells, whereas others are more likely to infect T cells.
3. Chemokine receptors have short extracellular domains (see Chapter 23), and binding draws gp120 closer to the host cell. Binding to a chemokine receptor also induces a change in the gp41 molecule, which normally has a structure similar to a closed zipper. When gp120 binds to a chemokine receptor, gp41 unzips and penetrates the cell membrane. (Fig. 32.1D)
4. The final step is that gp41 zips back up to its original length, effectively fusing the virus envelope and the cell membrane. (Fig. 32.1E)

Following sexual exposure to HIV, the virus uses the CCR5 chemokine receptor on dendritic cells and mucosal T cells present in the genital mucosa to gain entry into the body. Dendritic cells and mucosal T cells migrate to local

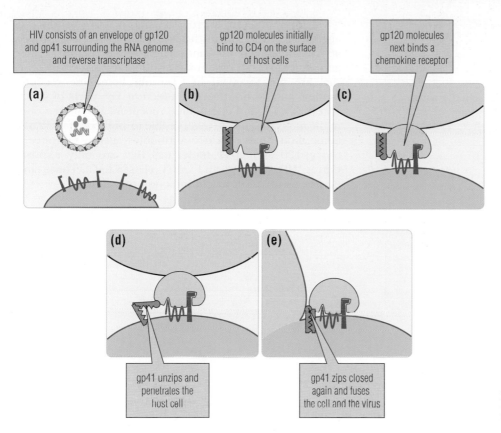

HIV consists of an envelope of gp120 and gp41 surrounding the RNA genome and reverse transcriptase

gp120 molecules initially bind to CD4 on the surface of host cells

gp120 molecules next binds a chemokine receptor

gp41 unzips and penetrates the host cell

gp41 zips closed again and fuses the cell and the virus

Figure 32.1 HIV uses CD4 and chemokine receptors to infect host cells. B–E are zoomed in views of HIV interacting with a target cell.

lymph nodes and infect other cells in the germinal center. Following nonsexual HIV transmission, for example, sharing needles during intravenous drug use, HIV can use either CXCR4 or CCR5 as receptors to gain entry to cells.

Reverse Transcription of the HIV Genome

The enzyme reverse transcriptase enters host cells along with the RNA genome. Reverse transcriptase uses the RNA genome to make a double-stranded DNA transcript, which inserts itself into the host genome (Fig. 32.2A,B). Reverse transcriptase is an error-prone enzyme and up to 1 in 10,000 bases mutate during the process. Furthermore, HIV has no mechanism for correcting these mutations. This means that 1 in 3 HIV life cycles leads to a virus containing a new mutation.

Because of this high mutation rate, within a few weeks of infection with a single HIV virus, many different strains of virus are detectable in most patients. The mutations affect the virus in several ways. For example, the gp120 molecule may mutate so that it switches its preference from the CCR5 chemokine receptor to the CXCR4 receptor, enabling it to infect a broad range of T cells.

HIV latency and Transcription

Once inserted into the host genome, the three HIV genes behave exactly like host genes. Most of the time the genes are silent and not transcribed. This is referred to as **viral latency**, and in the majority of infected cells, the virus remains latent. These latently infected cells provide a reservoir of infection, because in the absence of replication, no HIV peptides are expressed, and infected cells are not recognized by the immune system.

However, if the host cell becomes activated, transcription will commence. In infected T cells, HIV genes are regulated in exactly the same way as immune response genes. For example, the transcription factors nuclear factor (NF)-κB and NF-AT (see Chapter 11) generated during T-cell activation also promote transcription of HIV genes. New viral RNA is formed, and HIV precursor proteins are synthesized. A protease encoded by HIV cleaves the precursor proteins, forming a new virus (Fig. 32.2C,D).

High levels of viral replication destroy host cells, referred to as viral cytopathic effects, but this is only one of the ways that HIV damages CD4$^+$ T cells.

The Immune Responses to HIV

HIV is a very infectious virus, and there is evidence that most people exposed to it become infected. Once an individual has become infected, latent virus in long-lived cells make it almost impossible to eliminate the infection. Most research into the immune response has focused on mechanisms that limit the damage caused by HIV.

Plasmacytoid dendritic cells of the innate immune system secrete type I interferons in response to HIV (Fig. 32.3A). Although these cells are capable of inhibiting HIV replication *in vitro*, their function is often impaired in infected patients.

 MHC II

 Cytokine, Chemokine, etc.

 Complement (C')

 Signaling molecule

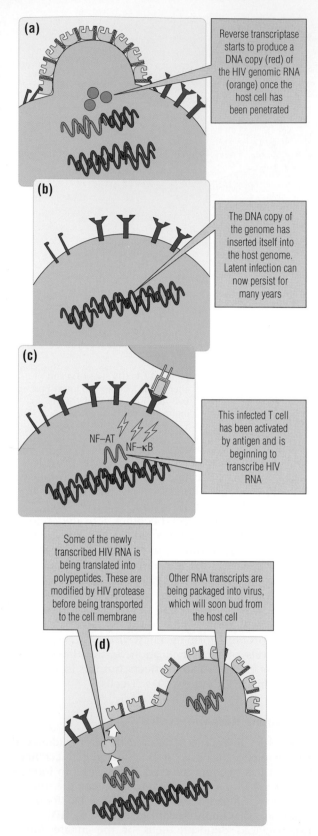

Reverse transcriptase starts to produce a DNA copy (red) of the HIV genomic RNA (orange) once the host cell has been penetrated

The DNA copy of the genome has inserted itself into the host genome. Latent infection can now persist for many years

This infected T cell has been activated by antigen and is beginning to transcribe HIV RNA

Some of the newly transcribed HIV RNA is being translated into polypeptides. These are modified by HIV protease before being transported to the cell membrane

Other RNA transcripts are being packaged into virus, which will soon bud from the host cell

Figure 32.2 Reverse transcription is an error-prone process. It enables HIV to mutate its antigenic structure, its affinity for different chemokine receptors, and its susceptibility to antiretroviral drugs.

Infected individuals produce high levels of antibodies against HIV. These form the basis of the HIV test (usually an enzyme-linked immunosorbent assay [ELISA]). These antibodies usually recognize epitopes of gp120 or gp41 that are not involved in CD4 or chemokine receptor binding and do not prevent infection. The parts of gp120 that bind CD4 and chemokine receptors are hidden deep in the molecule and are inaccessible to antibody (Fig. 32.3B). Some individuals produce antibodies against epitopes of the gp120 and gp41 molecules that are only exposed during HIV binding and entry (Fig. 32.3C). These antibodies are able to prevent infection of T cells.

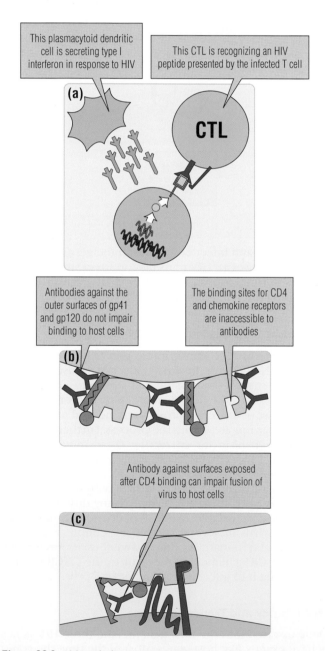

This plasmacytoid dendritic cell is secreting type I interferon in response to HIV

This CTL is recognizing an HIV peptide presented by the infected T cell

Antibodies against the outer surfaces of gp41 and gp120 do not impair binding to host cells

The binding sites for CD4 and chemokine receptors are inaccessible to antibodies

Antibody against surfaces exposed after CD4 binding can impair fusion of virus to host cells

Figure 32.3 Although there are innate immune system (type I interferon) and adaptive system responses to HIV (CTL and antibody), these rarely keep apace of mutations in HIV. CTL, cytotoxic T cell.

 T cell receptor (TCR)

 Immunoglobulin (Ig)

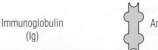 Antigen

 MHC I

Cytotoxic T cells (CTLs) have the most important role in HIV infection and are able to kill cells actively expressing and displaying HIV peptides (Fig. 32.3A). Thus, CTLs cannot kill cells in which infection remains latent. HIV is also able to overcome the CTL response by mutation. Previously generated CTLs cannot recognize cells expressing mutated HIV peptides.

An infected individual typically produces at least 10^5 new viruses each day. One in three will carry a new mutation; therefore, effectively, CTL and antibody have to contend with at least 3×10^4 new viral strains each day. Both immunoglobulin G (IgG) antibody production and CTLs require help from CD4$^+$ T cells. However, HIV infects and kills or damages CD4$^+$ T cells, and, therefore, the immune system is less able to produce new CTL or antibody responses. In these ways, HIV is able to keep one step ahead of immune system.

A final effect of the widespread activation of the immune system is apoptosis of CD4$^+$ T cells. Apoptosis usually occurs in the thymus and T cells that have been successful at eradicating invading pathogens. In HIV infection, CD4$^+$ T cells undergo apoptosis more readily. This is at least partly because the whole immune system is in an overactivated state. Excess apoptosis is the second way that CD4$^+$ T cells are destroyed.

The Clinical Features OF HIV Infection

Some newly infected patients have rashes, malaise, or a fever. This stage is referred to as **HIV seroconversion illness**, because it occurs at about the time antibodies to HIV appear. During this phase, there is a massive loss of CCR5 expressing mucosal CD4$^+$ T cells, but lesser damage to circulating CD4$^+$ T cells.

Over the next few weeks, the mechanisms described above bring viral replication under control. A lower level of viral replication then continues in lymph nodes, and a steady state of virus production and CD4$^+$ T-cell death is matched by equivalent rate CD4$^+$ T-cell production. During this phase, patients have no symptoms, although lymphadenopathy may be found. This **asymptomatic stage** of HIV infection may persist for several years.

During asymptomatic infection, up to 10^5 and 10^9 virions are produced each day, many of which contain mutated antigenic peptides or gp120. Viral replication is measured by viral load testing. In most individuals, HIV eventually escapes from antibody and CTL control. As a result of increased cytopathic effects and apoptosis, the **CD4 count** (the number of circulating CD4$^+$ T cells) begins to fall.

As the number of CD4$^+$ T cells declines, patients become susceptible to infection with virulent organisms such as *Candida albicans* (Fig. 32.4) and *Mycobacterium tuberculosis*. After further falls in the CD4 count, the patient becomes susceptible to opportunist organisms such as *Pneumocystis carinii* pneumonia (PCP) (Fig. 32.5). Finally, when little residual immune response remains, organisms such as low virulence mycobacteria and cytomegalovirus (CMV) cause infections. Tumors such as non-Hodgkin's lymphoma and Kaposi's sarcoma also occur.

Factors Affecting Outcome of Infection

The rate of diseased progression varies considerably from person to person and is affected by genetic factors. For example, some individuals inherit a polymorphism in the CCR5 chemokine receptor that reduces the ability of HIV

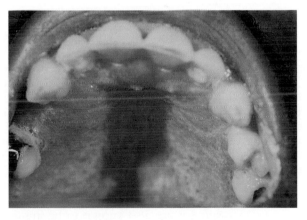

Figure 32.4 The white lesions on this man's palate are oral candidiasis, which is a marker of mild immunodeficiency, and it is often the first opportunistic infection in patients with HIV. Oral candidiasis is often seen in other mild secondary immunodeficiencies. (With permission from the Department of Medical Illustration, St. Bartholomew's Hospital, London.)

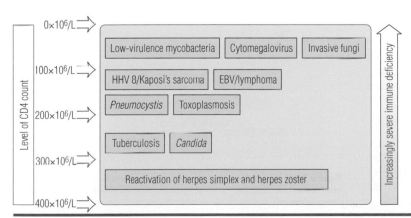

Figure 32.5 Different opportunistic infections occur after HIV has caused different levels of immunodeficiency. For example, infection with low-virulence mycobacteria requires much more severe immunodeficiency than tuberculosis.

 MHC II

 Cytokine, Chemokine, etc.

 Complement (C')

 Signaling molecule

to bind to and fuse with mucosal macrophages, dendritic cells, and T cells. Individuals who are homozygous for this polymorphism have a decreased risk for becoming infected with HIV after sexual exposure and a delayed rate of disease progression if they become infected—for example, by blood transfusion. Polymorphisms in CCR5 do not appear to cause any harmful effects on the immune system.

CTL responses to HIV vary between patients. For example, enhanced CTL responses protect some female sex workers against HIV, despite repeated unprotected intercourse, for up to 12 years. "Long-term nonprogressors" are patients remaining well at least 10 years after HIV infection, and they have stronger than usual CTL activity against HIV. The ability to produce CTL against HIV may be determined by human leukocyte antigen (HLA) polymorphisms in two different ways. First, the ability of different HLA alleles to bind HIV peptides and present them to CTL may vary. Second, individuals who are homozygous for all HLA alleles effectively have half as many different HLA molecules available for HIV peptide presentation as individuals who are heterozygous at all alleles. People who are heterozygous at all HLA alleles tend to have better outcomes after HIV infection (see Box 3.1).

Vaccines

An important question for HIV vaccine researchers is whether antibodies or T-cell responses give the best protection from infection. As described earlier, most antibody produced by infected people does not have beneficial effects. However, antibody may be effective in two special circumstances. The first is IgG against epitopes on gp120 and gp41 molecules that are only exposed during HIV binding and entry (Fig. 32.3C). The second type of antibody that appears to be protective in animal experiments is IgA, present in genital secretions. Most antibodies elicited by research vaccines so far do not protect from infection.

Strong CTL responses are also known to be important in protecting from HIV infection, as discussed earlier. However, to elicit these, vaccines would need to deliver antigen to the cytoplasm so that peptides from this vaccine are eventually expressed on major histocompatibility complex (MHC) class I. This has been achieved, in some experiments, with live recombinant vaccines constructed from canary pox and containing HIV genes.

The overwhelming problem for any vaccine is the vast antigenic variation seen in viral samples obtained from different geographic sites because of rapid HIV mutation. A vaccine that is effective in Thailand, for example, may not protect individuals in the United States. This remains the major problem for vaccine researchers.

Treatments for HIV Infection

Highly active antiretroviral therapy (HAART) has dramatically changed the prognosis in HIV infection. HAART consists of combinations of antiretroviral drugs. Three classes of drug are currently licensed (Fig. 32.6):

- **Reverse transcriptase inhibitors** are generally nucleoside analogues that are incorporated into the DNA transcript. These drugs then terminate the synthesis of the DNA strand because reverse transcriptase is unable to correct errors (Fig. 32.6B).
- **Protease inhibitors** inhibit the enzyme responsible for generating HIV structural proteins (Fig. 32.6C).
- **Fusion inhibitors** bound to gp41 prevent it from contracting and initiating fusion with the host cell (Fig. 32.6A).

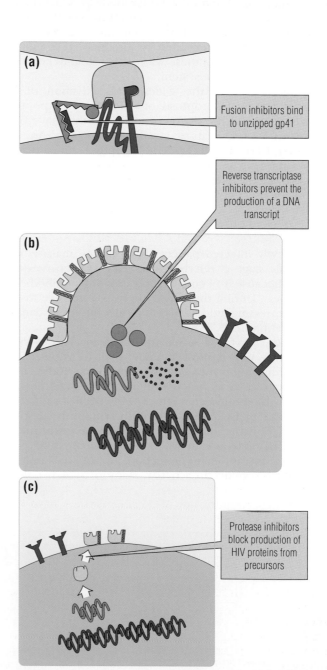

Fusion inhibitors bind to unzipped gp41

Reverse transcriptase inhibitors prevent the production of a DNA transcript

Protease inhibitors block production of HIV proteins from precursors

Figure 32.6 The three major classes of antiretroviral therapy are fusion inhibitors (one drug licensed), reverse transcriptase inhibitors (about 20 drugs licensed), and protease inhibitors (eight drugs licensed).

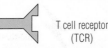 T cell receptor (TCR)   Immunoglobulin (Ig)   Antigen   MHC I

If only one drug is given at a time, HIV rapidly mutates and becomes resistant. For this reason, HIV antiretroviral drugs must be given in combination, usually as three drugs, to reduce the risk for the emergence of resistant strains. It is much less likely that a virus would mutate and become resistant to three different drugs at once. Following initiation of successful HAART, the viral load should fall, and the CD4$^+$ T-cell count should recover. Immune recovery is associated with reduced numbers of opportunist infections and improved outcomes. However, because latent virus can persist in long-lived cells, HAART would have to be given for at least 60 years before HIV infection is cleared.

Apart from HAART, there is also active research in treatments to boost the immune response in HIV infection. One interesting approach is to give Toll-like receptor binding drugs, such as imiquimod and CpG (see Chapter 20), in the hope that these will induce interferon secretion by plasmacytoid dendritic cells.

Interleukin-2 (IL-2) is a growth factor for T and B cells. Clinical trials suggest that administration of recombinant IL-2 along with HAART induces greater improvements in CD4 cell counts than drug therapy alone, and there is no increase in viral replication. One hope is that IL-2 will activate resting T cells harboring latent HIV. If this happened, there is a chance that these cells would be killed by CTLs and that sterilizing immunity from HIV could be achieved. The use of recombinant IL-2 is constrained by its side effects and its cost. You will learn more about recombinant cytokines in Chapter 35.

■ OTHER SECONDARY IMMUNODEFICIENCIES

A variety of other factors can cause secondary immunodeficiency. These factors often operate together. This can happen very easily during hospital admissions, when patients are exposed to stress, drugs, and possibly worse than usual nutrition.

Extremes of Age

The Immune System in the First Year of Life

Throughout the first year of life, the specific immune system remains immature. Although neonates have high numbers of T cells, these are all naive and so do not respond well to antigen (see Chapters 14 and 17).

Fetal antibody synthesis begins at 20 weeks, but adult levels of IgG are not reached until about 5 years. For the first few months of life, infants are reliant on maternal IgG. Pregnant women produce increased Igs under the effects of estrogens. IgG is transported across the placenta by specialized Fc receptors in the last 10 weeks of pregnancy. Breast milk is an additional source of protection in early life and protects against lung and gastrointestinal infection. Bottle-fed infants are 60 times more likely to develop pneumonia in the first 3 months of life.

Premature babies face the greatest problems with infection because they have had less time to receive maternal Ig

during the late stages of pregnancy. Immaturity of innate mechanisms such as lung surfactant (see Chapter 19) can increase the risk of respiratory infection.

Many infants develop low levels of antibody during the first year of life. **Transient hypogammaglobulinemia of infancy** is caused by a delay in maturation of Ig synthesis, especially IgG2, at a time when maternal antibody levels are falling.

The Aging Immune System

The elderly suffer more infections than younger patients. The mild immune deficiency that occurs with aging mainly affects T cells. T-cell memory is not long-lasting, and memory T cells only have a half life of about 50 days. Figure 24.7 illustrates just how quickly T-cell responses decline. Immune response requiring T-cell help often require newly generated T cells. There are three reasons why the generation of new memory T cells fails in the elderly (Fig. 32.7).

The thymus shrinks by about 3% a year throughout middle age, and there is a corresponding fall in the thymic production of naive T cells. Although thymic output can increase in response to specific circumstances (e.g., when circulating T cells have been destroyed by drugs), this cannot usually be sustained in old age.

Because fewer T cells emerge from the thymus in later life, proliferation of T cells in the periphery is mainly responsible for maintaining adequate T-cell numbers in adults. However, a biological clock is particularly important in limiting the number of occasions T cells can replicate. Each time a cell divides, there is a stepwise shortening of telomeric DNA. When telomere length is considerably shortened, cells can no longer divide. This **replicative senescence** affects T cells after about 40 divisions.

A third factor affecting T cells in old age is a herpesvirus family member called cytomegalovirus (CMV). CMV drives increasing numbers of T cells. In the elderly, the T-cell response becomes very oligoclonal, with disproportionate numbers of T cells having CMV specificity. These cells leave little room in the immune system for other specificities.

Consequences of impaired T-cell numbers and function in old age include poor response to vaccines, increased infections, and, possibly, increased risk for malignancy.

As you learned in Chapter 24, memory for preexisting antibody responses to effective vaccines may last for up to 50 or 60 years. So, for example, responses to smallpox vaccine remain effective for many decades. Aged B cells may show signs of a lifetime of exposure to microorganisms. Immunoglobulin synthesis is increased, and outgrowth of B-cell clones may lead to the presence of monoclonal immunoglobulin in the blood or B-cell malignancy (see Chapter 34). Autoantibodies are also more common in the elderly but are not usually associated with disease.

Miscellaneous Factors

Drugs

Drugs are a very common cause of secondary immunodeficiency, and eliminating the offending drug will usually

 MHC II

 Cytokine, Chemokine, etc.

 Complement (C')

 Signaling molecule

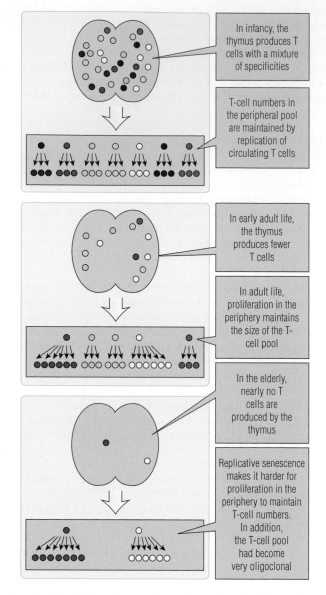

Figure 32.7 This figure shows why numbers of T cells decline in later life.

infection. Other drugs can cause antibody deficiency as an unexpected side effect. Among the most notorious are anticonvulsants, used to treat epilepsy.

B-cell Malignancy

Myeloma and chronic lymphocytic leukemia are malignancies of B cells (see Chapter 34). Although both may produce large amounts of monoclonal immunoglobulin (paraprotein), they are associated with low levels of antibody against pathogens. Myeloma and chronic lymphocytic leukemia are very common causes of secondary immunodeficiency in the elderly. Thymoma is a rare tumor that can cause immunodeficiency.

Kidney Disease

In nephrotic syndrome (see Chapter 28), there may be significant renal protein loss and a reduction in blood levels of IgG and IgA with normal IgM.

Igs can also be lost via the gut in severe diarrheal diseases. Renal failure and diabetes also cause secondary phagocyte defects, although the mechanism is not known.

Nutrition

Deficiency of zinc and magnesium impairs cell-mediated immunity, particularly T_H1-pattern cytokine secretion. This type of deficiency in micronutrients occurs in a wide range of situations, such as, in postoperative patients. Although vitamins, especially vitamins A and E, are required by the immune system, their role is less significant than mineral nutrients.

Physiologic Stress

Stress has potent affects on the adaptive immune system. Lymphocytes have receptors for both epinephrine (adrenaline) and corticosteroids. These hormones are secreted in response to stress, with epinephrine mediating rapid-onset, short-term effects and corticosteroids mediating longer-term effects. Physiologic stress, such as endurance training, can therefore inhibit immune responses to infection. Research has established that psychological stress can have negative effects on the immune system in the short and long term. How important this is clinically is unclear, but physiologic stress should be considered in patients with recurrent infection.

Infections

Infections can also cause immunodeficiency. Malaria and congenital rubella may cause antibody deficiency. Measles is well known for causing defects in cell-mediated immunity—sometimes enough to reactivate tuberculosis.

Many of these factors operate together in acutely ill patients (Box 32.2).

improve the immune response. Patients very often develop neutropenia during cytotoxic therapy for malignancy (see Box 20.1).

Damage to T and B cells is an expected side effect of corticosteroids, cytotoxic drugs, and the immunosuppressive regimens used in autoimmune disease and transplant rejection prophylaxis. Patients starting these drugs need to be aware that they are prone to opportunistic

 T cell receptor (TCR)   Immunoglobulin (Ig)   Antigen   MHC I

BOX 32.1 Monitoring HIV infection

A 29-year-old woman attends a general medical clinic with lumps in her neck. She has no other symptoms at all, notably no fevers or sweats. She had two normal pregnancies in her early twenties and an episode of pelvic inflammatory disease (caused by chlamydia infection) at age 26. She is a single parent, and her children are both well.

On examination, she is found to have generalized lymphadenopathy affecting her cervical, axillary, and inguinal nodes. Such generalized lymphadenopathy is not a feature of cancer or localized infection. HIV can cause generalized lymphadenopathy, and the patient gives consent for an HIV antibody test, which is positive. Further testing shows her CD4 count to be reduced to 310×10^6/L (normal above 500×10^6/L) and her viral load to be 2×10^5/mL. In spite of her lack of symptoms, these results are consistent with moderately advanced HIV infection. She is very concerned about her children, but when her antenatal records are checked, they confirm that her screening HIV test was negative during both pregnancies.

The CD4 count is repeated (because the first one could have been lowered by psychological stress), and this is found to be 290×10^6/L. She agrees to commence HAART and is prescribed a combination of three different reverse-transcriptase inhibitors. She tolerates these well, and there is a rapid fall in her viral load and a more gradual improvement in her CD4 counts (Fig. 32.8).

Patients with HIV infection require immunologic (CD4 counts) and virologic (viral load) monitoring. Different levels of CD4 cell count are associated with risks for different opportunistic infections. For example, patients with CD4 counts below 200×10^6/L have a high risk for PCP and should receive preventive medication (prophylaxis). Viral-load tests measure HIV viremia and reflect long-term risk for disease progression. Viral load and CD4 counts are used to determine the use of antiretroviral treatment. In the case history here, the patient had a very high viral load and evidence of significant CD4+ T-cell depletion.

CD4 cell counts are done by flow cytometry (see Fig. 5.7). They are affected by hormones. For example, because corticosteroid secretion has a diurnal pattern, so do CD4 counts—they are the lowest in the morning. Corticosteroid secretion in response to acute and chronic stress will suppress CD4 counts. Finally, they are affected by estrogen levels and vary at different stages of the menstrual cycle. These factors need to be taken into account when monitoring CD4 counts.

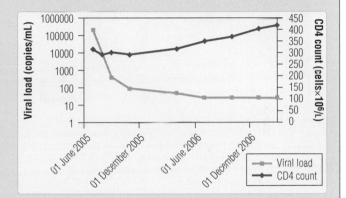

Figure 32.8 The effects of HAART on HIV viral load and CD4 count. The viral load falls rapidly after its replicative cycle is blocked. The CD4 count takes much longer to recover in adults. This is because at this age the thymus is no longer capable of producing many new CD4+ T cells. New CD4+ T cells are produced by proliferation of peripheral T cells.

 MHC II

 Cytokine, Chemokine, etc.

 Complement (C')

 Signaling molecule

BOX 32.2 Secondary Immunodeficiency in Acute Illness

A previously healthy 30-year-old man was admitted following a car crash. He is unconscious and has signs of cerebral edema. The patient has a tube inserted into his trachea, and a central venous line and urinary catheter are inserted. He is given high-dose corticosteroids in an attempt to reduce cerebral edema. After a series of convulsions, the anticonvulsant phenytoin is given intravenously (Fig. 32.9).

Two weeks later, he is recovering from his neurologic episode when he develops pneumonia (Fig. 32.10). In addition to physiologic stress and poor nutrition, this patient has his innate barriers penetrated at three different sites and is then exposed to two drugs that impair the immune system. It is no surprise his defenses against infection are impaired!

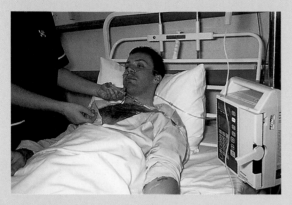

Figure 32.9 In acutely ill patients admitted to hospital, many factors interact to cause immunodeficiency. This is made worse when physical barriers are breached by cannulae and intravenous lines and because of the wide range of pathogens found inside hospitals. (With permission from the Department of Medical Illustration, St. Bartholomew's Hospital, London.)

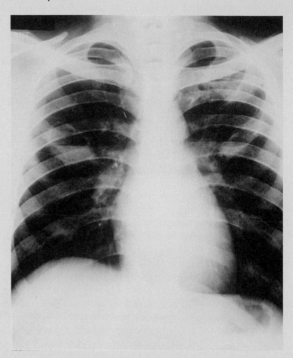

Figure 32.10 The patient's chest radiograph shows abscesses typical of staphylococcal pneumonia. This avoidable, life-threatening infection is a consequence of multiple factors in this patient. (With permission from the Department of Medical Illustration, St. Bartholomew's Hospital, London.)

LEARNING POINTS ... Can You Now ...

1. List the cells affected by HIV infection, and briefly describe their functions and roles in HIV infection?
2. Diagram the life cycle of HIV?
3. List how mutations benefit this virus?
4. Describe how you would monitor a patient with HIV infection?
5. List host factors that affect the course of HIV infection?
6. Make a list of the challenges to be overcome by effective HIV infection?
7. Explain which factors interact to predispose hospital patients to infection?

 T cell receptor (TCR)

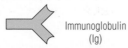 Immunoglobulin (Ig)

 Antigen

 MHC I

CHAPTER 33 Transplantation

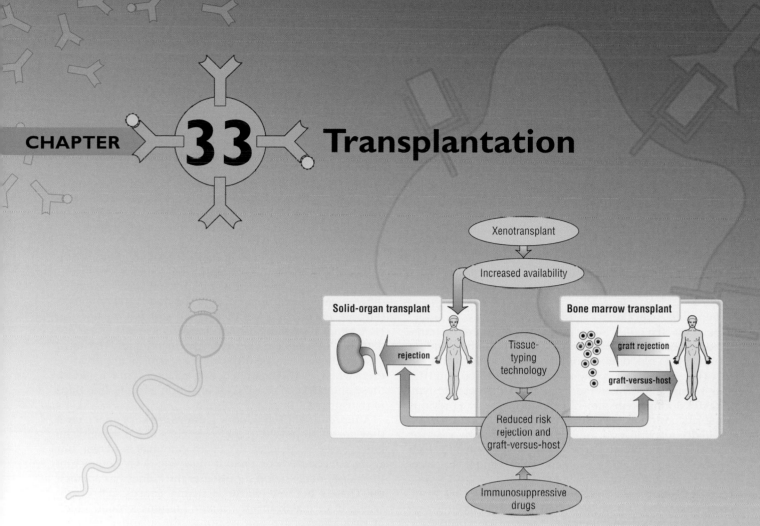

In this chapter, you will read about how graft rejection can complicate both solid-organ and stem cell transplantation. You will go on to read how graft-versus-host disease (GVHD) is an additional complication in stem cell transplantation. You will learn how tissue typing techniques and immunosuppressive drugs are used to reduce the risk of these complications. Finally, you will read about some of the problems that need to be overcome in order for xenotransplantation to become an effective alternative.

■ TRANSPLANTATION TERMINOLOGY

You first learned these terms in Chapter 8. Use this opportunity to check that you still understand these terms:

- **Rejection** refers to damage done by the immune system to a transplanted organ.
- **Autologous transplant** refers to tissue returning to the same individual after a period outside the body—usually in a frozen state.
- **Syngeneic transplant** refers to transplant between identical twins; there is usually no problem with graft rejection.
- **Allogeneic transplant** takes place between genetically nonidentical members of the same species; there is always a risk of rejection.

- **Xenogeneic transplant** takes place between different species, and this carries the highest risk of rejection.

■ SOLID-ORGAN TRANSPLANTATION

When Transplantation Is Indicated

Transplantation may be an option when a variety of solid organs stop functioning. Several criteria must be met before transplantation:

- There must be good evidence that the damage is irreversible or that alternative treatments are not applicable.
- The disease must not recur; for example, renal transplant is contraindicated in patients with Goodpasture's syndrome who have antiglomerular basement membrane antibodies (see Chapter 28).
- The chances of rejection must be minimized:
  - The donor and recipient must be ABO compatible.
  - The recipient must not have antidonor human leukocyte antigen (HLA) antibodies.
  - The donor should be selected with a close-as-possible HLA match to the recipient.
  - The patient must take immunosuppressive treatment.

The main problem with all solid-organ transplants is the risk for rejection, which we illustrate with renal transplant, the most common type of transplant. As shown in Figure 33.1, procedures vary for different organs. For example, because the cornea is not vascularized and is rarely exposed to the recipient immune system, corneal transplant recipients do not have to take immunosuppressive drugs. For reasons that are not well understood, liver transplantation can be done between HLA mismatched donor and recipients. Heart transplantation is almost always done when severe heart failure has developed very rapidly and the patient will die if they do not receive a transplant. There is not always time to wait for an HLA-matched donor for heart transplantation. The first heart that becomes available is often transplanted, and the recipient is treated with the most potent immunosuppressive drugs.

Mechanisms of Rejection

Hyperacute Rejection

Hyperacute rejection takes place within hours of transplantation and is caused by preformed antibodies binding to either ABO blood group or HLA class I antigens on the graft (Fig. 33.2). The recipient may have formed anti-HLA class I antibodies following exposure to allogeneic lymphocytes during pregnancy, blood transfusion, or a previous transplant. Antibody binding triggers a type II hypersensitivity reaction, and the graft is destroyed by vascular thrombosis. Hyperacute rejection can be prevented through careful ABO and HLA cross-matching and is now very rare.

Acute Rejection

Acute rejection is a type IV (cell-mediated) delayed hypersensitivity reaction and, therefore, takes place within days, and sometimes weeks, of transplantation. Acute rejection takes several days to develop because donor dendritic cells must first stimulate an allogeneic response in a local lymph node for responding T cells to proliferate and migrate into the donor kidney.

Acute rejection will take place if there is HLA incompatibility. Recipient T cells can respond to donor peptides presented by recipient major histocompatibility complex (MHC) or to donor MHC molecules themselves (Fig. 33.2). Although attempting to minimize any HLA mismatch of the donor and recipient can reduce acute rejection, the shortage of donor kidneys often means that a partially mismatched kidney is used. The survival of the kidney is related to the degree of mismatching, especially at the *HLA-DR* loci (Fig. 33.3).

Alternatively, the recipient may respond to "minor histocompatibility antigens" presented by donor or recipient cells (Box 33.1). Minor antigens are proteins that have different amino acid sequences in the donor and recipient; they are encoded by genes that are situated outside the HLA. Minor histocompatibility antigen mismatches are not detected by standard tissue-typing techniques. The term *minor* antigens may be misleading in terms of importance; even when an HLA-matched, live, related donor is found, these antigens can cause graft rejection in up to one third of transplants.

After removal from donors, kidneys are kept on ice until they are anastomosed to the recipient's blood vessels. The kidney can be held at 4°C with minimal ischemia, but acute rejection is worsened if there is a delay connecting the kidney to the blood supply after the kidney has warmed up. This is because warm ischemia causes cell death, which in turn activates the innate immune system, which in turn exaggerates any response the adaptive immune system is making to alloantigen.

FIG. 33.1 Transplant Procedures for Various Organs*

Organ	Characteristics	Type of Donor	Procedures per Million per Year	Graft Survival (%)
Cornea	No immunosuppression required because cornea does not become vascularized	Cadaveric	20	Over 90
Liver	Used for alcoholic liver disease, primary biliary cirrhosis, and virus-induced cirrhosis. Outcome not affected by degree of HLA matching	Live or cadaveric	10	Over 60
Kidney	Live related kidney donation often used. Graft survival optimized by HLA match; immunosuppression required	Live or cadaveric	50	Over 80
Pancreas	Usually transplanted along with kidneys in diabetics with renal failure. Separated islet cells have also been infused into the vena cava	Cadaveric	3	About 50
Heart	Used for coronary artery disease, cardiomyopathy, and some congenital heart disease. HLA matching not always possible and potent immunosuppression required	Cadaveric	10	Over 80
Stem cells	Used in malignancy, hematologic conditions, and some primary immunodeficiency. Best results when there is a match of HLA A, B, C, and DR	Live	100	Up to 80

*Transplantation of a variety of tissues is now possible. The examples at the top of this table are the most immunologically simple. As you work down to the bottom of the table, you encounter more complex types of transplantation. Stem cell transplantation is the most complex because graft-versus-host diseases can occur as well as graft rejection

 T cell receptor (TCR)

 Immunoglobulin (Ig)

 Antigen

 MHC I

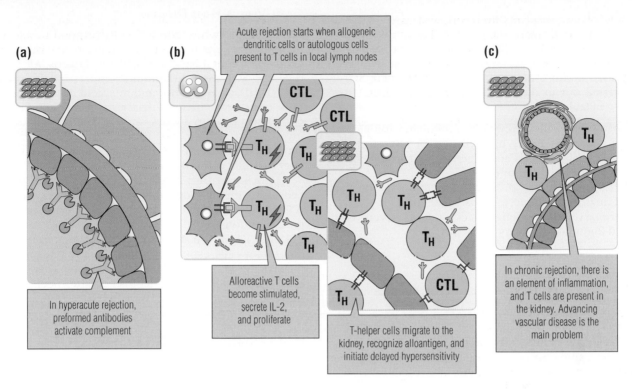

Acute rejection starts when allogeneic dendritic cells or autologous cells present to T cells in local lymph nodes

In hyperacute rejection, preformed antibodies activate complement

Alloreactive T cells become stimulated, secrete IL-2, and proliferate

T-helper cells migrate to the kidney, recognize alloantigen, and initiate delayed hypersensitivity

In chronic rejection, there is an element of inflammation, and T cells are present in the kidney. Advancing vascular disease is the main problem

Figure 33.2 Mechanisms of renal transplant rejection. Hyperacute (**A**) and acute (**B**) solid-organ graft rejection involves different mechanisms. The mechanism of chronic rejection (**C**) is not clear.

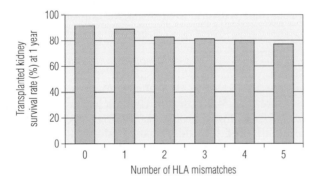

Figure 33.3 The impressive survival rates for mismatched kidneys would not be achievable without potent immunosuppressive drugs.

Chronic Rejection

Chronic rejection takes place months or years after transplant. There is often an element of allogeneic reaction mediated by T cells in chronic rejection, which can result in repeated acute rejection. In some cases, chronic rejection may be caused by recurrence of pre-existing autoimmune disease. In other cases, there is no direct evidence of damage caused by the adaptive immune system.

Tolerance

Tolerance is the state in which, following exposure to an antigen, specific T- and B-cell responses do not occur, although responses to other antigens remain normal (see Chapter 14). In central tolerance, self-reactive T and B cells are destroyed by apoptosis during negative selection in the thymus and bone marrow, respectively (see Chapter 15). In peripheral tolerance, T and B cells may become **anergic**; that is, they are not killed but become unable to respond to stimulation.

A state of tolerance of the foreign organ or cell is the clinical ideal in transplantation. However, tolerance of transplanted solid organs has not been achieved artificially in humans.

Immunosuppressive drugs prevent rejection if given at the time of transplantation, but once the drugs are stopped, rejection still takes place. Immunosuppressive drugs also lack the specificity of true tolerance and thus prevent immune responses to infectious agents. Opportunist infections are a major limit to the use of potent immunosuppressive drugs.

■ STEM CELL TRANSPLANT

In the future, pluripotent stem cells may be used to repair diseased neurologic or cardiac tissue. Currently, hematopoietic stem cells are used to restore myeloid and lymphoid cells in some clinical situations. In autologous stem cell transplant, marrow is removed, frozen, and reinfused after very potent chemotherapy has been given. Autologous transplants carry minimal immunologic risk. Allogeneic stem cell transplant (SCT) is a much riskier procedure than

 MHC II

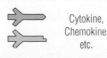 Cytokine, Chemokine, etc.

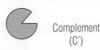 Complement (C′)

 Signaling molecule

most solid-organ transplants. Even with well-matched donors and in the best of circumstances, the mortality can be as high as 20% (Box 33.2). The additional risks are due to graft-versus-host-disease (GVHD), which you will read about later. Because of the high risks, allogeneic SCT is only carried out in dire situations when no other treatment is available:

- Hematologic malignancy: SCT is used after initial treatment if there is a very high chance for relapse. SCT is preceded by potent chemotherapy and irradiation to eradicate residual tumor cells.
- When myeloid cell production is reduced or very abnormal, for example, in aplastic anemia.
- In primary immunodeficiencies, such as severe combined immunodeficiency (SCID).

Source of Stem Cells

Following transplantation, myeloid cells are regenerated from hematopoietic stem cells. These can be obtained from a number of sources.

- Bone marrow is the usual source of stem cells. Harvesting requires aspiration of a considerable amount of donor marrow under general anesthetic.
- Peripheral blood stem cells are usually harvested after treating the donor with colony-stimulating factors to increase the numbers of circulating stem cells.
- Cord blood contains a large number of stem cells, which can be frozen prior to use. An advantage of cord blood is that the immature lymphocytes are less likely to cause GVHD (see later). Cord blood yields only enough stem cells to transplant in children or small adults.

Conditioning

Conditioning consists of high-dose chemotherapy or radiotherapy, which destroy the recipient's own stem cells, allowing donor stem cells to engraft. Apart from creating a physical space in the bone marrow for the donor marrow cells to engraft, it reduces the risk of the recipient immune system rejecting the allogeneic (donor) stem cells.

Graft-Versus-Host Disease

GVHD occurs when donor T cells respond to allogeneic recipient antigens. It occurs when there are mismatches in major or minor histocompatibility antigens. All patients receiving SCT are given immunosuppressive drugs to prevent GVHD, even if donor and recipient are HLA identical. This manoeuvre in itself has risks for infections. Acute GVHD occurs up to 4 weeks after SCT. There is widespread involvement of skin, gut, liver, and lungs; when severe, acute GVHD carries a 70% mortality. Chronic GVHD occurs later and affects the skin and liver.

Removing mature T cells from the source of the stem cells using immunological techniques reduces the risk for GVHD. T-cell depletion, however, increases the risk for graft rejection.

Donor T cells are also capable of reacting against recipient tumor cells, especially when there is a degree of HLA mismatch and mild GVHD is taking place. This beneficial **graft-versus-leukemia** effect is lost after T-cell depletion of stem cell preparations (Fig. 33.4).

■ TISSUE-TYPING TECHNIQUES

Prior to most allogeneic transplants, it is desirable to ensure that the donor and recipient have as closely matched as possible HLA alleles. It is also important to ensure that the donor has no antibodies against recipient cells, tested for using the cross-match procedure. Collectively, these tests carried out prior to allogeneic transplantation are referred to as "tissue typing" and are used to identify donor/recipient pairs with the lowest risk for complications.

HLA Typing

A patient who is being considered for a transplant is tissue-typed to identify HLA alleles. Over several million years, more than 500 different HLA alleles have evolved in humans. Specialized molecular biology techniques are required to precisely define any individual's HLA type (Fig 33.5A). If they have suitable siblings, a family search may be made for a live, related donor. However, any one

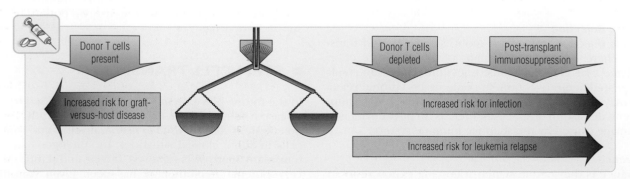

Figure 33.4 T-cell depletion has complex effects on stem cell transplant. The decision on whether or not to deplete T cells rests on the degree of donor matching and the condition being treated.

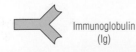 T cell receptor (TCR)

Immunoglobulin (Ig)

 Antigen

MHC I

sibling has only a one in four chance of being HLA-identical. If an identical sibling is found, he/she can act as a donor.

Otherwise, patients requiring solid-organ transplants, such as kidneys, go on a waiting list registry for a cadaveric organ (Fig 33.5B). When an organ becomes available, the donor is HLA-typed, and a search is made in tissue-typing registries for a suitable recipient (Fig 33.5C). Even when organ registries extend across many states or nations, it is possible to wait for many months before a well-matched organ becomes available.

Registries are also used for patients requiring SCT. In this case, registries consist of volunteers who have agreed to be potential donors and have been HLA-typed. Even when these registries include many millions of donors, it is possible that potential recipients will not find an HLA-identical donor.

HLA Cross-Matching

Cross-matching is performed to rule out preformed antibodies against donor HLA, which could cause hyperacute rejection (Fig 33.5D)

These antibodies could be produced by exposure to allogeneic HLA during pregnancy, blood transfusion, or a previous attempt at transplantation, as mentioned earlier. In the cross-match, donor B cells are incubated with recipient serum. Donor B cells are used in the cross-match, because they express HLA class I and class II molecules. The presence of antibodies to donor cells rules out the possibility of transplantation.

■ IMMUNOSUPPRESSIVE DRUGS

Immunosuppressive drugs are required to prevent and/or treat graft rejection and GVHD. The drugs tend to be used in combinations as part of defined regimens. For example, in renal transplant, combinations, such as corticosteroids, cyclosporin, and mycophenolate, may be used from the time of transplant. The exact combination of drugs used varies with the risk for rejection. If there is known to be an incomplete HLA match, a combination containing more potent drugs may be used. Corticosteroids are withdrawn gradually after several weeks and cyclosporin after a few months. Patients may stay on mycophenolate indefinitely. In the event of a rejection episode, stronger drugs may be given. All of these drugs carry the risk for infection as a consequence of immunosuppression. In addition, immunosuppressive drugs increase the risk for developing some tumors, as you will read in the next chapter.

Many of these drugs are also used in the treatment of autoimmune disease, and some familiarity with their modes of action is important (Fig. 33.6).

Corticosteroids

Corticosteroids inhibit synthesis of more than 100 proteins, but at low doses they predominantly act on antigen-presenting cells, preventing some of the early stages of graft rejection. Higher doses of corticosteroids have direct

effects on T cells, and these are used to treat episodes of rejection (see Chapter 30).

T-Cell Signaling Blockade

Cyclosporin and tacrolimus are discussed in Box 11.3. They work by interacting with proteins in the intracellular T-cell signaling cascade. Ciclosporin was the first to be discovered and improved the outcome of all types of transplant dramatically.

Interleukin-2 Blockade

Monoclonal antibodies against the IL-2 receptor can also be given (e.g., basiliximab and daclizumab). These antibodies completely block the most important growth factor for all types of lymphocyte and have very potent immunosuppressive effects. Because they are so potent, they are only used to *treat* episodes of acute graft rejection. Rapamycin is a drug that can be given orally and interacts with signaling events downstream of the IL-2 receptor. Rapamycin is less potent and easier to take than the monoclonal antibodies, so it is used to *prevent* graft rejection.

Antiproliferatives

Azathioprine, mycophenolate mofetil, and methotrexate inhibit DNA production. These drugs prevent lymphocyte proliferation, but they are not specific for T cells, and they can cause myelotoxicity.

■ XENOTRANSPLANTATION

The immunosuppressive drugs described have dramatically improved outcomes for transplantation. However, waiting lists for solid-organ transplants double every 10 years, whereas the number of transplants carried out remained static. This is because there are too few human organs available to meet the needs of patients. Currently, 10 patients die each day in the United States while on the waiting list to receive lifesaving vital organ transplants. Xenotransplants from other species may become an alternative in the future. But, before these provide a reliable source of organs, several problems need to be overcome:

- Primates assemble sugar side-chains different from other species. Galactose-α1,3-galactose (gal-α1,3-gal) is a sugar present on the cells of most nonprimate species. The immune system can recognize gal-α1,3-gal, and all humans possess antibodies against gal-α1,3-gal following exposure to, for example, gut bacteria. Similar **natural antibodies** have been mentioned in Chapter 27. Antibodies against gal-α1,3-gal bind onto xenotransplanted organs, activate complement, and trigger hyperacute rejection.
- Complement inhibitors from other species do not inhibit human complement. As a result of this molecular incompatibility, xenotransplanted organs activate complement (see Chapter 19).

 MHC II

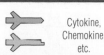 Cytokine, Chemokine, etc.

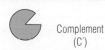 Complement (C')

 Signaling molecule

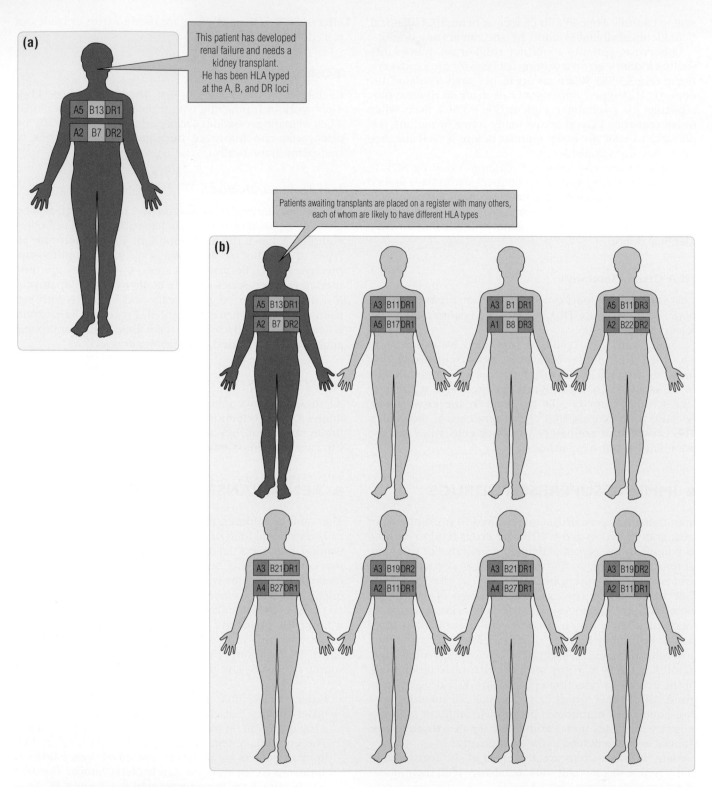

Figure 33.5 Patients requiring kidney transplants are human leukocyte antigen (HLA)-typed (**A**) and then placed on a register (**B**). If a brain-dead donor becomes available, for example, following a traffic accident, the relatives are asked for consent for transplantation. The donor is HLA-typed (**C**), and the organs are removed. The kidney is transported on ice, along with a blood sample, to hospitals where there are potential recipients with good HLA matches. B cells from the donor blood sample are used in a cross-match to detect antibodies against HLA and, potentially, other polymorphic alloantigens.

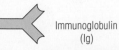 T cell receptor (TCR)

 Immunoglobulin (Ig)

 Antigen

 MHC I

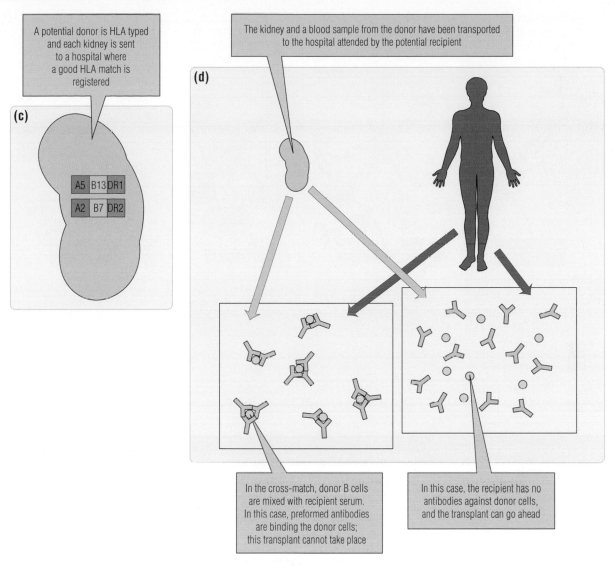

A potential donor is HLA typed and each kidney is sent to a hospital where a good HLA match is registered

The kidney and a blood sample from the donor have been transported to the hospital attended by the potential recipient

(c)

| A5 | B13 | DR1 |
| A2 | B7 | DR2 |

(d)

In the cross-match, donor B cells are mixed with recipient serum. In this case, preformed antibodies are binding the donor cells; this transplant cannot take place

In this case, the recipient has no antibodies against donor cells, and the transplant can go ahead

Figure 33.5 (*cont'd*)

Transgenic pigs are being developed with reduced gal-α1,3-gal expression to prevent natural antibody binding and with human complement inhibitors to bypass molecular incompatibility. Pigs are used because they are a similar size to humans and easy to rear in captivity. Two considerable theoretical problems remain.

• There may be acute rejection, because pig proteins elicit a T-cell response.

• Even pigs reared in microbe-free conditions are infected with endogenous retroviruses; these have never been known to infect humans, but they could do so following transplantation. Pig viruses are more likely to infect recipients taking immunosuppressive drugs.

 MHC II

 Cytokine, Chemokine, etc.

 Complement (C')

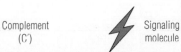 Signaling molecule

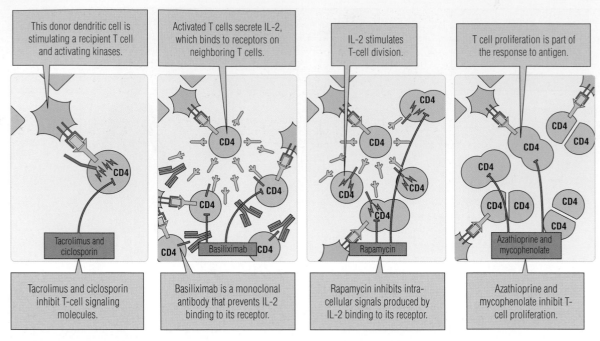

Figure 33.6 This figure illustrates the major immunosuppressive drugs (except corticosteroids). (From Helbert M: The Flesh and Bones of Immunology. London: Mosby, 2006.)

BOX 33.1 Acute Graft Rejection

A 43-year-old woman has polycystic kidney disease, a degenerative condition often leading to irreversible kidney failure. Three years ago her kidney failure became so severe that she started hemodialysis three times a week. She has now been referred to the renal transplant team. She is a good candidate for a transplant because her renal disease is unlikely to recur in a transplanted kidney. She has been HLA-typed, and although she has relatively common HLA alleles, she is told that there may be a long wait for a cadaveric kidney. This is because most kidney transplant schemes aim to match the donor and recipient as closely as possible and only about 1 in 5000 unrelated individuals have identical HLA types.

Live related donors are important in kidney transplantation, provided they are not affected by the same genetic disease! Our patient has three brothers, none of whom are affected by polycystic kidney disease. Because of the long potential wait, the patient's brothers decide to undergo tissue typing, and one of them is found to be an exact HLA and blood group match. The patient's serum did not react with her brother's lymphocytes during cross-match, and following transplantation, there was no evidence of hyperacute rejection. With current technology, it is not possible to match minor histocompatibility antigens, and it is possible that these can trigger graft rejection, even in live, related donors with HLA-matched organs. For this reason, our patient was given post-transplant rejection prophylaxis with ciclosporin, mycophenolate mofetil, and corticosteroids.

The transplant appeared to be going well, but on day eight, the patient started to feel unwell and feverish. On palpation, the transplanted kidney was swollen, and blood tests showed her renal function had deteriorated.

A renal biopsy showed acute rejection as a result of minor antigen mismatch (Fig. 33.7). Initial treatment with high-dose corticosteroids was ineffective. The patient was treated for 5 days with a monoclonal anti-IL-2 receptor antibody, during which time renal function improved, and there were no further episodes of rejection.

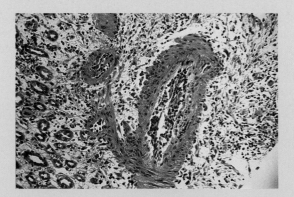

Figure 33.7 This is a biopsy of the kidney transplant described in the clinical box. There is a lymphocytic infiltration in the graft consistent with acute rejection.

 T cell receptor (TCR)   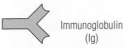 Immunoglobulin (Ig)   Antigen   MHC I

BOX 33.2 Infection Following Stem Cell Transplant

A 36-year-old woman with lymphoma is at high risk for relapse following initial chemotherapy. Neither of her two siblings is HLA-identical. Following an extensive search on a registry, a donor is found. Although the donor is HLA-identical, there is a risk for graft-versus-host disease (GVHD) because of minor antigen incompatibility. Prophylaxis with ciclosporin is used for 6 weeks following stem cell transplant. Fortunately, her lymphoma does not relapse, and she does not develop GVHD. She does, however, have a series of infections.

   Conditioning, GVHD prophylaxis, and stem cell transplant itself cause severe immunosuppression, and infection is the most common cause of death in these patients. Figure 33.8 shows how immune reconstitution takes place and the specific infections likely to occur.

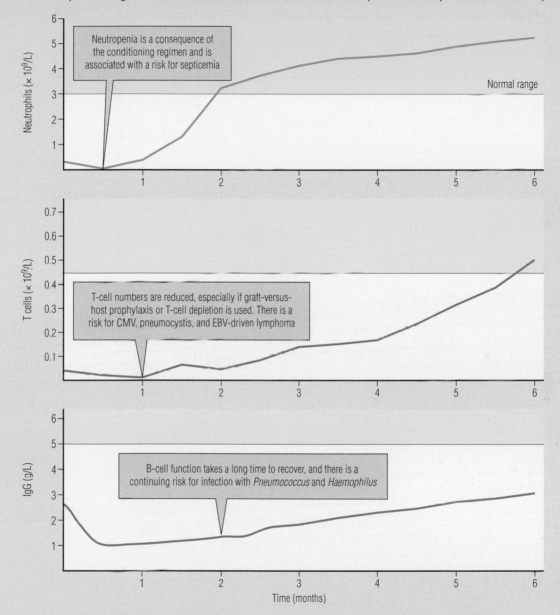

Figure 33.8 Risk of infection following bone marrow transplantation. CMV, cytomegalovirus; EBV, Epstein-Barr virus.

 MHC II

 Cytokine, Chemokine, etc.

 Complement (C')

 Signaling molecule

LEARNING POINTS Can You Now ...

1. List the different types of transplants and the organs that are transplanted?

2. Describe the three phases of rejection of solid organs?

3. Describe the two laboratory procedures designed to reduce the risk for infection?

4. Explain how stem cell transplant differs from solid-organ transplant?

5. List the problems that need to be overcome to make xenotransplantation safe?

 T cell receptor (TCR)

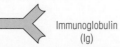 Immunoglobulin (Ig)

 Antigen

 MHC I

34 Tumor Immunology

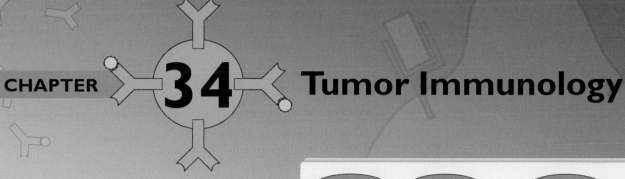

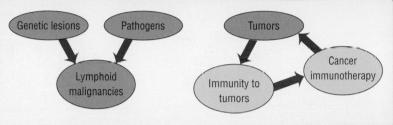

In this chapter, you will read about the two main strands of tumor immunology. You will read about how genetic events and interactions with pathogens lead to tumors of lymphoid cells themselves, and you will read how the immune system can respond to tumors and how this knowledge is being turned into new tumor immunotherapies.

■ LYMPHOID TUMORS

The malignancies affecting the adaptive immune system originate from a single lymphocyte or plasma cell. Each cell of the malignant population has undergone identical immune receptor gene rearrangements and expresses identical immunoglobulin or T-cell receptor molecules. The identical nature of the cells is referred to as **monoclonality**.

The cellular origins of lymphoid malignancy are shown in Figure 34.1 and the characteristics of tumor cells in Figure 34.2. The characteristics of each type of tumor are dictated by the biology of the originating cell. For example, acute lymphoblastic leukemia (ALL) is derived from rapidly dividing pre–B cells and is extremely aggressive. Untreated ALL can kill within weeks of diagnosis. Myeloma is derived from mature, slow-growing plasma cells, which secrete monoclonal immunoglobulin. Myeloma patients can survive for years without treatment.

Because cells from lymphoid malignancies are easy to remove and grow in vitro, we know a lot about how they arise. This is usually the result of oncogene activation by chromosomal translocations or the effects of pathogens.

Oncogenesis

Chromosomal Translocations
During immune-receptor gene recombination, chromosomal breaks may not be correctly repaired. In B cells, chromosomal breaks can also occur during class switching. Occasionally, segments of different chromosomes are brought together. This will often have lethal consequences for the lymphocyte. However, some rare chromosomal translocations have positive effects on cell survival. This may happen because translocation of an oncogene with an immunoglobulin gene promoter or enhancer may result in permanent activation of the oncogene.

In lymphoma, the oncogenes c-*myc* (chromosome 8) and *bcl-2* (chromosome 18) are commonly translocated to the immunoglobulin heavy chain gene on chromosome 14. Activated c-*myc* stimulates lymphocyte proliferation. In normal lymphocytes, proliferation is always balanced by apoptosis. Activated Bcl-2 protein protects against apoptosis, and this allows unrestrained proliferation of lymphocytes.

Oncogene translocations are more likely to occur after exposure to radiation. Myeloma was common in survivors of the Hiroshima atomic bombings.

Pathogens
Herpesvirus family members and retroviruses infect cells without killing them. It is in the interest of viruses to stimulate uncontrolled growth of these infected cells.

Epstein-Barr virus (EBV) causes infectious mononucleosis/glandular fever (see Chapter 15), lymphoma, and nasopharyngeal carcinoma. Unlike many other viruses, EBV does not convert the cellular machinery to virus production and destruction of the cell (see Box 15.4). Instead, EBV immortalizes cells by producing proteins that drive B-cell proliferation and inhibit apoptosis. EBV proteins also help infected cells to evade the immune response by blocking proteosome-mediated antigen degradation.

EBV causes lymphoma, particularly in two situations. In regions where malaria is endemic, Burkitt's lymphoma occurs in up to 1 in 1000 children. Burkitt's lymphoma is a consequence of polyclonal activation of B cells by both

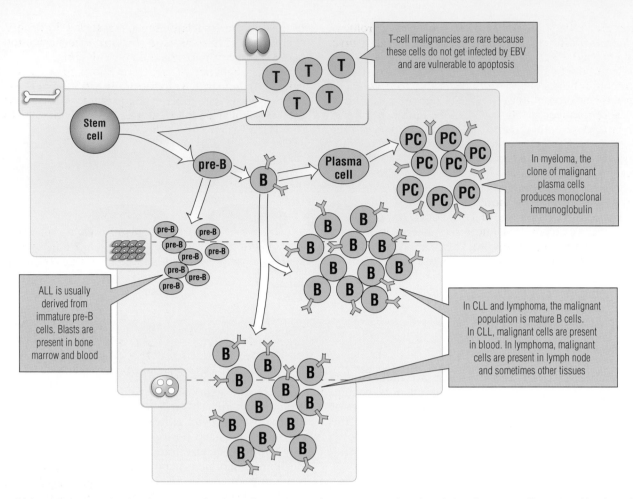

Figure 34.1 Origins of lymphoid malignancies. Clonal populations arise in bone marrow or lymph node but they may spill over into blood or other tissues. ALL, acute lymphoblastic leukemia; CLL, chronic lymphocytic leukemia; EBV, Epstein-Barr virus.

FIG. 34.2 Lymphoid Malignancies and Their Characteristics

Malignancy	Cell Type	Special Characteristics	Diagnosis
Acute lymphoblastic leukemia (ALL)	Immature pre–B cells or B cells	Rare. Affects young people. Aggressive disease with replacement of bone marrow and invasion of tissues (e.g., brain)	Characteristic cells on examination of blood or marrow. Flow cytometry may be required to distinguish ALL from acute myeloid leukemia.
Chronic lymphocytic leukemia (CLL)	Mature B cells	Relatively common in the elderly. May be very nonaggressive	Lymphocytosis on blood film. CLL lymphocytes express characteristic surface molecules detected by flow cytometry.
Lymphoma	Mature B cells	Frequently associated with EBV or infection and chromosomal translocation. Tend to cause solid lesions, often beginning in lymph nodes or mucosa associated lymphoid tissue	Biopsy of affected tissue. Heavy-chain rearrangement (Box 6.1). Chromosomal analysis
Multiple myeloma	Plasma cells	Relatively common in the elderly	Detection of monoclonal immunoglobulin in blood or light chains in urine. Presence of plasma cells in marrow and osteolytic lesion on radiograph
T-cell malignancy	T cells	Rare. May be caused by HTLVI infection	Can behave either as leukemia (with blood involvement) or lymphoma (with solid-tissue involvement)

 T cell receptor (TCR)

 Immunoglobulin (Ig)

Antigen

 MHC I

malaria and EBV. The marked polyclonal B-cell prolifera-tion increases the risk for translocations involving *myc*, leading to the growth of a malignant population.

In immunodeficient patients, the normal response to EBV-infected B cells is lost, and EBV is able to drive B-cell growth. B-cell proliferation is initially polyclonal and pre-sents as a prolonged glandular fever-like illness with fever and lymphadenopathy. Translocations involving *myc* then occur and promote the growth of a malignant monoclonal population. Infection with another herpes virus, human herpes virus 8 (HHV8), can cause Kaposi's sarcoma in immunodeficient individuals.

Helicobacter pylori is another organism that can con-tribute to the development of lymphoma. *H. pylori* is a bacterium that triggers chronic inflammation in the sto-mach. This commonly causes stomach ulcers. More rarely, the inflammation caused by *H. pylori* causes lymphomas

to arise in the associated mucosa-associated lymphoid tis-sue. Importantly, treatment of the *H. pylori* infection can lead to the lymphoma going into remission.

T-cell malignancy is rare, but when it occurs, it is often caused by human T lymphotrophic virus 1 (HTLV1). This is a retrovirus that encodes Tax protein, which has effects that are similar to interleukin-2 (IL-2) (T-cell growth fac-tor). HTLV1 is rare in the developed world.

Cancers are usually a consequence of at least two events affecting gene expression. Figure 34.3 illustrates this principle.

Diagnosing Lymphoid Malignancy

In some types of lymphoid malignancy, abnormal cells can be recognized by their appearance. For example, in acute leukemia, the presence of high numbers of very immature

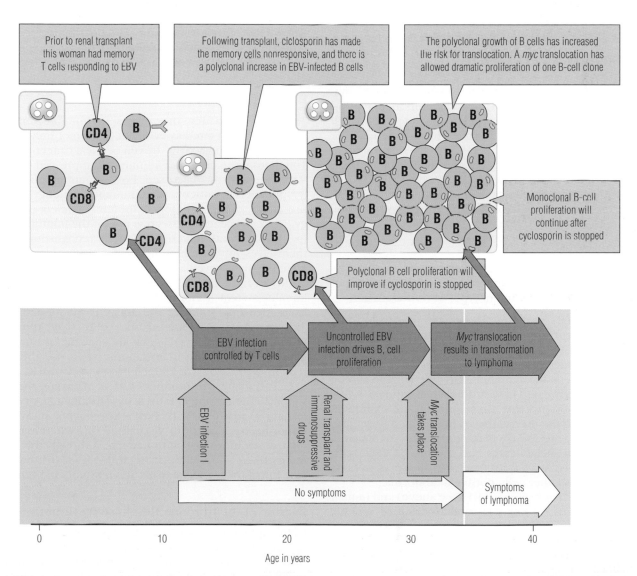

Figure 34.3 A sequence of events is usually required in oncogenesis. In this case, Epstein-Barr virus infection, post-transplant immunosuppression, and then a gene translocation lead to monoclonal B-cell proliferation. Compare this to the multistage process required for autoimmune disease (see Fig. 27.4).

 MHC II   Cytokine, Chemokine, etc.   Complement (C')   Signaling molecule

cells ("**blasts**") in the blood and marrow is diagnostic. Flow cytometry may then be used to distinguish between acute myeloid leukemia (AML) arising from neutrophil precursors and acute lymphoblastic leukemia (ALL) arising from immature B-cell precursors.

In other situations, the malignant cells look very similar to their normal counterparts. For example, in chronic lymphocytic leukemia (CLL), the abnormal cells look very similar to normal, mature lymphocytes. As described in the first clinical box (Box 34.1), flow cytometry can be used to show the presence of abnormal molecules on the surface of the leukemia cells.

Malignancy of plasma cells (myeloma) is a special case. In the second clinical box in this chapter (Box 34.2) you will read how the monoclonal immunoglobulin secreted by these cells acts as a marker of malignancy. In the case of B-cell lymphoma, immunoglobulin is not necessarily secreted. In this case, monoclonality can be determined using molecular techniques that assess heavy chain gene rearrangement (see Box 6.1).

■ IMMUNITY TO TUMORS

We have discussed how cells of the adaptive immune system may give rise to tumors. However, components of the immune system may also recognize and, sometimes, kill malignancies arising in other tissues. This is potentially of great importance, because it has been hoped that immunotherapy would offer hope to patients with cancer, most types of which remain incurable. To understand this, it is important to know how malignant cells may become antigenic or, in other words, express **tumor antigens**.

Tumor Antigens

Tumor antigens are molecules produced by tumor cells that can potentially be recognized by the immune system. There are a number of different types of tumor antigen.

- Developmental proteins. These are normally only transiently expressed during development but may be re-expressed by tumor cells. For example, carcinoembryonic antigen is normally expressed on many tissues during fetal life. Carcinoembryonic antigen can be abnormally expressed in gastrointestinal cancer.
- Lineage-specific proteins. These proteins are expressed in cancers and the normal tissues from which they arise. For example, melanoma is a skin cancer of melanocytes. Normal melanocytes and melanoma cells both express the enzyme tyrosinase. Tyrosinase is not expressed in any other cells, normal or abnormal.
- Viral proteins. For example, EBV (see above) and human papilloma virus (in cervical cancer) produce specific proteins.
- Proteins produced through translocations. For example, the Bcr-Abl fusion protein is the product of the *bcr/abl* translocation.

Developmental and lineage-specific proteins are poorly immunogenic because they are expressed on normal tissues. T cells with receptors capable of recognizing these proteins are deleted through tolerance induction. The same system that protects from autoimmunity thus impairs tumor recognition by the immune system. For example, carcinoembryonic antigen present in colon cancer does not elicit a strong immune response. Nonetheless, tests to detect carcinoembryonic antigen are sometimes used to screen for this type of cancer.

Viral and fusion proteins tend to be more immunogenic because they are never present in the normal individual. Each of these has been investigated for its possible clinical role in diagnosing, preventing, and treating cancer.

The greatest victory so far in preventing tumors is an indirect one. In some parts of the world, the risk for hepatoma caused by hepatitis B virus has been dramatically reduced following the introduction of hepatitis B vaccine. There are hopes that new vaccines based on papilloma virus and EBV antigens will decrease the incidence of cervical cancer and lymphoma.

Immunotherapy for cancer remains experimental. Knowledge of tumor immunity and how tumors evade the immune system is necessary to understand the problems immunologists face in developing useful therapy for cancer.

Evidence for Tumor Immunity

The high frequency of cancers in immunosuppressed patients is often cited as evidence for tumor immunity, for example, papilloma virus–driven cervical cancer (which is 100 times more common in immunosuppressed patients). We have already discussed how common EBV–driven lymphoma is in patients with immunodeficiency. The high prevalence of these tumors in immunodeficient patients is evidence of the more effective role of the immune system in clearing viral infection than in recognizing tumors themselves. Immune surveillance for viruses is much more effective than surveillance for cancers.

However, there is also good evidence that the human immune system attempts to eradicate other types of tumor by recognizing some of the antigens mentioned earlier. Most research has focused on T cells (e.g., tumor-infiltrating lymphocytes [TIL]) that are specific for tumor antigens (e.g., tyrosinase in melanoma). TILs use their T-cell receptors to recognize antigen presented by MHC.

Occasionally, the immune system damages the blood supply to tumors and kills them by starving them of oxygen, leading to necrosis. Very early experiments showed that tumor necrosis factor (TNF) can do this when injected at high doses into mice with cancers. Although this is how the cytokine's full name arose, it is not clear how important any of these mechanisms are in tumors in humans.

Evasion of the Immune Response By Tumors

Unlike infections, tumors very rarely produce danger signals and do not directly activate the innate immune system through Toll-like receptors or other pattern-recognition molecules. Apart from natural-killer cells (see later), this means that the innate immune system does not usually attempt to kill tumor cells or alert the adaptive immune

 T cell receptor (TCR)

 Immunoglobulin (Ig)

 Antigen

⊢⊣ MHC I

response to the presence of danger. This can lead to T-cell anergy—failure to respond to antigen.

Some tumors evade the adaptive immune system by decreasing expression of MHC and losing the ability to present antigen to T cells. Mutations in the MHC genes themselves are not unusual in these tumors. Cells expressing low levels of MHC make excellent targets for killing by natural-killer cells, which may act as a back-up system in this situation.

In most tumors, the malignant cells successfully evade the immune response using various mechanisms (Fig. 34.4). Rapidly dividing malignant cells may mutate and acquire one or more of these evasion mechanisms. This will give this clone of cells an advantage over nonmutated cells.

Immunotherapy

Attempts at using immunotherapy have been based on the idea that the immune system could eradicate existing tumors. Many approaches at tumor immunotherapy have been attempted, and most have failed. We only mention some of the immunotherapy approaches that have been of some success. Although most tumor-immunity research has focused on T cells, two of the most successful drugs developed to date are monoclonal antibodies.

Passive Cancer Immunotherapy

Passive cancer immunotherapy relies on the use of monoclonal antibodies to destroy malignant cells. At the time of this writing, two different sets of monoclonal antibody have achieved widespread use for cancer immunotherapy. Anti-CD20 is a monoclonal antibody with a variety of uses in oncology. CD20 is expressed on normal B cells and on lymphoma cells. Infusion of anti-CD20 can reduce or cure up to 50% of B-cell lymphomas. Anti-CD20 destroys malignant B cells by activating antibody-dependent complement and cell-mediated cytotoxicity. Anti-CD20 also triggers B-cell signaling, which induces apoptosis. Anti-CD20 has been engineered in a number of ways (see Chapter 35). Anti-CD20 molecules have been conjugated to radioiodine to deliver high doses of radioactivity directly to the site of the tumor. Antibodies such as CD20 against normal antigens will damage normal cells, in this case nonmalignant B cells. Radiolabeled anti-CD20 can also be used to determine the spread of lymphoma in the body.

The second important monoclonal antibody used for cancer chemotherapy is trastuzumab (Herceptin™). Trastuzumab is a humanized monoclonal antibody that is specific for a cell-surface molecule called HER-2. HER-2 is the human epidermal growth factor receptor 2 and is essential for initiating and maintaining tumor growth and progression in about 30% of breast cancers. Breast cancer cells from these cases show much higher levels of HER-2 expression than is ever found in normal tissues, making this molecule an ideal target for a monoclonal antibody.

Trastuzumab binds to and inactivates the HER-2 molecule, thus inhibiting tumor cell growth. Furthermore, trastuzumab activates antibody-dependent cellular cytotoxicity by natural-killer cells and macrophages. These combined mechanisms are very effective, at least in patients whose tumors express the HER-2 receptor. In these cases, trastuzumab can induce remission in up to 30% of patients who have already relapsed on conventional chemotherapy.

Active Cancer Immunotherapy

Active immunotherapy aims to overcome the anergy of T cells. Anergy could develop if a tumor cell presents antigen to a T-helper cell without the necessary costimulatory molecules.

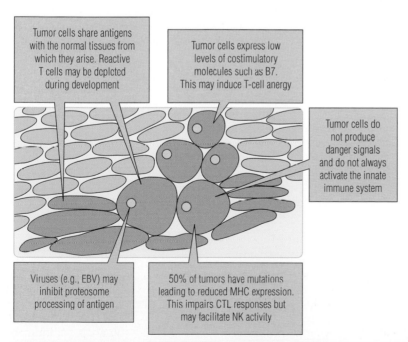

Tumor cells share antigens with the normal tissues from which they arise. Reactive T cells may be depleted during development

Tumor cells express low levels of costimulatory molecules such as B7. This may induce T-cell anergy

Tumor cells do not produce danger signals and do not always activate the innate immune system

Viruses (e.g., EBV) may inhibit proteosome processing of antigen

50% of tumors have mutations leading to reduced MHC expression. This impairs CTL responses but may facilitate NK activity

Figure 34.4 Malignant cells use various mechanisms to evade the immune system. Compare these with some of the mechanisms used by viruses (discussed in Chapters 21, 22, and 23). CTL, cytotoxic T lymphocytes; EBV, Epstein-Barr virus; NK, natural killer.

 MHC II

 Cytokine, Chemokine, etc.

 Complement (C')

Signaling molecule

One way of providing costimulatory signals is to use Toll-like receptor ligands. Unmethylated cytosine and guanosine sequences (CpG motifs) bind to TLR9, and imiquimod, a synthetic drug that mimics single-stranded RNA, binds TLR7. These drugs provide a danger signal for the innate immune system, which subsequently activates the adaptive immune system. As mentioned in Box 20.2 in Chapter 20, there are drugs that have been shown to be successful in the treatment of some tumors.

Another way of providing costimulation is to infuse the patient with cytokines. IL-2 treatment activates T cells (and natural-killer cells) directly. Unfortunately, IL-2 is pleiotropic and has many different effects on the immune system. High-dose IL-2 causes severe side effects, the most dreaded of which is the capillary leak syndrome, in which fluid shifts to the extravascular space, causing edema and hypotension.

Systemic use of interferon (IFN), both IFN-α and IFN-β, increases MHC class I expression, enabling improved tumor antigen presentation. IFNs also have direct antiproliferative effects on tumor cells, although systemic use of these cytokines also causes side effects.

BOX 34.1 Chronic Lymphocytic Leukemia

An elderly man presents with unusually severe shingles (herpes zoster infection), suggesting a mild secondary immunodeficiency state. On examination, he has generalized lymphadenopathy. These clinical features are consistent with chronic lymphocytic leukemia or lymphoma. Laboratory testing shows a raised lymphocyte count (5.6×10^6/mL when the normal range is 1.5–3.0×10^6/mL). As an approximating guide, in a normal blood film, the numbers of neutrophils visible should exceed the number of lymphocytes. In the blood film in the figure, although six lymphocytes are visible, there are no neutrophils. The lymphocytes have normal morphology, without any features enabling the diagnosis of leukemia of lymphoma to be diagnosed (Fig. 34.5). Flow cytometry was carried out to characterize the molecules on the surface of the abnormal cells. Figure 34.6 shows that the lymphocytes were abnormal B cells expressing the CD5 molecule. The shingles was caused by immunodeficiency secondary to B-cell chronic lymphocytic leukemia.

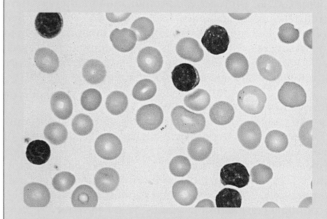

Figure 34.5 This blood sample shows a striking lymphocytosis.

Continued

 T cell receptor (TCR)

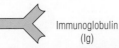 Immunoglobulin (Ig)

 Antigen

 MHC I

BOX 34.1   Chronic Lymphocytic Leukemia—cont'd

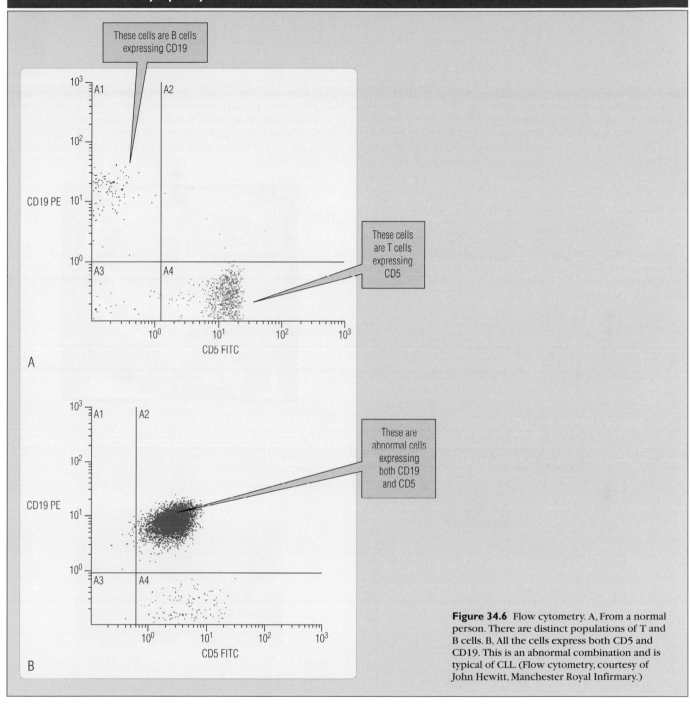

Figure 34.6 Flow cytometry. A, From a normal person. There are distinct populations of T and B cells. B, All the cells express both CD5 and CD19. This is an abnormal combination and is typical of CLL. (Flow cytometry, courtesy of John Hewitt, Manchester Royal Infirmary.)

 MHC II

 Cytokine, Chemokine, etc.

Complement (C')

 Signaling molecule

BOX 34.2 Myeloma

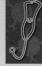

A woman presents with fatigue and bone pain. Electrophoresis showed a band in the serum (Fig. 34.7) that represented mono-clonal IgGk in the serum. There are also free k light chains in the urine-referred to as **Bence Jones protein**. The presence of serum monoclonal immunoglobulin and urinary monoclonal light chains with lytic bone lesions confirms the diagnosis of myeloma.

A series of radiographs are done, and they show she has multiple lytic bone lesions (Fig. 34.8). Additionally, a bone-marrow aspirate is taken and confirms the presence of excessive numbers of plasma cells in the bone marrow (Fig. 34.9).

Monoclonal immunoglobulins can be produced in response to some infections, and they are seen in some healthy elderly people: so-called **monoclonal gammopathy of uncertain significance** (MGUS). However, monoclonal immunoglobulin is also produced by malignant plasma cells in myeloma, in which case the number of marrow plasma cells is dramatically increased. Bone destruction (osteo-lytic lesions) is seen in some patients with myeloma but never in MGUS, which helps to distinguish the two conditions.

The patient was started on cytotoxic chemotherapy for her myeloma, and initially she made a good response. However, she developed *Haemophilus* pneumonia, a consequence of her secondary antibody deficiency, and died.

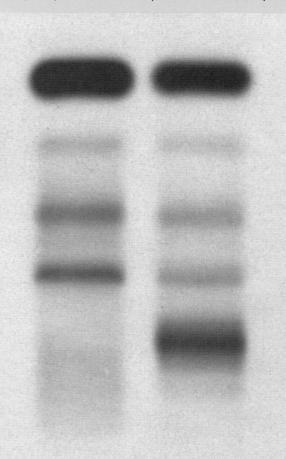

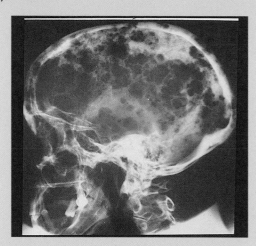

Figure 34.8 A skeletal survey showed that this patient had multiple lytic lesions. Hypercalcemia occurs as a result of increased bone resorption and contributes to renal failure. (With permission from the Department of Medical Illustration, St. Bartholomew's Hospital, London.)

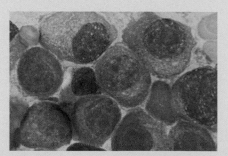

Figure 34.9 This figure shows a bone marrow aspirate from the patient in the box. All the cells in this field are plasma cells, secreting the monoclonal immunoglobulin seen in Figure 34.6.

Figure 34.7 The serum electrophoresis strip on the *left* is from a normal control. The strip on the *right* shows a band in the γ region, reflecting a monoclonal immunoglobulin. Compare with Figure 4.4. (Electrophoresis courtesy of Karen Sneade, Manchester Royal Infirmary.)

 T cell receptor (TCR)

 Immunoglobulin (Ig)

 Antigen

 MHC I

LEARNING POINTS Can You Now ...

1. Describe the different lymphoid malignancies?
2. List the techniques used to diagnose lymphoid malignancies?
3. Explain how host and viral oncogenes interact to cause cancer?
4. Describe the different types of tumor antigen and explain how tumors evade the immune response?

5. List several approaches to cancer immunotherapy?
6. Describe two different examples of therapeutic monoclonal antibodies used to treat malignancies?

 MHC II

 Cytokine, Chemokine, etc.

 Complement (C')

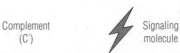 Signaling molecule

35 Monoclonal Antibodies and Recombinant Cytokines

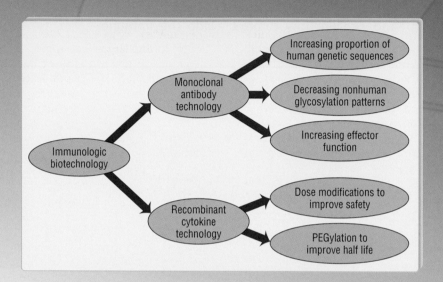

Monoclonal antibodies (mAbs) and recombinant cytokines are increasingly being used to treat patients (use is doubling every 4 years currently). In this chapter, you will learn about some of the ways that biotechnology is being used to improve mAbs and cytokines for use in clinical medicine (see overview figure above). Our enhanced understanding of biotechnology has been used to improve mAbs, for example, by reducing the amount of murine genetic sequence and increasing the amount of human genetic sequence while preserving the original specificity of the mAb ("humanized" mAbs). Genetic approaches have also been used to alter the oligosaccharide side chains of mAbs to make them less "murine-like" and less likely to react with anticarbohydrate antibodies that recognize species-specific differences (see Chapter 33).

Recombinant cytokines have also been altered by derivatization with polyethylene glycol (PEG) to make them less likely to induce anticytokine antibodies and to increase their half-life in serum. This chapter will aid in review of some material presented in Chapters 4 and 5 and illustrates some practical uses of biotechnology applied to immunology for clinical medicine.

■ MONOCLONAL ANTIBODIES

Two key regions of antibodies have made them attractive molecules for biotechnologists to develop as drugs (Fig. 35.1):

- The Fab region (see Chapter 4) of any given antibody confers specificity for antigen and could act as a "magic bullet," directing its effects against pathogens or tumor cells. This specificity results in predictable therapeutic effects and reduced side effects, compared to other drugs, which cannot be directed to specific target cells.
- The Fc region of antibody is the effector region. For IgG, the physiologic effects of the Fc region include activation of the complement cascade and of macrophages, natural killer (NK), and mast cells. The Fc region can also be altered to deliver drugs and toxins to specific cells.

Historical Approaches to Antibody Therapy

During the past 100 years, various biotechnologic approaches to antibody treatments have been tried (Fig. 35.2). Animal polyclonal immunoglobulin, given as injections of serum, was previously used to treat infections and to neutralize snake venom (antivenom). Horse serum was frequently used, but frequently induced antihorse antibodies, which formed immune complexes with the horse proteins. The circulating immune complexes trigger a type III hypersensitivity reaction, leading to serum sickness (see Chapter 29).

Polyclonal human immunoglobulin is sometimes given as a form of passive immunity. You have already read how antirabies virus immunoglobulin is used to protect people exposed to this virus (see Chapter 4) and immunoglobulin replacement therapy is given to patients with antibody deficiency (see Chapter 31). Anti-D immunoglobulin is given to rhesus-negative women pregnant with rhesus-positive fetuses, to prevent hemolytic disease of the newborn (see Chapter 28). However, obtaining large quantities of human immunoglobulin from donors is expensive and always carries a risk for transmitting blood-borne infection. Additionally, because human volunteers cannot be deliberately immunized with infectious agents or with tumor cells, the scope of therapeutic antibodies available from human sources is limited.

Monoclonal Antibody Technologies

Mouse monoclonal antibodies (murine mAbs) were invented in 1975 with the specific aim of developing large quantities of very specific antibody that could be given cheaply and safely. Murine mAbs also have the advantage that they can be raised against antigens that could not be used to deliberately immunize humans, for example, dangerous pathogens or tumor cells.

The conventional approach to making murine mAbs has been to fuse spleen cells from immunized mice with mouse myeloma cells (see Box 4.3). This leads to production of high levels of murine mAb. The development of *in vitro* diagnostic procedures, such as flow cytometry and enzyme-linked immunosorbent assay (ELISA), both described in Chapter 5, would not have been possible before murine mAbs with very well-defined specificities, high affinity, and purity became available.

Murine mAbs have mouse Fc regions and do not always interact well *in vivo* with human complement molecules or Fc receptors on human macrophages and NK cells. In addition, when murine mAbs are used in vivo, they invoke the production of antimouse antibodies. These antimouse antibodies can recognize the unique oligosaccharide side chains expressed on mouse proteins or the amino acid sequence of the constant regions of the mouse immunoglobulin chains. Antimouse antibodies can cause immune complex disease (IgG antimouse antibodies; see Chapter 29) or anaphylaxis (IgE; see Chapter 26). Antimouse IgG antibodies also neutralize the effects of the murine mAb and are produced in about 40% of patients. To overcome these problems, several approaches have been used to increase the proportion of human genetic sequences used in manufacturing mAbs (Fig. 35.3).

1. **Chimeric mAbs** use mouse immunoglobulin variable region gene sequences (derived from immunized mice) and human constant region gene sequences, both cloned into mammalian cells, which then express a chimeric immunoglobulin molecule. Chimeric mAbs contain only about 30% mouse amino acid sequence but still tend to elicit antibodies when used therapeutically.
2. **Humanized mAbs** use a technique similar to chimeric antibodies, but only the mouse hypervariable region gene sequence is used. Only about 10% of the amino acids are derived from mouse sequences.
3. **Transgenic mice** can be manufactured to make human-like mAbs. At least two strains of mice have been created by knocking out mouse constant region genes and inserting synthetic minichromosomes containing human heavy-chain and γ and λ light-chain loci. After immunization, these mice process the human genes almost exactly as you have read in Chapter 6, leading to the synthesis of human-like antibodies.
4. A very different technique is to avoid immunizing an animal altogether and to use **phage libraries**. These are libraries of random and slightly differing V_H and V_L

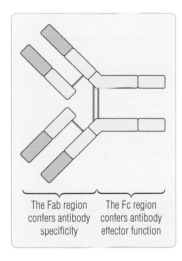

The Fab region confers antibody specificity

The Fc region confers antibody effector function

Figure 35.1 You can use this opportunity to review what you learned about immunoglobulin structure in Chapter 4.

FIG. 35.2 Types of Therapeutic Antibody Currently Available

Source	Example	Problems
Horse serum	Antivenom, Infections	Antihorse antibodies leading to serum sickness
Human immunoglobulin	Used in antibody deficiency, infection prevention, and prevention of hemolytic disease in newborns	Expense, risk of infection, cannot deliberately immunize humans
Mouse monoclonal antibodies	Extensively used in vitro, increasingly used in vivo to treat cancer, inflammation, transplant rejection, and in many other situations	Antimouse antibodies leading to loss of efficacy
Humanized and chimeric monoclonal antibodies		Decreased risk of antimouse antibodies
Monoclonal antibody derived from phage libraries or transgenic mice		Low risk of antimouse antibodies

 MHC II    Cytokine, Chemokine, etc.   Complement (C')   Signaling molecule

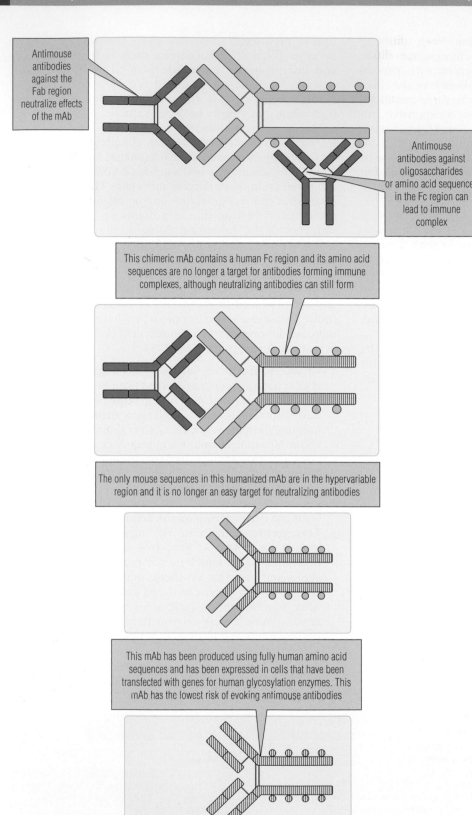

Antimouse antibodies against the Fab region neutralize effects of the mAb

Antimouse antibodies against oligosaccharides or amino acid sequences in the Fc region can lead to immune complex

This chimeric mAb contains a human Fc region and its amino acid sequences are no longer a target for antibodies forming immune complexes, although neutralizing antibodies can still form

The only mouse sequences in this humanized mAb are in the hypervariable region and it is no longer an easy target for neutralizing antibodies

This mAb has been produced using fully human amino acid sequences and has been expressed in cells that have been transfected with genes for human glycosylation enzymes. This mAb has the lowest risk of evoking antimouse antibodies

Figure 35.3 This figure shows modifications aimed at reducing the risk of antimouse antibodies being produced against mAbs. The small circles represent oligosaccharide molecules on the surface of the immunoglobulin.

 T cell receptor (TCR)   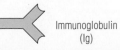 Immunoglobulin (Ig)   Antigen   MHC I genes expressed in bacteriophages. Many different phages can be produced, each of which express different variable region molecules. These can be screened for binding to the antigen of interest and then cloned into a mammalian cell (along with constant–region genes) for expression.

New genetic sequences produced by chimeric, humanized, transgenic, or phage library techniques can be expressed in different ways. The oldest technology relies on growing large quantities of hybridoma cells in vats. This was a low-yield technology, and the cost of mAbs produced in this way has prevented the widespread use of mAbs in some parts of the world. A new high-yield approach is to manufacture transgenic animals that express the mAb in breast milk. The mAb-containing milk can be collected in a dairy and then purified at reduced cost. Plants have also been transfected with genes to produce high levels of mAbs and may provide low-cost mAbs in the future.

These technologies have been used to develop mAbs with human-like amino acid sequences and reduce the risk of evoking antimouse responses. A further complication is provided by the differences in glycosylation of immunoglobulin produced in human and nonhuman cells. Glycosylation refers to the addition of oligosaccharide side chains to proteins. The structure of these side chains has species specificity due to species-specific enzymes involved in their synthesis. In Chapter 33, you learned how different mammals have different glycosylation patterns and antibodies can recognize these. When mAbs are expressed in nonhuman cells, there is a tendency for them to be recognized by anticarbohydrate antibodies.

Increasing the Effects of Monoclonal Antibodies

The technology described so far has been used to produce mAbs that elicit fewer problematic immune responses in humans. In many cases, these simple antibodies are very effective. For example, mAbs that block the effects of cytokines have already been widely used. These include antitumor necrosis factor mAbs used in rheumatoid arthritis (see Chapter 30) and anti interleukin-2 receptor mAbs used to treat transplant rejection (see Chapter 33).

However, in cancer immunotherapy, only a minority of mAbs tested so far have been effective at killing target cells through complement activation and ADCC. These include the anti-CD20 and anti-HER-2 mAbs mentioned in Chapter 34. In most other cancers, simple mAbs do not deliver potent enough effects. Various approaches have been used to increase the effects of mAbs, which we illustrate here with cancer immunotherapy (Fig. 35.4):

Bispecific Antibodies

These combine the specificities of two different antibodies. In the case of cancer immunotherapy, these have been manufactured against the T-cell receptor on cytotoxic T cells (CTLs) and target antigens on tumor cells. The bispecific antibody brings the CTL and target cell together and activates the CTL to initiate cell killing.

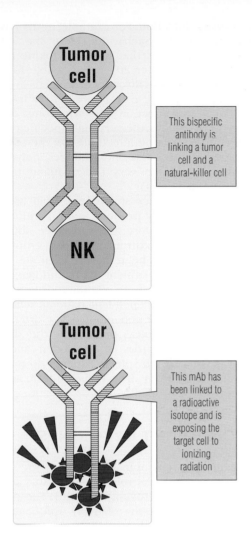

Figure 35.4 This figure shows how modifications to the Fc region of mAbs can enhance effector function.

Conjugates

mAbs can be combined with substances that would otherwise be too toxic when administered at higher concentration alone. For example, mAbs can be conjugated to toxins or radioactive isotopes to deliver them to the target cells. Conjugation thus increases the specificity of the toxin or isotope for the target cells.

Some Successes and Failures in mAb Therapy

mAbs have already gained an important place in the treatment of several common diseases (Fig 35.5). It is interesting that mAbs are beginning to provide useful therapy in cancer, where there is little evidence that antibodies are part of the normal human immune response to cancer. On the other hand, although antibody has a very clear role in the physiologic defense against infection, mAbs have so far proved to be rather unsuccessful. Much research has been carried out on using passive immunotherapy with

 MHC II   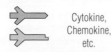 Cytokine, Chemokine, etc.   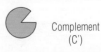 Complement (C')   Signaling molecule

mAbs to combat infection. For example, mAbs have been raised against lipopolysacharide (LPS), the substance released from organisms that trigger cytokine release in septic shock (see Chapter 20). It is possible to produce mAbs against LPS, but the diversity of antigens in wild-type organisms means that these mAbs are not always effective in a strain causing infection and symptoms. Similar to other types of pathogens, the very high specificity of mAbs limits their use in treating infections. On the other hand, active immunity using vaccines induces polyclonal responses that have been very successful at preventing infection (see Chapter 24).

mAbs have been successful in one final area where humans do not normally produce helpful antibodies; the treatment of drug overdose and substance abuse. Some drugs, for example, digoxin are very dangerous in overdose but cannot easily be removed from the body by conventional means. Treatment with antidigoxin mAbs leads to rapid clearance of the offending drug. mAbs have also been used in drug-dependent patients who wish to reduce or eliminate their dependence. The drug and mAb form an immune complex, preventing the drug from reaching specific receptors in the brain and instead directing the drug to the spleen. Patients do not receive the normal reward from drug consumption, and hence dependency can be broken.

■ RECOMBINANT CYTOKINES

Most research on recombinant immunologic cytokines has been on the potential role of stimulatory or growth factor cytokines on improving immunity. The two major immunologic cytokines in relatively frequent use are interferon-α (IFN-α) and IL-2.

Interferon-α

IFN-α is used to treat some forms of viral hepatitis. Treatment needs to be continued for up to a year to be successful. IFN-α induces a mild acute-phase response, and this makes most patients feel slightly unwell during treatment. Some patients produce anti-IFN-α which neutralize the effects of the treatment. The major problem has been

the cost of treatment, up to $15,000 per year. This cost is at least in part attributable to the very short, 4-hour half-life of IFN-α, which means that infusions have to be given on a daily basis.

Some of these problems can be overcome by adding polyethylene glycol (PEG) molecules to the IFN-α structure. During so-called PEGylation, PEG molecules are covalently joined onto the IFN-α molecule. This increases the half-life of the molecule by increasing its molecular weight so that it is not filtered at the kidney. PEGylation also effectively surrounds the IFN-α molecule so that it is not digested by proteases (Fig. 35.6). Together, these effects increase the half-life to 40 hours, meaning treatment can be given weekly in stead of daily. PEGylation also protects the IFN-α molecule from the patient's immune system and reduces the risk for inducing anti- IFN-α antibodies. When PEGylation is carried out appropriately, it does not affect binding to the IFN-α receptor.

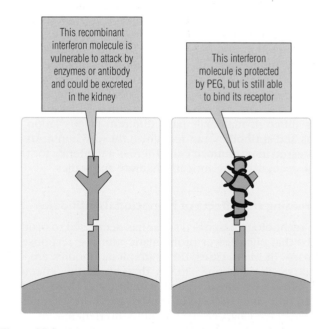

Figure 35.6 PEGylation can be used to increase the biologic half-life of some recombinant molecules. PEG, polyethylene glycol.

FIG. 35.5 Clinically Important mAbs			
Example of mAb	**Target Antigen**	**Type of mAb**	**Clinical use**
Rituximab	CD20 on B Cells	Chimeric	Treatment of lymphoma (Chapter 34)
Trastuzumab (Herceptin) Basiliximab	HER2 receptor on breast cancer cells IL2 receptor on activated T cells	Humanized Chimeric	Treatment of advanced breast cancer (Chapter 34) Potent immunosuppression, for example, in kidney transplant rejection (Chapter 33)
Daclizumab	IL2 receptor on activated T cells	Humanized	Anti-inflammatory used in rheumatoid
Infliximab	TNF	Chimeric	arthritis (Chapter 30)

*The presence of "xi" in the name of an mAb denotes a chimeric origin, whereas "zu" denotes a humanized mAb.

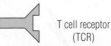 T cell receptor (TCR)

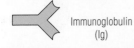 Immunoglobulin (Ig)

 Antigen

 MHC I

Interleukin-2

Unlike IFN-α, the biological activity of IL-2 is lost when it is PEGylated. Whenever this cytokine is used, it has to be given as a daily intravenous infusion.

Recombinant IL-2 has been used in HIV infection in combination with HAART (see Chapter 32). Compared with HAART alone, the use of IL-2 results in faster and greater restoration of T-cell numbers. IL-2 induces production of Bcl-2 and thus has antiapoptotic effects (see Chapter 21). IL-2 thus helps prevent destruction of CD4+ T cells through apoptosis in HIV infection. In addition, IL-2 boosts T-cell proliferation and thus helps T-cell numbers recover in HIV infection. One final hope for HIV infection is that IL-2 will stimulate T cells latently infected with HIV. These cells then express HIV peptides and are subject to cytotoxic T-cell killing. In this way, it is hoped, IL-2 may "flush out" HIV in latently infected cells.

You will recall from Chapter 23 that cytokines such as IL-2 are pleiotropic; they affect many different cell types. To achieve the benefits described above in HIV infection, IL-2 has to be given at moderate daily doses on weekly cycles, for several months. At these doses IL-2 affects multiple cell types and triggers a low-grade acute phase reaction (see Chapter 19). Hence, patients being treated in this way with IL-2 experience low-grade fevers, fatigue, and muscle ache, mimicking the symptoms of chronic infection. For these reasons, IL-2 treatment is reserved for HIV infected patients in whom CD4 counts have not recovered during virologically effective HAART.

IL-7 is another growth factor for T cells. It appears to be less pleiotropic, and some initial data suggest that it may help increase T-cell numbers in HIV with fewer side effects.

IL-2 also has effects in some cancers. It is thought to act by overcoming anergy or apoptosis in tumor-specific T cells (see Chapter 34) and by activating NK cells. IL-2 is licensed for use in renal cancer and in melanoma. In cancer treatment, IL-2 works most effectively when given at very high doses. However, at high doses, IL-2 has effects on the endothelium leading to the capillary leak syndrome. This in turn can cause severe pulmonary edema and hypotension. High dose IL-2 is, therefore, a risky drug to give and is always administered in intensive care units.

These dose-limiting effects mean that some patients cannot benefit from high-dose systemic IL-2. An alternative approach is to deliver IL-2 directly into lesions when these are accessible. Intralesional IL-2 activates T cells and NK cells that have already entered the tumor. An experimental approach is to transfect tumor cells with IL-2 genes so that the tumor cells themselves can activate T cells.

LEARNING POINTS Can You Now ...

1. List the problems encountered with early therapeutic antibodies derived from horse or human plasma?

2. List several strategies to reduce the antigenicity of murine mAbs?

3. Describe with diagrams two ways in which the Fc region of mAbs can be modified to enhance effector function?

4. List several examples of where mAbs have proven successful and where they have been so far disappointing in clinical medicine?

5. Explain how PEGylation makes some cytokine therapies more feasible?

6. List at least two diseases where treatment with IL-2 may be helpful, and explain the mechanism of action of IL-2 in these examples?

 MHC II

 Cytokine, Chemokine, etc.

 Complement (C')

 Signaling molecule

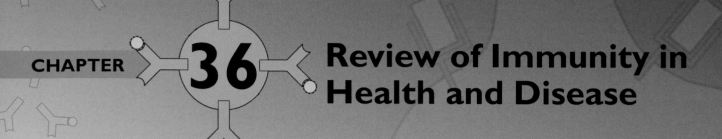

36 Review of Immunity in Health and Disease

In this chapter, we review the contents of this last section, which covered vaccines and clinical problems involving the immune system.

To illustrate the kinds of health problems the immune response can aid with or contribute to, we follow the life of a physician born in England in 1942. None of the problems encountered by her friends and family are particularly rare. This chapter illustrates how immunopathology frequently causes diseases, affecting all ages, which are part of everyday experience.

Most infections can be dealt with by the innate and adaptive immune systems working in unison. Some infections, for example, measles (Box 36.1), are usually cleared by the immune system and only cause trivial problems in most cases. But even measles can be life-threatening in some individuals. Other infections (e.g., hepatitis B) are much harder for the immune system to clear and can cause life-long infection. Either type of infection can be prevented by the use of vaccines.

Vaccines stimulate components of the adaptive immune system to produce immunologic memory (see Chapter 24). Specific antibodies either prevent infection from taking place or bind to toxins produced by pathogens, reducing the severity of the disease.

Vaccines produced from killed pathogens or recombinant proteins are very safe but tend to produce weak responses. Adjuvants are often used to boost the effects of killed or subunit vaccines. Other vaccines use live patho-gens that have been attenuated. Live vaccines are often more effective than killed or subunit vaccines, but there is a higher risk of side effects.

Newer technologies aim to stimulate the immune system in novel ways, for example, by inserting the gene for an antigen using DNA vaccines.

Hypersensitivity reactions are an important cause of disease and are caused by the immune system reacting to a range of antigens (see Chapter 25). These antigens can include peptides produced by microbes. It is possible that

---

BOX 36.1 Infancy

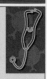

At the age of 7, our patient developed a widespread blotchy rash and high fever. Her family recognized the characteristic rash of measles. However, she deteriorates over the next 2 days and develops signs of pneumonia. Luckily, she gradually improves without specific treatment.

Measles pneumonia is an unusual complication of this viral infection. Measles also causes brain inflammation (encephalitis) from time to time. A vaccine for measles has been in routine use in the developed world since the 1970s and has largely prevented these infrequent, but potentially life-threatening, complications. In the developing world, measles remains a major cause of death of young children.

in some infections (e.g., forms of leprosy) the immune response causes at least as much damage as the pathogen itself.

Atopy is an immediate hypersensitivity reaction to environmental antigens, mediated by immunoglobulin E (IgE) (type I hypersensitivity; see Chapter 26). We use the term allergy synonymously. Allergic diseases are one of the most common forms of hypersensitivity and are thought to be increasing in prevalence in the developed world. This increase in allergy is occurring, although immunity mediated by T helper 2 (T_H2) cells, IgE, and mast cells, which was originally developed to fend off worm infestations, is less required, as these are now rare in the developed world. There is also a decline in bacterial infections in developed countries; the hygiene hypothesis suggests that this may skew the immune system toward T_H2 responses.

The most widely recognized forms of allergy occur immediately after patients have been exposed to allergens and are caused by the effects of mast cell degranulation after IgE cross-linking (Box 36.2). Allergy can also have a late phase, mediated largely by eosinophils. The late phase accounts for many of the symptoms of diseases such as asthma.

Apart from infections and allergens, hypersensitivity can also occur in response to autoantigens (see Chapter 27). Although a degree of autoimmunity is normal, autoimmune mechanisms can cause disease through three mechanisms: direct effects of antibodies (type II hypersensitivity; see Chapter 28), immune complexes (type III; see Chapter 29), or delayed hypersensitivity (type IV; see Chapter 30). Autoimmunity has complex genetic and environmental origins and reflects the breakdown of normal self-tolerance. It is not unusual for these diseases, especially organ-specific autoimmune disease, to run in families.

In type II hypersensitivity, antibodies bind to cells, causing a number of effects. In Chapter 28, we described how antibodies binding to red cells can fix complement or stimulate opsonization. In either instance, hemolytic anemia is the result. Antibodies can also mimic the effects of trophic hormones, as in Graves' disease (Box 36.3). Detection of these autoantibodies with a variety of techniques is used to help make the diagnosis.

Type III hypersensitivity is caused by immune complexes. These can form in the tissues (e.g., farmer's lung) or circulate in the blood. Although circulating immune complexes can be the consequence of autoimmune disease, they can also be the result of exogenous antigens, such as infections or drugs, as in Box 36.4. Immune complexes activate the innate immune system and cause inflammation. The kidneys are very often the targets for this process.

Type IV hypersensitivity can also be the result of infection (e.g., tuberculosis, leprosy) or autoimmunity. In the autoimmune diseases, insulin-dependent diabetes, rheumatoid arthritis, and multiple sclerosis, T-cells infiltrate the target organs and cause chronic inflammation (Box 36.5). The damage in each case is mediated by cytokines. Tumor necrosis factor is probably the most important of these. Each of these autoimmune diseases is associated with specific autoantibodies. Although these may be useful in making the diagnosis, they are not strongly implicated in damaging the target organs.

Transplantation is used to replace diseased organs. In all types of allogeneic transplant, except for corneal trans-

---

BOX 36.3 Adolescence

Our subject has now progressed to high school, but her family begins to notice weight loss and irritability. At first her family thinks she is simply studying too hard in her efforts to get a place at medical school (in England one can enter medical school from high school). Her condition deteriorates, and eventually she goes to see a physician. He finds she has hyperthyroidism, and a diagnosis of Graves' disease is made (see Chapter 28). She responds very well to drug treatment.

BOX 36.4 Life As a Student

Our subject is successful in getting into medical school. During her undergraduate medical training, she sees a number of patients with severe infection being treated with horse antiserum. This was an early attempt at immunotherapy and was in quite widespread use until the 1960s. Unfortunately, horse antiserum induces antihorse antibodies, which are capable of triggering immune complex disease—serum sickness. In our subject's lifetime, improvements in technology saw the introduction of monoclonal antibodies. As you read in Chapter 35, these have been successful in treating inflammation and some cancers, but are still not very successful in treating infection.

BOX 36.2 Childhood

As an 11-year-old, our subject goes on a picnic with family friends. A few minutes after eating a peanut butter sandwich, one young boy develops rapid-onset swelling of the face and breathlessness. The boy is taken to the emergency department and gradually improves. Relatively little was known about peanut-induced anaphylaxis in the 1950s, and skin prick and specific immunoglobulin E testing were not widely available. The experience kindles an interest in medicine in our subject.

BOX 36.5 The Family

Our subject's younger sister has been unwell with fatigue for several weeks. On a visit home, our subject decides her sister may have diabetes, remembering that organ-specific autoimmune disease tends to run in families. The sister's blood sugar is high, confirming the diagnosis.

 MHC II   Cytokine, Chemokine, etc.   Complement (C')   Signaling molecule

plant, rejection is a major problem (see Chapter 33). At its most severe, hyperacute rejection takes place when antibodies bind allogeneic human leukocyte antigen (HLA) antibodies, destroying the transplanted organ within minutes. Acute rejection is caused by T cells responding to allogeneic antigens in the donor organ. These two types of rejection are similar to type II and type IV hypersensitivity, respectively. The fetus resembles a transplanted organ but it is not rejected by the mother because T-cell responses are dampened down by systemic factors (estrogens and cytokines), and natural killer cells are inhibited by local factors in the uterus.

Bone marrow transplant is a special case because T cells arising from the donor can attack the recipient, giving rise to graft-versus-host disease. The risks of graft rejection and graft-versus-host disease are minimized by tissue typing techniques (Box 36.6).

Immunodeficiency can occur as a result of primary defects within the immune system or secondary to external factors. Primary immunodeficiencies usually have genetic components (see Chapter 31). Severe secondary immunodeficiencies occur in patients infected with HIV, malignancies, or after specific drug treatments (see Chapter 32). Mild secondary immunodeficiencies occur in patients with poor nutrition and during physiologic stress.

Immunodeficiencies cause either recurrent infection or opportunist infections with low-virulence organisms. They need to be recognized because, if left untreated, infections can cause irreversible damage or death. The type of infection often gives important clues to the severity and type of immunodeficiency operating (Box 36.7).

Cells of the innate immune system quite often form malignancies (see Chapter 34). This is especially true of B cells because they can be infected with Epstein-Barr virus and because they undergo somatic hypermutation. Much is known about the genetic basis of these lymphoid malignancies.

The immune system also has a role in fighting cancers, although more often than not the immune system recognizes oncogenic viruses rather than tumor antigens themselves. Many tumors have developed molecular mechanisms for evading the immune system. Tumor immunotherapy aims to reverse some of these mechanisms.

BOX 36.6 The Family

After a further 15 years, our subject's sister has developed chronic renal failure as a result of the diabetes. Our subject is unable to act as a donor because of her history of viral hepatitis. One of their other siblings is found to be an exact human leukocyte antigen match and donates his kidney. The transplant goes ahead without any signs of rejection. This is lucky, because even in the early 1980s, many of the potent antirejection drugs, for example, ciclosporin, were not available.

BOX 36.7 Retirement

Our subject is now 64 and planning her retirement. Unfortunately, she has had two very painful bouts of shingles, caused by reactivation of the chickenpox virus, herpes varicella zoster. She has also suffered from a series of chest and sinus infections. Tests for immunodeficiency are carried out, and her T-cell, immunoglobulin G (IgG), and IgA levels are found to be low. Her blood also contains a monoclonal IgM protein. A sample of bone marrow is taken and shows multiple myeloma. A diagnosis of immunodeficiency secondary to myeloma is made.

  T cell receptor (TCR)

 Immunoglobulin (Ig)

 Antigen

 MHC I

GLOSSARY

Activation phase. Phase of the immune response when a lymphocyte divides to give many more of the same cell (clonal expansion).

Active immunity. Active immunity is protective immunity that develops after exposure to infection or vaccination.

Acute phase response. A systemic reaction to infection or inflammation, mediated by cytokine production and characterized by fever and production of acute phase proteins.

Adaptive (acquired) immune system, response. Part of the immune system in which genetic recombination is used to recognize specific molecules. Slow to respond, but produces lasting memory.

Adjuvant. Substance that increases the immunogenicity of a vaccine, usually by activating the innate immune system.

Affinity. Strength of binding between antigen and antibody, or T- or B-cell receptor.

Affinity maturation. Process by which B cells undergo somatic hypermutation and increase the affinity of the B-cell receptor.

Allele. Normal genetic variants, occurring in more than 1% of the population. For example, eye color or different HLA types.

Allelic exclusion. Any one B cell expresses only immunoglobulin of one allotype in a heterozygous individual.

Allergen. An environmental substance capable of eliciting an immediate hypersensitivity reaction.

Allergy. Immediate hypersensitivity reaction to an otherwise harmless environmental substance, mediated by immunoglobulin E.

Allogeneic. Immune reactions to a genetically different member of the same species.

Allogeneic transplant. Transplant between genetically different members of the same species.

Allotype. Genetic polymorphisms (different alleles) of both heavy- and light-chain immunoglobulin genes that can be detected by antibodies.

Alternative pathway. Activation of the complement cascade by exposure to a solid surface lacking complement inhibitors.

Anaphylatoxin. Low-molecular-weight product of complement activation that increases capillary permeability and attracts leukocytes.

Anergy. State of dormancy induced by exposure to antigen in certain circumstances. For example, T cells become anergic during tolerance induction.

Antibody. Protein produced in response to and capable of binding specifically with an antigen. Antibodies have an immunoglobulin structure.

Antigen. Molecules specifically recognized by receptors of the adaptive immune system.

Antigen recognition molecules (ARMs). The ARMs are the B- and T-cell receptor molecules and the proteins encoded by the major histocompatibility complex.

Antigen-binding site. The portion of the antibody that makes contact with antigen.

Antigenemia. High levels of antigen circulating in the bloodstream.

Antigenic drift. Gradual change in an organism's antigens, consequent to acquisition of mutations.

Antigen-presenting cells (APCs). Cells that can process antigen and present antigen to T cells.

Apoptosis. Deliberate, programmed cell death.

Asthma. Transient airflow limitation due to bronchial smooth muscle constriction and mucus secretion.

Atopy. Genetic predisposition to allergy.

Attenuated vaccine. Vaccine produced by genetically modifying a pathogenic organism.

Autoantibody. Antibody produced against self antigen.

Autoimmune disease. Disease caused by hypersensitivity reactions occurring as exaggerated autoimmunity.

Autoimmunity. Recognition of normal components of the body by the adaptive immune system. Occurs in healthy individuals but can also cause autoimmune disease.

Autologous transplant. Tissue returning to the same individual after a period outside the body—usually in a frozen state.

B-cell receptor (BCR). The cell surface–located receptor for antigen on B cells.

B lymphocytes. Subset of white blood cells that can secrete antibody molecules.

Bence Jones protein. Monoclonal light chain present in the urine in myeloma.

Blasts. Immature, rapidly proliferating cells.

Bone marrow. The major hematopoietic organ in humans. Particularly important in B-cell generation, but all the blood cell types except mature T cells are generated in the bone marrow.

Caspase. Proteolytic enzymes involved in triggering apoptosis.

CD. Cluster of differentiation nomenclature system for cell surface molecules (and thus for cell subsets).

CD4 count. Number of circulating $CD4^+$ T cells; used to monitor HIV infection.

Cell-mediated immunity. Refers to the function of T cells as opposed to humoral or antibody-mediated immunity.

Central tolerance. Tolerance induced in immature T or B cells in the thymus and bone marrow, respectively.

Chemokines. Chemotactic cytokines; attract cells to the site of infection.

Chemotaxis. Directed movement of cells, often to the site of infection.

Chimeric monoclonal antibody. Monoclonal antibody using mouse immunoglobulin variable regions and human immunoglobulin constant regions.

Class switching. The process by which an individual B cell can, during maturation, switch immunoglobulin heavy-chain usage, while retaining the same variable genes and antigen specificity.

Classical pathway. Activation of the complement cascade by exposure to aggregated immunoglobulin.

Clonal selection theory. The idea that each lymphocyte expresses a unique antigen receptor and that this pre-existing cell divides on exposure to antigen and gives rise to many daughter cells (clones).

Clone. In immunology, a series of genetically identical lymphocytes, all derived from one B cell or T cell after receptor recombination.

Cognate antigen. The precise antigen that a given antigen receptor has specificity for.

Cognitive phase. Phase of an active immune response during which antigen is recognized by a cell bearing a receptor that is specific for the antigen.

Collectin. Molecules forming part of the innate immune system, containing lectin (carbohydrate-binding) domains and collagen-like domains.

Colony-stimulating factor (CSF). Growth factors that induce differentiation of specific cell lineages during hematopoiesis.

Combinatorial diversity. Refers to immunoglobulin or T-cell receptor variable-region gene segments recombining in multiple combinations, e.g., $30V_\kappa \times 5J_\kappa = 150$ different variable regions.

Complement. Cascade of serum enzymes activated by the presence of pathogens.

C-reactive protein (CRP). Acute-phase protein produced at high levels during inflammation.

Cross-reactivity. Occasionally, an antigen-recognition molecule is specific for a particular antigen but a different antigen fits well enough for stable binding to occur.

Cytokine. Soluble molecules used to transmit messages from cell to cell. Interferons and chemokines are types of cytokines.

Cytokine network. System of cytokines used to regulate interactions between cells of the innate and adaptive immune systems.

Danger signals. Molecular signals indicating damage, either because of infection or physical or chemical injury to cells.

Defensin. Low-molecular-weight peptides capable of damaging bacteria.

Degranulating cell. Innate immune system cells that release toxic granules on activation.

Delayed hypersensitivity. Reaction taking several days to develop, involving antigen-presenting cells and T cells.

Dendritic cell. Irregularly shaped cell with many branchlike processes that is critical in antigen capture and presentation to T cells.

Desensitization. Type of treatment for allergy involving increasing doses of antigen.

Diapedesis. Term used to describe lymphocyte passage through the tight junction between adjacent endothelial cells into the tissues.

Effector cell. Effector B cells are the plasma cells that secrete antibody molecules, and effector T cells are the T-helper and cytotoxic T-lymphocyte populations.

ELISA. Enzyme-linked immunosorbent assay.

Eosinophil. Short-lived degranulating cells.

Eotaxin. Chemokine that attracts eosinophils to the site of inflammation.

Epithelioid cell. Type of mature macrophage.

Epitope. Area of an antigen with which an antibody reacts/binds specifically.

False positive. Erroneous positive test result, for example, produced by a cross-reacting antibody.

Fas. Cell-surface molecule that, when bound, can trigger apoptosis.

Flow cytometry. The process of enumerating live cells that express an antigen that can be recognized with an antibody (usually a monoclonal antibody).

Follicular dendritic cell. Antigen-presenting cell found only in lymphoid follicles. They may have a different origin from bone marrow–derived dendritic cells. Antigen-antibody complexes are retained on their surface attached to Fc and complement receptors.

Germinal centers. Area of lymphoid follicles containing chiefly activated B cells.

Germline diversity. Term that refers to the multiple copies of *V*, *D*, and *J* gene segments.

Giant cell. Type of mature macrophage.

Glial cell. Type of mature macrophage.

Glomerulonephritis. Inflammation of the glomerulus.

Graft-versus-leukemia effect. Beneficial effects of stem cell transplant against malignancy in recipient.

Granuloma. A localized area of chronic inflammation, usually produced in response to a pathogen that is hard to clear.

Granzyme. Protein in granules found in cytotoxic T cells and natural-killer cells.

Haplotype. A block of alleles that are inherited together, e.g., in the major histocompatibility complex.

Hapten. Small molecule, only capable of acting as antigen after combining with host proteins.

Heaf test. Skin test for exposure to *Mycobacterium tuberculosis*.

Heat shock protein (HSP). Stress-induced proteins found in a wide range of organisms.

Hematopoietic stem cells. Pluripotential, self-renewing stem cells that give rise to all blood cell types.

Hemolysis. Damage to red cells.

Herd immunity. High levels of immunity sufficient to prevent epidemics in a given community.

Histamine. Mediator produced by activated mast cells.

Histiocyte. Type of mature macrophage.

HLA. Human leukocyte antigen—also referred to as major histocompatibility complex. Genetically polymorphic proteins whose function is to bind and present antigen to T cells.

HLA cross-matching. Laboratory procedure to rule out reactions between patient or donor cells, prior to transplantation.

HLA typing. Laboratory procedure to determine patient or donor HLA type, prior to transplantation.

Human immunodeficiency virus (HIV). Virus capable of infecting cells and damaging the immune system.

Humanized monoclonal antibody. Monoclonal antibody in which only the mouse hypervariable region is used. The rest of the molecule uses human amino acid sequences.

Humoral (antibody-mediated) immunity. Antibody-mediated immunity.

Hygiene hypothesis. Hypothesis that exposure to organisms, particularly mycobacteria, early in life prevents allergies from developing.

Hypermutation. A process of rapid mutation of sequences that encode the binding site for antigen in antibody molecules.

 T cell receptor (TCR)

 Immunoglobulin (Ig)

 Antigen

 MHC I

Hypersensitivity. Inflammation caused by an exaggerated response to an antigen. The immune response, rather than the antigen, causes disease.

Hypervariable region (hv). Amino acids that are part of the binding site for antigen and are also contact residues for the antigen.

Idiosyncratic adverse drug reactions. Unpredictable reactions to drugs, often with an immunologic basis.

IL (generic). Interleukin (IL) is an old name for cytokine. The IL abbreviation is used as a naming system for cytokines.

Immediate hypersensitivity. Reaction occurring within a few minutes after a response to a trigger, usually mediated by immunoglobulin E.

Immune complex. Lattices of antibody and antigen formed in the body.

Immunofluorescence. Laboratory techniques used to show the presence of a substance in a tissue (direct immunofluorescence) or antibody in the blood (indirect immunofluorescence).

Immunogen. An immunogen is a substance that by itself causes an immune response, e.g., antibody production.

Immunoglobulin. A soluble molecule composed of variable and nonvariable domains with antibody function.

Immunoglobulin domain. Parallel β-sheet structure folded into globular domains that are held together by disulfide bonds.

Immunoglobulin superfamily. A family of molecules with domain structure similar to that of immunoglobulin. Each has a different role in the immune system. For example, immunoglobulin, T-cell receptor, and major histocompatibility complex molecules.

Immunological synapse. The area of close binding between an antigen-presenting cell and a T cell that involves multiple receptor-ligand interactions and facilitates cell activation.

Inflammation. Defined clinically as the presence of redness, swelling, and pain. Histologically, inflammation is defined as the presence of edema and white cells in a tissue.

Innate (nonadaptive) immune system, response. The older part of the immune system, which responds rapidly to infection, but with exactly the same response each time.

Insertional mutagenesis. Mutations caused in the genome after random insertion of a therapeutic gene, for example.

Interferon. A cytokine with antiviral effects.

Invariant chain. A nonpolymorphic protein that facilitates "loading" of major histocompatibility complex class II molecules with antigen.

Junctional diversity. Different sequences created by random addition of nucleotides during formation of junctions between gene segments, e.g., *V* and *J*, leads to greater antibody diversity.

Killer immunoglobulin-like receptors (KIRs). Receptor on the surface of natural-killer cells.

Kupffer cells. Type of mature macrophage.

Lactoferrin. Bactericidal protein produced by neutrophils and macrophages.

Late-phase response. Follows immediate hypersensitivity in some allergic reactions and is mediated by T cells and eosinophils.

Lectin pathway. Activation of the complement cascade by mannan-binding lectin.

Lymph nodes. Lymph nodes function to concentrate and survey lymph-borne antigens for presentation to T and B cells.

Lymphocyte homing. Effector and memory T lymphocytes migrate and lodge in selected tissue sites, e.g., peripheral tissues, where they may remain for some time. The process is controlled by interactions between several adhesion molecules.

Lymphocyte recirculation (trafficking). Most mature lymphocytes are in constant circulation (trafficking) from one tissue to another. A lymphocyte may make a complete circuit of the body once or twice a day.

Lymphoid tumors. Tumors derived from cells of the adaptive immune system.

Macrophage. Large phagocytic cells with many granules that function as a critical link between the innate and adaptive systems since these cells are active in antigen processing and presentation.

Major histocompatibility complex (MHC). Major Histocompatibility Complex. Gene cluster containing genes for cell surface proteins that present antigens to T cells. The human version of MHC is referred to as HLA.

Mantoux test. Skin test for exposure to *Mycobacterium tuberculosis*.

Mast cell. Mast cells are resident in tissues and able to release granules during some types of infections.

Membrane attack complex. Final part of the complement cascade, capable of damaging cells or pathogens.

MHC polymorphism. Polymorphism refers to the existence of allelic alternatives, and the MHC with a large number of allelic determinants is the most polymorphic locus known.

MHC restricted. T lymphocytes recognize antigen in association with MHC class I or II molecules, and their antigen recognition is therefore said to be "MHC restricted."

Molecular mimicry. Idea that infections may trigger autoimmunity when pathogen antigens cross-react with autoantigens.

Monoclonal. A population of B cells or T cells with identical immunoglobulin molecules or receptors. Monoclonal populations are often neoplastic.

Monoclonal antibody. A homogeneous immunoglobulin of defined specificity generally prepared using hybridoma technology for biomedical research, diagnostic use, or therapy.

Monocyte. Immature, circulating macrophage.

Mucociliary escalator. Innate defenses of the airways.

Mucosa-associated lymphoid tissue (MALT). Lymphoid tissue in the respiratory and gastrointestinal tracts that is enriched in immunoglobulin A-producing plasma cells and specialized epithelial cells—M cells—that take up antigen by pinocytosis.

Naive lymphocyte. A lymphocyte that is mature but has not yet encountered the nonself antigen that it has specificity for.

Natural antibody. IgM antibody produced without previous exposure to antigen.

Natural-killer (NK) cell. These large granular lymphocytes have two major roles: (1) killing some virally infected cells, e.g., Herpes virus infected cells, and (2) helping to activate the adaptive immune response.

Negative selection. The deletion of lymphocytes capable of recognizing and damaging normal host components.

Nephritis. Kidney inflammation.

Neutrophil. Short-lived phagocytic cell.

NKG2/CD94. Receptor on the surface of natural-killer cells.

Opsonization. Particles that have been opsonized become targets for phagocytosis.

Osteoclast. Type of mature macrophage.

Passive immunity. Transfer of effector components (e.g., immunoglobulin, T cells) from one individual to another.

Pathogen. Disease-causing organism.

Pattern-recognition molecules. Molecules of the innate immune system capable of recognizing molecules characteristic of infection, for example, double-stranded RNA and some sugars.

 MHC II

  Cytokine, Chemokine, etc.

 Complement (C')

 Signaling molecule

Perforin. A protein found in the granules of NK and cytotoxic T cells that can polymerize and form a pore in the membrane of target cells.

Periarteriolar lymphoid sheath (PALS). Concentric cuffs of lymphocytes (chiefly T cells) found around central arterioles in the spleen.

Peripheral tolerance. Tolerance induced in mature T or B cells in the nonlymphoid tissues.

Phage libraries. Collections of genetic sequences expressed in bacteriophages.

Phagocyte. Cells capable of engulfing and destroying particulate matter.

Plasma cell. Terminally differentiated B cell capable of secreting large quantities of immunoglobulin.

Polyclonal. A population of B cells or T cells producing a complex mixture of immunoglobulin molecules or T-cell receptors.

Polygenic disorder. Disorder caused by a combination of several genetic and environmental factors.

Polymorphism. Slight genetic differences between members of a population.

Positive selection. The ability of T cells to recognize self major histocompatibility complex with moderate affinity, and so survive in the thymus.

Pre–B-cell receptor. At the early pre-B cell stage of B-cell development, two invariant proteins associate to create a light chain–like structure and associate with μ_H to form a receptor complex called the Pre-BCR.

Primary immunodeficiency. Immune deficiency caused by genetic defects.

Primary lymphoid organs. The organs in which lymphocytes are produced (the bone marrow and thymus in adult humans).

Prion. Infectious particle containing no genetic sequences.

Prostaglandin. Mediator released from mast cells and eosinophils.

Proteosome. A cytoplasmically located complex of proteases involved in creating peptides that may bind to major histocompatibility complex class I molecules.

Pyogenic. Pus-forming.

Receptor editing. The process in certain immature B cells of reinitiating *V(D)/J* rearrangement to attempt to alter the B-cell receptor specificity and create a receptor with no self-reactivity.

Rejection. Ability of the host immune response to destroy transplanted tissue.

Replicative senescence. Loss of ability to proliferate by aged lymphocytes.

Respiratory burst. Production of toxic molecules by activated phagocytes.

Retrovirus. Virus that transcribes a DNA genomic sequence from an RNA template.

Reverse transcriptase. Enzyme capable of translating RNA to DNA.

Rhinitis. Nasal inflammation.

Secondary immunodeficiency. Immune deficiency caused by disease after birth.

Secondary lymphoid organs. These are the organs in which lymphocytes come into contact with antigen, clonally expand, and mature into effector cells, i.e., the spleen and lymph nodes.

Selectins. Family of adhesion proteins that bind sugars on the surface of cells, for example, to selectively attract the cells to specific tissues.

Self-restriction. Refers to T cells that are capable of recognizing antigen only if presented on self major histocompatibility complex molecules.

Septic (endotoxic) shock. Hypotension caused by exposure to substances released from bacteria.

Serum sickness. Disease caused by circulating immune complexes.

Skin prick testing. Test for allergy.

Somatic recombination. This is the process of gene segment rearrangement that occurs to create a repertoire of antigen receptors.

Spleen. A secondary lymphoid organ that functions as a "filter" for the blood and as the main site of immune responses to blood-borne antigens.

Subcapsular zone. An area of the thymus containing the earliest progenitor thymocytes.

Subunit vaccine. Vaccine using parts of a pathogen.

Syngeneic transplant. Transplant between genetically identical individuals.

T-cell receptor (TCR). The receptor for antigen on T lymphocytes.

T-cell tolerance. Tolerance is the process of preventing the immune response to autoantigens. T cells are initially tolerant to self antigens in the thymus, and only those T-cell receptors with appropriate specificity for self–major histocompatibility complex and nonself peptides are selected.

T_H1 cell. T-helper cell that provides help for cytotoxic T cells, macrophages, and IgG production.

T_H2 cell. T-helper cell that provides help for immunoglobulin E secretion and eosinophil activation.

Thymocytes. Progenitor T cells.

Thymus. A bilobed organ found in the anterior mediastinum that is responsible for T-cell development.

Thymus-dependent antigen. Antigens that require B-T cell cooperation to produce an immune response.

Thymus-independent antigen. Antigens that can activate B cells without T-cell help, e.g., certain common bacterial cell wall components such as lipopolysaccharide.

Transgenic mice. Genetically altered mice.

Tumor antigens. Antigen expressed on a tumor and either absent or present at only very low levels on healthy cells.

Vasculitis. Inflammation of the blood vessels.

Viral latency. Part of a viral life cycle when there is no active replication or host cell damage.

Wegener's granulomatosis. A relatively rare disease that involves a type II hypersensitivity reaction leading to vasculitis affecting the nose, lungs, and glomeruli. Patients with this disease develop autoantibodies to an enzyme found in neutrophils called proteinase 3.

Western blotting. An immunoblotting technique used to characterize complex mixtures of antigens biochemically.

Wild-type organism. Unaltered (native) organism used to manufacture vaccines.

Xenogeneic transplant. Transplant between members of a different species.

 T cell receptor (TCR)

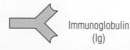 Immunoglobulin (Ig)

 Antigen

 MHC I

INDEX

Note: Page numbers followed by the letter f refer to Figures; those followed by t refer to tables; and those followed by b refer to boxed material.